Advances in Glaucoma Surgery

Advances in Glaucoma Surgery

Editors

Michele Figus
Karl Mercieca

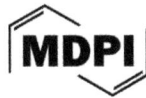

Basel • Beijing • Wuhan • Barcelona • Belgrade • Novi Sad • Cluj • Manchester

Editors
Michele Figus
University of Pisa
Pisa, Italy

Karl Mercieca
University Hospital Eye Clinic
Bonn, Germany

Editorial Office
MDPI
St. Alban-Anlage 66
4052 Basel, Switzerland

This is a reprint of articles from the Special Issue published online in the open access journal *Journal of Clinical Medicine* (ISSN 2077-0383) (available at: https://www.mdpi.com/journal/jcm/special_issues/glaucoma_surgery_clinical).

For citation purposes, cite each article independently as indicated on the article page online and as indicated below:

Lastname, A.A.; Lastname, B.B. Article Title. *Journal Name* **Year**, *Volume Number*, Page Range.

ISBN 978-3-0365-8868-1 (Hbk)
ISBN 978-3-0365-8869-8 (PDF)
doi.org/10.3390/books978-3-0365-8869-8

© 2023 by the authors. Articles in this book are Open Access and distributed under the Creative Commons Attribution (CC BY) license. The book as a whole is distributed by MDPI under the terms and conditions of the Creative Commons Attribution-NonCommercial-NoDerivs (CC BY-NC-ND) license.

Contents

About the Editors . . . . **ix**

Karl Mercieca and Michele Figus
Advances in Glaucoma Surgery
Reprinted from: *J. Clin. Med.* **2023**, *12*, 828, doi:10.3390/jcm12030828 . . . . **1**

Leonardo Mastropasqua, Lorenza Brescia, Francesca D'Arcangelo, Mario Nubile, Giada D'Onofrio, Michele Totta, et al.
Topical Steroids and Glaucoma Filtration Surgery Outcomes: An In Vivo Confocal Study of the Conjunctiva
Reprinted from: *J. Clin. Med.* **2022**, *11*, 3959, doi:10.3390/jcm11143959 . . . . **3**

Afrouz Ahmadzadeh, Line Kessel, Bo Simmendefeldt Schmidt and Daniella Bach-Holm
Steroid Response after Trabeculectomy—A Randomized Controlled Trial Comparing Dexamethasone to Diclofenac Eye Drops
Reprinted from: *J. Clin. Med.* **2022**, *11*, 7365, doi:10.3390/jcm11247365 . . . . **15**

Yantao Wei, Yihua Su, Lei Fang, Xinxing Guo, Stephanie Chen, Ying Han, et al.
Effect of Combined Surgery in Patients with Complex Nanophthalmos
Reprinted from: *J. Clin. Med.* **2022**, *11*, 5909, doi:10.3390/jcm11195909 . . . . **23**

Faisal A. Almobarak, Abdullah S. Alobaidan and Mansour A. Alobrah
Outcomes of Deep Sclerectomy for Glaucoma Secondary to Sturge–Weber Syndrome
Reprinted from: *J. Clin. Med.* **2023**, *12*, 516, doi:10.3390/jcm12020516 . . . . **35**

Pedro P. Rodríguez-Calvo, Ignacio Rodríguez-Uña, Andrés Fernández-Vega-Cueto, Ronald M. Sánchez-Ávila, Eduardo Anitua and Jesús Merayo-Lloves
Plasma Rich in Growth Factors as an Adjuvant Agent in Non-Penetrating Deep Sclerectomy
Reprinted from: *J. Clin. Med.* **2023**, *12*, 3604, doi:10.3390/jcm12103604 . . . . **43**

Aleksandra K. Kicińska, Monika E. Danielewska and Marek Rekas
Safety and Efficacy of Three Variants of Canaloplasty with Phacoemulsification to Treat Open-Angle Glaucoma and Cataract: 12-Month Follow-Up
Reprinted from: *J. Clin. Med.* **2022**, *11*, 6501, doi:10.3390/jcm11216501 . . . . **55**

Peter Szurman
Advances in Canaloplasty—Modified Techniques Yield Strong Pressure Reduction with Low Risk Profile
Reprinted from: *J. Clin. Med.* **2023**, *12*, 3031, doi:10.3390/jcm12083031 . . . . **69**

Marta Orejudo de Rivas, Juana Martínez Morales, Elena Pardina Claver, Diana Pérez García, Itziar Pérez Navarro, Francisco J. Ascaso Puyuelo, et al.
Descemet's Membrane Detachment during Phacocanaloplasty: Case Series and In-Depth Literature Review
Reprinted from: *J. Clin. Med.* **2023**, *12*, 5461, doi:10.3390/jcm12175461 . . . . **85**

Chiara Posarelli, Michele Figus, Gloria Roberti, Sara Giammaria, Giorgio Ghirelli, Pierpaolo Quercioli, et al.
Italian Candidates for the XEN Implant: An Overview from the Glaucoma Treatment Registry (XEN-GTR)
Reprinted from: *J. Clin. Med.* **2022**, *11*, 5320, doi:10.3390/jcm11185320 . . . . **97**

Matteo Sacchi, Antonio M. Fea, Gianluca Monsellato, Elena Tagliabue, Edoardo Villani, Stefano Ranno and Paolo Nucci
Safety and Efficacy of Ab Interno XEN 45 Gel Stent in Patients with Glaucoma and High Myopia
Reprinted from: *J. Clin. Med.* **2023**, *12*, 2477, doi:10.3390/jcm12072477 107

Charlotte Evers, Daniel Böhringer, Sara Kallee, Philip Keye, Heiko Philippin, Timothy Piotrowski, et al.
XEN®-63 Compared to XEN®-45 Gel Stents to Reduce Intraocular Pressure in Glaucoma
Reprinted from: *J. Clin. Med.* **2023**, *12*, 5043, doi:10.3390/jcm12155043 117

Yuri Kim, Myungjin Kim, Dai Woo Kim and Seungsoo Rho
XEN Gel Stent for Conjunctiva with Minimal Mobility Caused by Scleral Encircling: A Case Report
Reprinted from: *J. Clin. Med.* **2023**, *12*, 4293, doi:10.3390/jcm12134293 129

Constance Weber, Sarah Hundertmark, Michael Petrak, Elisabeth Ludwig, Christian Karl Brinkmann, Frank G. Holz and Karl Mercieca
Clinical Outcomes of XEN45®-Stent Implantation after Failed Trabeculectomy: A Retrospective Single-Center Study
Reprinted from: *J. Clin. Med.* **2023**, *12*, 1296, doi:10.3390/jcm12041296 135

Giorgio Enrico Bravetti, Kevin Gillmann, Harsha L. Rao, André Mermoud and Kaweh Mansouri
Outcomes of Deep Sclerectomy following Failed XEN Gel Stent Implantation in Open-Angle Glaucoma: A Prospective Study
Reprinted from: *J. Clin. Med.* **2022**, *11*, 4784, doi:10.3390/jcm11164784 145

Carlo Enrico Traverso, Roberto G. Carassa, Antonio Maria Fea, Michele Figus, Carlo Astarita, Benedetta Piergentili, et al.
Effectiveness and Safety of Xen Gel Stent in Glaucoma Surgery: A Systematic Review of the Literature
Reprinted from: *J. Clin. Med.* **2023**, *12*, 5339, doi:10.3390/jcm12165339 159

Kazuyoshi Kitamura, Yoshiko Fukuda, Yuka Hasebe, Mio Matsubara and Kenji Kashiwagi
Mid-Term Results of Ab Interno Trabeculectomy among Japanese Glaucoma Patients
Reprinted from: *J. Clin. Med.* **2023**, *12*, 2332, doi:10.3390/jcm12062332 181

Jens Julian Storp, Friederike Elisabeth Vietmeier, Ralph-Laurent Merté, Raphael Koch, Julian Alexander Zimmermann, Nicole Eter and Viktoria Constanze Brücher
Long-Term Outcomes of the PRESERFLO MicroShunt Implant in a Heterogeneous Glaucoma Cohort
Reprinted from: *J. Clin. Med.* **2023**, *12*, 4474, doi:10.3390/jcm12134474 197

Michael X. Fu, Eduardo M. Normando, Sheila M. H. Luk, Mira Deshmukh, Faisal Ahmed, Laura Crawley, et al.
MicroShunt versus Trabeculectomy for Surgical Management of Glaucoma: A Retrospective Analysis
Reprinted from: *J. Clin. Med.* **2022**, *11*, 5481, doi:10.3390/jcm11185481 211

Shigeo S. M. Pawiroredjo, Wichor M. Bramer, Noemi D. Pawiroredjo, Jan Pals, Huub J. Poelman, Victor A. de Vries, et al.
Efficacy of the PRESERFLO MicroShunt and a Meta-Analysis of the Literature
Reprinted from: *J. Clin. Med.* **2022**, *11*, 7149, doi:10.3390/jcm11237149 225

Xiaotong Ren, Jie Wang, Xuemin Li and Lingling Wu
Long-Term Changes in Corneal Endothelial Cell Density after Ex-PRESS Implantation: A Contralateral Eye Study
Reprinted from: *J. Clin. Med.* **2022**, *11*, 5555, doi:10.3390/jcm11195555 . . . . **237**

Yitak Kim, Won Jeong Cho, Jung Dong Kim, Hyuna Cho, Hyoung Won Bae, Chan Yun Kim and Wungrak Choi
Tube–Iris Distance and Corneal Endothelial Cell Damage Following Ahmed Glaucoma Valve Implantation
Reprinted from: *J. Clin. Med.* **2022**, *11*, 5057, doi:10.3390/jcm11175057 . . . . **245**

Faisal A. Almobarak, Ahmed Alrubean, Waleed Alsarhani, Abdullah Aljenaidel and Essam A. Osman
Outcomes and Predictors of Failure of Ultrasound Cyclo Plasty for Primary Open-Angle Glaucoma
Reprinted from: *J. Clin. Med.* **2022**, *11*, 6770, doi:10.3390/jcm11226770 . . . . **259**

About the Editors

Michele Figus

Prof. Figus was born in Siena, Italy. He has served as an Associate Professor in Ophthalmology and as Chairman in the Residency School in Ophthalmology at the University of Pisa, Italy, since 2018. He became Head of the Ophthalmology Unit at Azienda Ospedaliero Universitaria Pisana and Head of the Center for Vision Education and Rehabilitation of Pisa in 2021. He has worked at Azienda Ospedaliero-Universitaria Pisana since 2001 in various areas of interest, including glaucoma, cataract surgery, ocular surface diseases, uveitis and retinal diseases. He has also acted as a National Expert in ophthalmic diagnosis (2010-2020) for the Italian Ophthalmology Society. Prof. Figus is an eye surgeon (cataract, glaucoma). He is the author of 160 JCR-indexed articles in ophthalmology and visual sciences, as well as 5 books. He has been the Principal Investigator in many clinical trials, and serves as an Associate Editor in three indexed journals. He has been a Fellow of the European Board of Ophthalmology (FEBOphth) since 2016 and serves as a Faculty member of the European School for Advances Studies in Ophthalmology (ESASO) and as an Advisor in the Ocular Disease Patients Association. He has been a guest speaker at lectures and delivered invited presentations at numerous international meetings and clinical courses. He is member of the American Academy of Ophthalmology, European Glaucoma Society and World Glaucoma Association.

Karl Mercieca

Karl Mercieca is a Senior Consultant Ophthalmologist and the Glaucoma Clinical Lead at the University Hospital Eye Clinic in Bonn, Germany. He is also an Honorary Senior Lecturer and the MSc IOVS glaucoma co-lead at the University of Manchester, UK, and the co-chair of the European Glaucoma Society (EGS) Sub-Speciality Training and Examinations Committee. Mr Mercieca has authored over 75 peer-reviewed publications to date and his research interests include CSF pulsatility, vascular biomarkers, non-penetrating glaucoma surgery and uveitic glaucoma. Mr Mercieca has also been the Primary Investigator for several large multi-centre trials on novel glaucoma surgery devices and drug delivery systems. He has also received many academic prizes throughout his career, including the Peter Watson Medal for the highest score in the FEBOS-GL glaucoma sub-speciality exam and the prize for the best poster presentation, awarded by the American Academy of Ophthalmology. Mr Mercieca is passionate about post-graduate medical education and improving ophthalmology and glaucoma teaching across Europe, with a particular interest in novel methods of learning, such as serious games and interactive visual learning.

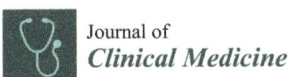

Editorial

Advances in Glaucoma Surgery

Karl Mercieca [1,2,*] and Michele Figus [3]

1. Glaucoma Unit, University Hospital Eye Clinic, 53127 Bonn, Germany
2. Faculty of Biology, Medicine and Health, University of Manchester, Manchester M13 9PL, UK
3. Department of Surgical, Medical, Molecular Pathology and Critical Care Medicine, University of Pisa, 56126 Pisa, Italy
* Correspondence: karl.mercieca@ukbonn.de

Glaucoma is one of the leading causes of irreversible sight loss worldwide, with a prevalence of 64.3 million in 2013 and an estimated increase to 111.8 million by 2040 [1]. The initial treatment for glaucoma usually comprises topical medication, but further procedures depend on the type of glaucoma, disease stage and severity, and several individual factors, including age, life expectancy, treatment adherence, quality of life, and both patients' and clinicians' personal choices. Irrespective of all these factors, surgical intervention may still be required in those patients with significant progression and uncontrolled disease despite maximum medical therapy [2].

Since its inception over 50 years ago, trabeculectomy has been the most common glaucoma surgery performed globally [3], although studies from the United States have demonstrated a decreasing trend in trabeculectomy cases in favor of newer surgical techniques such as minimally invasive or less invasive glaucoma surgical devices [4]. These span a large variety of true microinvasive invasive glaucoma surgeries or MIGS, defined by an 'ab interno' intracameral microincisional approach [5–7], and bleb-forming subconjunctival drainage devices such as the PreserFlo™ Microshunt (Santen, Miami, FL, USA) and Xen-45™ (Abbvie/Allergan, Irvine, CA, USA). The former can further be subdivided into 'cutting' MIGSs such as the Kahook Dual Blade™ (KDB, New World Medical, Rancho Cucamonga, CA, USA) and Trabectome™ (NeoMedix Corp., San Juan Capistrano, CA, USA), 'Trabecular Meshwork stent bypass' MIGSs such as the iStent™ (Glaukos, Aliso Viejo, CA, USA) and Hydrus™ (Alcon, Fort Worth, TX, USA), and 'Canaloplasty' MIGS techniques such as the OMNI™ (Sight Sciences, Menlo Park, CA, USA) and iTrack Advance™ (Nova Eye, Lakes Creek, Queensland, Australia) systems. These techniques have become more popular, particularly in patients who need a reduction in medication burden and also to potentially avoid some of the postoperative complications attributed to conventional glaucoma filtration surgery [8,9]. Additionally, and particularly in Europe, non-penetrating glaucoma surgeries (NPGS), such as deep sclerectomy and canaloplasty, have been developed to provide safer yet still effective ways of reducing intraocular pressure (IOP) in patients with more advanced glaucoma where target eye pressures are significantly lower [10–12]. The use of these procedures is increasing significantly compared to conventional trabeculectomy due to the drawbacks of risk of hypotony, intensive post-operative management, the need for proper training, and a significant learning curve. Finally, a further group of glaucoma surgeries, in the form of glaucoma drainage devices (GDDs) or 'tubes', have been around for a while as options for complex disease, including secondary glaucoma due to neovascularization and uveitis, congenital and juvenile glaucoma, aphakic glaucoma, etc. [13–15]. Although not that new in concept, new GDDs have been developed over the last few years, offering different lumen sizes and plate designs, which can further alter the outcomes we expect from these devices [16–18].

Advances in glaucoma surgery have therefore been happening for over the last five decades. However, there has never been such an exciting time to work in the field of glaucoma surgical therapy as the spectrum of options available has become so wide, dense,

Citation: Mercieca, K.; Figus, M. Advances in Glaucoma Surgery. *J. Clin. Med.* **2023**, *12*, 828. https://doi.org/10.3390/jcm12030828

Received: 11 January 2023
Accepted: 17 January 2023
Published: 20 January 2023

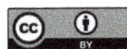

Copyright: © 2023 by the authors. Licensee MDPI, Basel, Switzerland. This article is an open access article distributed under the terms and conditions of the Creative Commons Attribution (CC BY) license (https://creativecommons.org/licenses/by/4.0/).

and varied. Big Pharma is acquiring more and more start-ups that have developed, tried, and tested their products with ever-increasing amounts of evidence building over the last few years. This trend will only increase the drive to seek the best devices and to utilize them to their best capacity in individualized ways. Ultimately, this can only benefit the patient, as long as sound evidence, real-life experience, and cost-effectiveness are also available and considered simultaneously. The evolution of older surgeries such as more modern and innovative ways of performing trabeculectomy and NPGS, and the dissemination of more recent techniques and devices, including their use beyond the original indications for which they were developed, can only boost our chances of effectively lowering IOP and reducing glaucoma visual disability for our patients. We truly hope that this Special Issue, entitled "Advances in Glaucoma Surgery", can truly capture the essence of these new, exciting, and creative ways of enhancing the effectiveness and safety of our glaucoma surgical armamentarium.

Conflicts of Interest: The authors declare no conflict of interest.

References

1. Tham, Y.C.; Li, X.; Wong, T.Y.; Quigley, H.A.; Aung, T.; Cheng, C.Y. Global prevalence of glaucoma and projections of glaucoma burden through 2040: A systematic review and meta-analysis. *Ophthalmology* **2014**, *121*, 2081–2090. [CrossRef] [PubMed]
2. Musch, D.C.; Gillespie, B.W.; Lichter, P.R.; Niziol, L.M.; Janz, N.K.; Investigators, C.S. Visual field progression in the Collaborative Initial Glaucoma Treatment Study the impact of treatment and other baseline factors. *Ophthalmology* **2009**, *116*, 200–207. [CrossRef] [PubMed]
3. Mansouri, K.; Medeiros, F.A.; Weinreb, R.N. Global rates of glaucoma surgery. *Graefes Arch. Clin. Exp. Ophthalmol.* **2013**, *251*, 2609–2615. [CrossRef] [PubMed]
4. Edmunds, B.; Thompson, J.R.; Salmon, J.F.; Wormald, R.P. The National Survey of Trabeculectomy III: Early and late complications. *Eye* **2002**, *16*, 297–303. [CrossRef] [PubMed]
5. Saheb, H.; Ahmed, I.I. Micro-invasive glaucoma surgery: Current perspectives and future directions. *Curr. Opin. Ophthalmol.* **2012**, *23*, 96–104. [CrossRef] [PubMed]
6. Nichani, P.; Popovic, M.M.; Schlenker, M.B.; Park, J.; Ahmed, I.I.K. Microinvasive glaucoma surgery: A review of 3476 eyes. *Surv. Ophthalmol.* **2021**, *66*, 714–742. [CrossRef] [PubMed]
7. SooHoo, J.R.; Seibold, L.K.; Radcliffe, N.; Kahook, M.Y. Minimally invasive glaucoma surgery: Current implants and future innovations. *Can. J. Ophthalmol.* **2014**, *49*, 528–533. [CrossRef] [PubMed]
8. Chen, D.Z.; Sng, C.C.A. Safety and Efficacy of Microinvasive Glaucoma Surgery. *J. Ophthalmol.* **2017**, *2017*, 3182935. [CrossRef] [PubMed]
9. Conlon, R.; Saheb, H.; Ahmed, I.I. Glaucoma treatment trends: A review. *Can. J. Ophthalmol.* **2017**, *52*, 114–124. [CrossRef] [PubMed]
10. Fyodorov, S.N. Nonpenetrating deep sclerectomy in open angle glaucoma. *Ophthalmosurgery* **1989**, *3*, 52–55.
11. Mendrinos, E.; Mermoud, A.; Shaarawy, T. Nonpenetrating glaucoma surgery. *Surv. Ophthalmol.* **2008**, *53*, 592–630. [CrossRef] [PubMed]
12. Rabiolo, A.; Leadbetter, D.; Alaghband, P.; Anand, N. Primary Deep Sclerectomy in Open-Angle Glaucoma: Long-Term Outcomes and Risk Factors for Failure. *Ophthalmol. Glaucoma* **2021**, *4*, 149–161. [CrossRef] [PubMed]
13. Aref, A.A.; Gedde, S.J.; Budenz, D.L. Glaucoma Drainage Implant Surgery. *Dev. Ophthalmol.* **2017**, *59*, 43–52. [PubMed]
14. Christakis, P.G.; Kalenak, J.W.; Tsai, J.C.; Zurakowski, D.; Kammer, J.A.; Harasymowycz, P.J.; Mura, J.J.; Cantor, L.B.; Ahmed, I.I.K. The Ahmed Versus Baerveldt Study: Five-Year Treatment Outcomes. *Ophthalmology* **2016**, *123*, 2093–2102. [CrossRef] [PubMed]
15. Rockwood, E.J. The Ahmed Baerveldt Comparison (ABC) Study: Long-Term Results, Successes, Failures, and Complications. *Am. J. Ophthalmol.* **2016**, *163*, xii–xiv. [CrossRef] [PubMed]
16. Koh, V.; Chew, P.; Triolo, G.; Lim, K.S.; Barton, K. Treatment Outcomes Using the PAUL Glaucoma Implant to Control Intraocular Pressure in Eyes with Refractory Glaucoma. *Ophthalmol. Glaucoma* **2020**, *3*, 350–359. [CrossRef] [PubMed]
17. Vallabh, N.A.; Mason, F.; Yu, J.T.S.; Yau, K.; Fenerty, C.H.; Mercieca, K.; Spencer, A.F.; Au, L. Surgical technique, perioperative management and early outcome data of the PAUL® glaucoma drainage device. *Eye* **2022**, *36*, 1905–1910.
18. Roy, S.; Villamarin, A.; Stergiopulos, C.; Bigler, S.; Guidotti, J.; Stergiopulos, N.; Kniestedt, C.; Mermoud, A.J. Initial Clinical Results of the eyeWatch: A New Adjustable Glaucoma Drainage Device Used in Refractory Glaucoma Surgery. *J. Glaucoma* **2019**, *28*, 452–458. [CrossRef] [PubMed]

Disclaimer/Publisher's Note: The statements, opinions and data contained in all publications are solely those of the individual author(s) and contributor(s) and not of MDPI and/or the editor(s). MDPI and/or the editor(s) disclaim responsibility for any injury to people or property resulting from any ideas, methods, instructions or products referred to in the content.

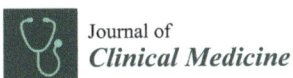

Article

Topical Steroids and Glaucoma Filtration Surgery Outcomes: An In Vivo Confocal Study of the Conjunctiva

Leonardo Mastropasqua [1,†], Lorenza Brescia [1,*], Francesca D'Arcangelo [1,‡], Mario Nubile [1], Giada D'Onofrio [1], Michele Totta [1], Fabiana Perna [1,2], Raffaella Aloia [1] and Luca Agnifili [1,†]

1 Ophthalmology Clinic, Department of Medicine and Aging Science, University G. d'Annunzio of Chieti-Pescara, 66100 Chieti, Italy; mastropa@unich.it (L.M.); francescadarcangelo@gmail.com (F.D.); m.nubile@unich.it (M.N.); giada01.88@hotmail.it (G.D.); michetto135@gmail.com (M.T.); f.perna@iapb.it (F.P.); raffaellaaloia77@gmail.com (R.A.); l.agnifili@unich.it (L.A.)
2 International Agency of Prevention of Blindness, 00185 Rome, Italy
* Correspondence: brescia.lorenza@gmail.com; Tel.: +39-0871-358-489; Fax: +39-0871-358-794
† These authors contributed equally to this work.
‡ F.D. passed away during the manuscript preparation.

Abstract: (1) Background: The purpose of this study is to investigate the effects of topical steroids on conjunctiva in patients undergoing filtration surgery (FS) for glaucoma by using confocal microscopy (CM); (2) Methods: One hundred and four glaucomatous patients were randomized to fluorometholone or lubricants four weeks before FS. CM was performed before treatments and pre-operatively. Dendritic and goblet cell densities (DCD, GCD), stromal meshwork reflectivity (SMR), vascular tortuosity (VT), and intra-ocular pressure (IOP) were the main outcomes. By evaluating treatments and outcomes (12-month success/failure) as categorical variables, patients were grouped into Group 1, 2, 3, or 4 (success/failure with fluorometholone, or lubricants); (3) Results: Twelve-month IOP was reduced in Groups 1 and 3 ($p < 0.001$). After treatments, DCD and SMR were reduced in Groups 1 and 2 ($p < 0.01$), and 1 and 3 ($p < 0.05$), respectively. Pre-operative DCD was lower in the steroid compared to lubricant group ($p < 0.001$), whereas SMR was lower in successful (1 and 3) compared to failed groups (2 and 4) ($p = 0.004$). There were no significant differences between the fluorometholone and lubricant groups for success percentages. The number of bleb management procedures and IOP lowering medications were lower in Group 1 compared to Groups 2–4 ($p < 0.05$); (4) Conclusions: Topical steroids mitigate conjunctival inflammation and lower the stromal density in patients undergoing FS. These modifications lead to less intensive post-operative management.

Keywords: glaucoma filtration surgery; surgery outcome; steroids; conjunctiva; ocular surface preparation; in vivo confocal microscopy

1. Introduction

More than fifty years after its introduction, filtration surgery (FS) still represents the most diffuse surgical procedure to reduce the intra-ocular pressure (IOP) in patients with medically uncontrolled glaucoma. FS works by creating an intra-scleral fistula that drains aqueous humor (AH) from the anterior chamber toward the sub-conjunctival space, thus forming a resorption structure known as a filtration bleb [1–3]. However, the filtration bleb may fail in its function over time for different reasons.

As widely demonstrated, glaucoma therapy-related conjunctival modifications may significantly affect the bleb filtration capabilities after FS, since IOP lowering medications damage, disturb, or stimulate components that are involved in the AH outflow through the bleb-wall [4–11]. These components include goblet cells (GCs), stromal collagen bundles, inflammatory dendritic cells (DCs), and blood or lymphatic vessels. In detail, GCs work as carriers of the AH, whereas stromal collagen hinders AH resorption by increasing the bleb-wall resistivity to fluids outflow. On the other hand, DCs and blood vessels stimulate

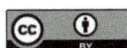

inflammation, affecting the AH carriers and stimulating collagen deposition [3,8,9,11]. The progressive alterations of these structures increase the risk of inadequate AH drainage and surgical failure [4–7,12]. Therefore, the need to manage the ocular surface before FS, especially by mitigating inflammation, is keenly felt by surgeons [13,14].

To date, very few studies have investigated whether pre-operative strategies aimed at mitigating ocular surface disease (OSD) can favorably affect the FS outcome. In a randomized placebo-controlled trial, the use of topical ketorolac or fluorometholone one month before trabeculectomy reduced the likelihood of post-operative bleb needling or the need for IOP lowering drugs, with better results in patients receiving steroids compared to those taking ketorolac [15]. In another study, Lorenz et al. found that a simplified pre-operative medication regimen, which comprised only a preservative-free (PF) fixed combination of dorzolamide/timolol, reduced the ocular surface inflammation and was as effective as topical steroids and systemic acetazolamide in terms of surgical outcomes [16]. Nevertheless, though the reduction of pre-operative conjunctival inflammation is believed to limit scarring within the bleb-wall after FS, studies evaluating the conjunctival changes induced by steroids at the site of FS at a cellular level are still lacking.

In vivo confocal microscopy (IVCM) has been widely used to describe the conjunctiva in patients with glaucoma, either during the medical management of the disease or in the pre-operative period [7–9,11]. In fact, IVCM is able to evaluate the above-mentioned components involved in the AH outflow after surgery, which can be considered as potential indicators of surgical outcomes. This is crucial, because a pre-operative assessment may guide the clinician in adopting personalized peri-operative strategies.

The aims of the present study were to evaluate, using IVCM, the impact of topical steroids on conjunctival GCs, DCs, stromal density, and blood vessels on FS outcomes, and to evaluate whether confocal features could play a role in predicting success or failure in patients undergoing FS.

2. Materials and Methods

2.1. Study Population

This prospective, placebo-controlled, single center study adhered to the tenets of the Declaration of Helsinki and was approved by the Institutional Review Board of Department of Medicine and Aging Sciences, University G. d'Annunzio of Chieti and Pescara, Italy. All eligible patients who agreed to participate in the study signed an informed consent form before enrollment, after receiving an explanation of the nature and possible consequences of the study. Consecutive patients scheduled for first-time FS (trabeculectomy) were enrolled at the Ophthalmology Clinic, National High-Tech Eye Center (NHEC) of the University G. d'Annunzio of Chieti and Pescara, Chieti, Italy.

Inclusion criteria were: open angle glaucoma with uncontrolled IOP under maximal tolerated medical therapy (three active compounds, comprising the short-term use of systemic oral acetazolamide when required); progression of visual field (VF; Humphrey Field Analyzer (HFA), Guided Progression Analysis software) damage, as confirmed on three consecutive reliable tests; and IOP lowering therapy regimen unmodified in the last three months. Exclusion criteria were: secondary glaucoma; history of concomitant intra-ocular or ocular surface disease that could potentially contraindicate the use of topical steroids; known allergy to steroids; bulbar trauma; systemic or topical therapies in the last 6 months, potentially affecting the ocular surface; any previous ocular surgery (excluding cataract); use of contact lenses; and pregnancy. If both eyes were eligible for the study, only the eye with the more advanced perimetric stage was included.

2.2. Pre-Operative Treatments and Peri-Operative Considerations

After enrollment, patients were randomized (by a computer-based randomization program in a double-blinded fashion) to receive fluorometholone 0.1% (Fluaton, Bausch & Lomb-IOM SpA, Aci Sant'Antonio, Catania, Italy; Group A) or lubricants (Hyalistil BIO, SIFI, Aci Sant'Antonio, Catania, Italy; Group B). All study medications contained benzalkonium chloride (BAK) as a preservative. The labels of the study medication bottles were concealed from the patient as well as the physician.

In the 4 weeks preceding the date of surgery, patients were instructed to administer in the eye scheduled for FS one drop of their assigned medication four times daily, and to continue unmodified their IOP-lowering medical therapy. Two weeks after the initiation of pre-operative treatment, a safety check with IOP measurement was scheduled.

All patients underwent a 0.02% mitomycin-C (3 min, in soaked sponges) augmented trabeculectomy, as previously described [17]. All surgical procedures were performed using a standardized technique, which required the creation of a fornix-based conjunctival flap and a 4 × 4 mm, 300-µm thick scleral flap, which was sutured down with four 10-0 nylon sutures. To limit post-operative inflammation, the conjunctival flap was sutured down using 10-0 nylon sutures.

As per protocol, the post-surgical therapy required the use of PF dexamethasone eye drops four times daily (tapered in 12 weeks) and PF levofloxacin four times daily (discontinued after 2 weeks).

Patients were examined weekly during the first month; then, the frequency of controls was scheduled in accordance with the post-operative course, considering as clinical indicators the filtration bleb features at slit lamp (Mainz Bleb Appearance Grading System) and IOP [18]. The last follow-up was planned at 12 months.

Each decision on the timing for additional procedures was made according to post-operative IOP and bleb morphology. If IOP progressively increased and was not considered at target for the patient [19], and bleb features tended to become encapsulated or flat, management strategies including laser suture lysis, bleb needling with 5-fluorouracil, or bleb revision with mitomycin-C were sequentially adopted. When all management strategies failed to control IOP, anti-glaucoma therapy was restarted.

At the 12-month visit, surgery was considered successful when baseline IOP was reduced by at least 30%, with or without anti-glaucoma medications; otherwise, it was considered to have failed. In case of failure, patients abandoned the study and received additional glaucoma surgery.

2.3. Examinations

At baseline, before initiating treatments, patients underwent a complete examination, with the determination of the best corrected visual acuity, slit lamp ocular surface and lid assessment, IOP measurement (Goldmann applanation tonometry, AT900®, Haag Streit Diagnostics, Koeniz, Switzerland), anterior and posterior segment evaluation, and VF test (HFA 24-2 test, SITA-standard). Twenty-four hours later, patients underwent IVCM of the conjunctiva, which was repeated at the same site after four weeks, i.e., the day before the FS.

2.4. IVCM of the Bulbar Conjunctiva

IVCM (HRT III Rostock Cornea Module, diode-laser 670 nm; Heidelberg Engineering, Heidelberg, Germany) was performed at the upper bulbar conjunctiva, with particular attention at the site corresponding to the bleb formation after FS, to evaluate the structures involved in AH resorption, that is, epithelial GCs and DCs, stroma, and blood vessels. GCs and stroma can be considered as pre-surgical indicators of further trans bleb-wall AH flow and resistivity, respectively. DCs and blood vessels can be considered as indicators of glaucoma therapy-related ocular surface inflammation and can be used to estimate the post-surgical fibrotic reaction of the conjunctiva [9]. Two masked investigators (LB, investigator 1; MT, investigator 2) independently calculated the GCD and DCD to assess the interobserver variability.

2.5. Confocal Parameters

(i) Goblet cell density (GCD): in accordance with the definition and images provided in previous confocal studies, GCs had to appear as oval-shaped and hyperreflective cells, dispersed within the epithelium (or crowded in groups), larger than the surrounding epithelial cells, and located at a depth of 10–30 μm [7–9,11]. As documented, GCs act as carriers of the AH through the bleb-wall epithelium after filtration surgery [8,9,11]. The cell count software (Heidelberg Engineering GmbH) of the confocal microscope was used to determine the GCD (cells/mm^2 ± SD) in manual mode.

(ii) Dendritic cell density (DCD): the definition and features of DCs had to be consistent with those reported in literature [9,11,20]. DCs can appear mature and activated (hyper-reflective and elongated body, with membrane processes and frequently crowded in clusters) or immature and silent (large body with rare membrane processes, if any). They are located within the epithelium and the basal membrane of the conjunctiva (10–30 μm to 30–50 μm of depth) and act as peripheral effectors of the immune system, stimulating inflammation and fibrosis in response to toxic stimuli [20,21]. As for GCD, the cell count software was used to determine the DCD (cells/mm2 ± SD) in manual mode.

(iii) Stromal meshwork reflectivity (SMR): as for GCs and DCs, the characteristics of the conjunctival stroma at IVCM had to be consistent with those reported in previous studies [9,22]. This layer (50–150 μm of depth) appears loosely arranged with thin collagen fibers and some blood vessels in the external portion but presents a denser, fibrous network with bundles of collagen fibers—occasionally hosting blood vessels, cystic spaces, and inflammatory cells—in the internal portion [22–24]. The tissue reflectivity represents an indirect confocal indicator of the amount of collagen fibers contained within the stroma and, thus, is a surrogate measure of the conjunctival resistivity to fluid movement. SMR was calculated as previously described, i.e., by determining the average gray value of a selected high-quality image, using the Image J software (http://imagej.nih.gov/ij/ accessed on 21 September 2021; provided in the public domain by the National Institutes of Health, Bethesda, MD, USA) [9]. SMR was graded as follows: normal (Grade 0: average gray value <90), mild (Grade 1: gray value between 90.01 and 105), moderate (Grade 2: gray value between 105.01 and 125), and high (Grade 3: >125.01), reflectivity; according to this grading scale, grades 0 to 3 corresponded to a loosely, mildly, densely, and very densely arranged stromal networks, respectively.

(iv) Vessel tortuosity (VT): conjunctival vessels are located in the sub-epithelium or superficial stroma, and less frequently in the deep fibrotic portion of the stroma. They appear as broad black linear or slightly curved structures with parallel sides, frequently showing hyper-reflective and round-shaped cells within the lumen [22–24]. VT was assessed according to a previously adopted grading scale with four grades: straight (0), mild (1), moderate (2), and severe (3) [22]. Vessel tortuosity is an indirect indicator of stromal fibrosis and a direct indicator of chronic local inflammation [25].

2.6. Confocal Microscopy Procedure

The details of the confocal microscopy procedure to analyze the upper bulbar conjunctiva in patients undergoing FS have been previously described [9]. Briefly, with the patient instructed to direct the gaze downward, the entire upper bulbar conjunctiva (superior nasal, superior central, and superior temporal portions) was analyzed.

Images were acquired at the epithelium (10–30 μm of depth) to evaluate GCs, at the sub-epithelium (10–30 μm) to evaluate DCs, and from the stroma (50–150 μm) to evaluate the SMR. The automatic brightness mode was selected during all examinations.

Sixty images (20 images per each portion; field of view of 400 × 400 μm) were acquired in both the pre-and post-treatment sessions; among all the acquired images, 15 randomly selected, high-quality scans per case (five per portion) without motion blur or compression lines were selected for the analysis. Two different, experienced IVCM operators performed the confocal examinations and selected the images (LB and MT); a second experienced operator evaluated the images (GDO). All the operators were masked regarding the patient history and group assignment.

2.7. Outcomes of the Study

Pre- and post-treatment sessions, and 12-month data were considered the time points for the statistical analyses. The main outcome measures were the modification of GCD, DCD, SMR, and VT, and the success or failure at 12 months based on the relative IOP reduction as compared with baseline IOP. Differences among treatments for post-operative bleb management procedures (laser suture lysis, needling, needling revision) and IOP lowering medications, and correlations between post-surgical procedures, IOP lowering medications, and 12-months IOP and group classification were also evaluated.

2.8. Statistical Analysis

The sample size was determined based on a success rate of 100% in the group treated with steroids (Group 1) and 76% in the control group (Group 2) [15]. The alpha level was set to 0.05 and the power to 80%. To minimize the number of patients with the worse outcome, the enrollment ratio was set to 0.6, i.e., 3 out of every 5 patients were assigned to the group that would receive steroid therapy prior to surgery. The required sample size was determined to be 53 patients: 33 in the steroid group and 20 in the non-treated group. Enrolled patients were assigned to treatment groups using a block (size = 5) design.

The two treatment groups (A, steroid and B, lubricant) and the two possible outcomes (success or failure at 12 months) were evaluated as categorical variables and further grouped in the following manner: Group 1 and 2, success or failure after steroid treatment; Group 3 and 4, success or failure without steroid treatment. Patient characteristics for the treatment groups were evaluated using chi squared and student's *t*-test, as appropriate. Variations from baseline to pre-operative values of IOP, DCD, GCD, and SMR were evaluated using an ANOVA with post-hoc Tukey HSD test, and VT with a Kruskal-Wallis Test.

Moreover, the canonical discriminant analysis (CDA) was used to discern the four groups using the percentage variation between baseline and pre-operative clinical and confocal microscopy parameters, and to estimate the impact of steroid treatment on the surgical outcomes. Statistical significance for backward selection was determined using an $\alpha = 0.05$. Leave-one-out cross-validation was used to validate the predictive model.

Spearman's non-parametric coefficient was used to investigate the correlations between post-surgical procedures, IOP lowering medications, and 12-month IOP and group classification.

Statistical analyses were performed using SPSS software (version 26, International Business Machines Corp., Armonk, NY, USA). MedCalc Statistical Software version 16 (MedCalc Software Ltd., Ostend, Belgium) was used to determine sample size.

3. Results

3.1. Clinical Results

All patients completed surgery without complications, and none was lost to follow-up. Table 1 reports the demographic and clinical characteristics of the four groups. Pre-operative IOP did not significantly change compared to baseline in any of the groups and did not differ among groups at both time points. Significant differences were found between baseline and 12 months IOP for Groups 1 and 3 ($p < 0.001$).

There were no significant differences between groups treated with fluorometholone (1 and 2) and control groups (3 and 4) with regard to the percentage (%) of patients with complete success ($p = 0.08$) or qualified success ($p = 0.37$). Conversely, the numbers of post-operative bleb management procedures and IOP lowering medications were lower in Group 1 compared to Groups 2–4 ($p < 0.05$). Figure 1 shows the jittered distribution of overall bleb management procedures among groups.

3.2. IVCM Results

The four treatment groups did not present statistically significant differences in baseline DCD, GCD, SMR, and VT, or in pre-operative, GCD, and VT. Compared to baseline, DCD was significantly reduced in Groups 1 and 2 ($p < 0.001$ and $p < 0.01$, respectively), whereas SMR was slightly reduced in Groups 1 and 3 ($p < 0.05$). Pre-operative DCD was significantly lower in Groups 1 and 2 compared to control groups ($p < 0.001$), whereas SMR was significantly lower in successful (1 and 3) compared to failed groups (2 and 4) ($p = 0.004$). VT and GCD did not change between baseline and pre-operative time points in any of the groups, but pre-operative GCD was significantly higher in Groups 1–3 compared to Group 4 ($p < 0.001$) (Table 2). GCD (28.72 ± 2.14 and 28.91 ± 3.21, respectively), and DCD (58.22 ± 7.32 and 58.97 ± 6.99, respectively) estimated by investigator 1 (LB) were not significantly different ($p > 0.05$) from that estimated by the investigator 2 (MT).

Table 1. Demographic and clinical data.

	Gender (M/F)	Age (Years $\pm$ SD)	Time on Therapy (Months $\pm$ SD)	Baseline IOP (mmHg $\pm$ SD)	Pre-OP IOP (mmHg $\pm$ SD)	12 Months IOP (mmHg $\pm$ SD)	Post-OP Procedures ($n \pm$ SD)	Post-OP IOP Lowering Medications ($n \pm$ SD)
Group 1	13/16	68.34 ± 7.97	72.5 ± 3.2	29.55 ± 5.32	28.24 ± 4.57	15.51 ± 2.28 †‡	1.28 ± 1.01 *#	0.93 ± 0.88 *
Group 2	10/13	72.65 ± 7.23	75.2 ± 4.1	31.55 ± 7.62	30.22 ± 5.69	26.11 ± 1.76	2.61 ± 1.23	1.36 ± 1.01 §
Group 3	15/11	65.54 ± 6.24	68.7 ± 3.1	28.93 ± 5.07	27.08 ± 4.51	14.10 ± 2.49 †‡	3.23 ± 2.10	1.92 ± 0.81
Group 4	12/14	74.76 ± 8.47	70.7 ± 2.9	30.22 ± 6.48	28.89 ± 5.11	25.67 ± 3.16	3.87 ± 1.71	2.15 ± 1.15

IOP: (mmHg $\pm$ SD, standard deviation), intraocular pressure; M: males; F: females. * $p < 0.001$ vs. Groups 3 and 4; # $p < 0.05$ vs. Group 2; § $p < 0.05$ vs. Groups 3 and 4; † $p < 0.001$ vs. Baseline IOP; ‡ $p < 0.01$ vs. failure Groups (2 and 4).

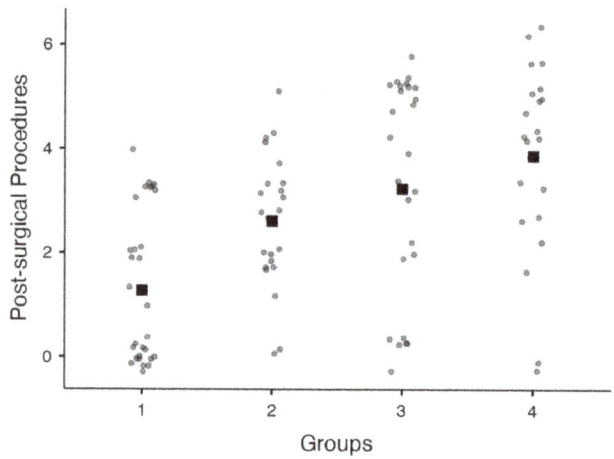

Figure 1. Graphical distribution of jittered data (values are plotted as dots along each axis) among groups representing post-surgical bleb management procedures. Median value is representing by squares along axes.

3.3. Canonical Discriminant Analysis

CDA was used to distinguish groups using two discriminant functions, based on DCD and SMR, which were the highly significative variables found between baseline and pre-operative time points. Specifically, the standardized CDA was based on the percentage variation of DCD and SMR, where the coefficients were 0.957 and 0.334 for function 1 and −0.294 and 0.943 for function 2 (Figure 2). Both functions were able to discriminate the four groups (Wilks's lambda < 0.001), while each function alone did not perform as well (Wilks's lambda = 0.001). Functions 1 and 2 correctly classified 90.6% of the original grouped patients. Leave-one-out cross-validation, where each case was classified by the functions derived from all other cases, correctly classified 86.8% of cases, thus validating the results of predictive correlation between the modification of DCD and SMR in the 4 weeks before surgery and the success/failure of trabeculectomy at 12 months.

The number of post-surgical procedures and the number of post-operative IOP lowering medications positively correlated with 12-month IOP ($p < 0.001$, rho = 0.406) and group classifications ($p < 0.001$, rho = 0.518). Figure 3 is a mosaic of confocal frames taken from two representative patients, showing the modification of the confocal parameters between baseline and the pre-operative time point in successful (Group 1) vs. failed cases (Group 4).

Table 2. Confocal microscopy parameters.

	Baseline DCD	Baseline GCD	Baseline SMR	Baseline VT	Pre-OP IOP	Pre-OP DCD	Pre-OP GCD	Pre-OP SMR	Pre-OP VT
Group 1	57.57 ± 8.69	28.09 ± 2.82	104.68 ± 8.28	1.72 ± 0.92	28.24 ± 4.57	35.04 ± 7.40 *	30.63 ± 2.78	94.99 ± 11.85 #	1.38 ± 0.82 #
Group 2	59.26 ± 5.04	29.36 ± 4.22	100.68 ± 8.70	1.55 ± 0.73	30.22 ± 5.69	41.98 ± 4.42 ^	28.61 ± 4.07	104.29 ± 9.68 ¥	1.33 ± 1.12
Group 3	59.35 ± 9.44	29.52 ± 4.12	103.21 ± 10.65	1.54 ± 0.93	27.08 ± 4.51	55.78 ± 10.65 §	29.15 ± 4.41	96.59 ± 10.57 #	1.15 ± 0.88 #
Group 4	58.27 ± 4.78	28.39 ± 4.79	100.72 ± 9.31	1.55 ± 0.88	28.89 ± 5.11	66.67 ± 4.48 §	24.93 ± 4.43 °	109.11 ± 5.18 ¥	1.67 ± 0.71

DCD (cells/mm^2 ± SD), dendritic cell density; GCD (cells/mm^2 ± SD), goblet cell density; SMR, stromal meshwork reflectivity (arbitrary grading scale); VT, vascular tortuosity (arbitrary grading scale). * $p < 0.001$ vs. Baseline; ^ $p < 0.01$ vs. Baseline; # $p < 0.05$ vs. Baseline; § $p < 0.001$ vs. steroid Groups (1 and 2); ° $p < 0.001$ vs. Groups 1–3; ¥ $p = 0.004$ vs. successful Groups (1 and 3).

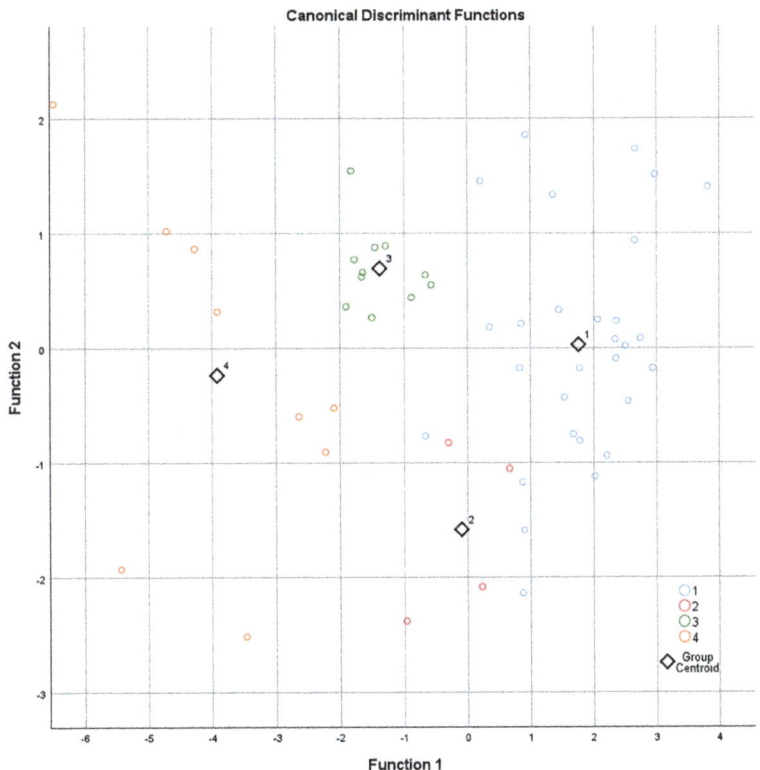

Figure 2. Scatter plot generated with the two functions obtained with the canonical discriminant analysis of patients belonging to the four treatment-outcome groups. Function 1: +0.957 (delta DCD) and +0.334 (delta SMR). Function 2: −0.294 (delta DCD) and +0.943 (delta SMR). These functions correctly classified 90.6% of the original grouped patients and validation with leave-one-out cross-validation correctly classified 86.8%.

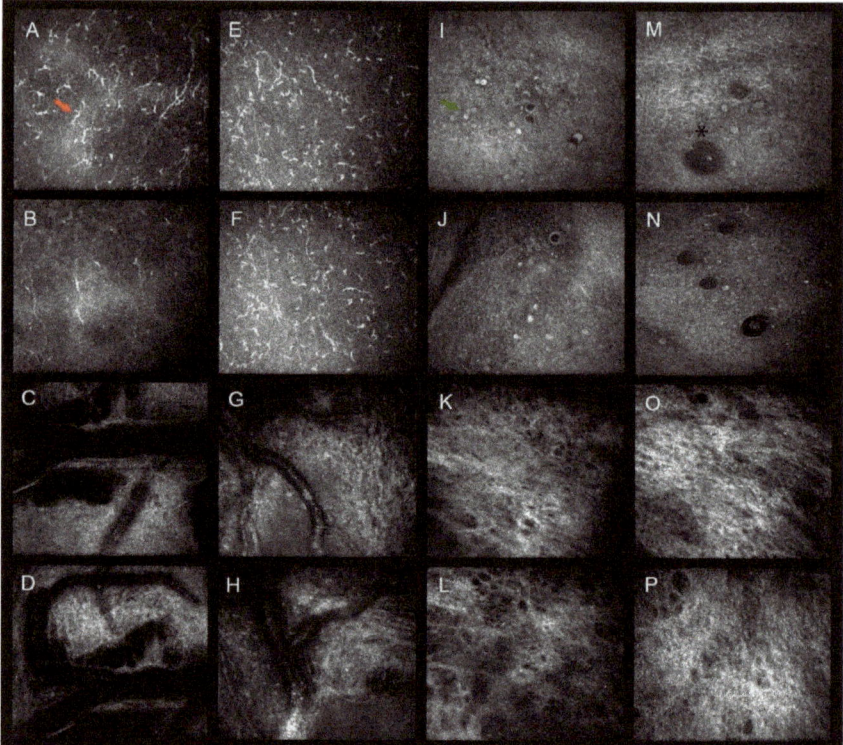

Figure 3. Baseline and post-treatments confocal frames of the conjunctival epithelium and stroma in representative patients that received topical fluorometholone (**A–D,I–L**; Group 1) or lubricants (**E–H,M–P**, Group 4). Compared to baseline (**A**), fluorometholone significantly reduced sub-epithelial DCs (red arrow) four weeks after treatments (**B**), whereas lubricants did not (**E,F**). Epithelial GCs (green arrow) did not change their baseline density neither in patients receiving steroids (**I,J**) nor in controls (**M,N**) with an intra-epithelial conjunctival microcyst surrounded by goblet cells recognizable (asterisk, **M**). The baseline vessel tortuosity did not change after steroid (**C,D**) or lubricant (**G,H**) treatments. The stromal meshwork reflectivity presented a mild reduction compared to baseline in patients receiving fluorometholone (**K,L**) while this was not observed in patients receiving lubricants (**O,P**).

4. Discussion

The bulk of the literature clearly demonstrates that the pre-operative features of the ocular surface and the outcomes of glaucoma filtration surgery have a strong mutual relationship [6,14,26]. Therefore, improving the ocular surface quality plays a critical role in the management of patients who are candidates for surgery [13,14].

In the present study, IVCM was, for the first time, used to evaluate the effects of topical steroids on the most crucial conjunctival structures involved in the AH resorption through the bleb-wall. In detail, we found that unpreserved fluorometholone reduced pre-operative DCD by 40% and 30%, in successful and failed surgeries (Groups 1 and 2), respectively. Moreover, fluorometholone slightly reduced (9%) SMR only in patients that underwent a successful FS (Group 1). Interestingly, these modifications were not associated with an increase in the success rate of surgery, but showed a significantly reduced need for post-operative bleb manipulation procedures or the use of IOP lowering eyedrops.

These results are in agreement with previous findings, highlighting that the ocular surface improvement induced by low-potency steroids such as fluorometholone was associated with less intensive post-operative management [15,27]. The novelty of our study lies in the fact that we investigated, in vivo and at a microscopic level, the cellular modifications underlying the clinical effects of topical steroids.

DCs represent a key cellular population in patients with glaucoma; their activation and proliferation were shown to contribute to ocular surface inflammation and to increase the risk of bleb dysfunction over time [7,9,20]. Similarly, the presence of a pre-operative, dense conjunctival stroma was found to exert a negative influence on the surgery outcome [9]. Therefore, the pre-operative reduction of DCD and SMR induced by topical steroids may positively affect bleb functionality after surgery by mitigating inflammation and limiting tissue fibrosis.

These results agree with the findings of Baudouin et al., who observed a significant reduction of a key inflammatory marker, human leukocyte antigen (HLA)-DR, after one month of therapy with fluorometholone, and with the observation that steroids have significant anti-proliferative activity on Tenon's fibroblast cell line cultures, reducing collagen deposition [27,28].

As stated above, fluorometholone-related DCD and SMR reductions led to less intensive post-operative management. Specifically, this was documented only in patients who had the greatest inflammation reduction and a partial improvement of the stromal density of the conjunctiva (Group 1). In fact, Group 1 presented a 10% higher DCD reduction compared to Group 2, with a decrease in SMR of almost 10% (SMR did not change in Group 2). On this basis, one may hypothesize that steroid treatment may influence surgery outcomes only if the inflammation mitigation surpasses a certain threshold (at least one third reduction in the tested parameters) and when the inflammation mitigation is coupled with a slight decrease in tissue fibrosis. These considerations appear to be in line with a pioneer study in which Broadway and co-workers found that the pre-operative use of fluorometholone 1% increased success rates by reducing both the density of inflammatory cells and fibroblasts within the conjunctiva [29].

A critical interpretation of these observations is that the inflammation mitigation induced by steroids, when under a certain limit, is only useful to reduce the need for post-operative management, rather than to increase the likelihood of surgical success [15]. It is likely that in order to achieve an increase in the success rate of FS, the reduction of pre-operative inflammation and of stromal density should be greater than 40% and 10%, respectively. This could be obtained with longer duration treatments or by using more potent steroids.

The results observed in Group 3 raise different considerations. This group that received topical lubricants had the same percentage of successful surgeries compared to Group 1, without DCD reduction and with mild SMR improvement. On the other hand, Group 3 required a higher number of bleb manipulation procedures and post-operative IOP lowering medications compared to Group 1 (3 times more).

Based on these findings, one cannot completely rule out a potential impact of sodium hyaluronate on surgical outcomes. As is known, the use of sodium hyaluronate represents one potential strategy to prepare patients for FS, since it mitigates dry eye and, thus, may contribute to reducing inflammation [13,14]. In addition, sodium hyaluronate seems to stimulate GCs, which play an active role in the aqueous humor resorption through the bleb-wall after FS [8,9,11]. Nonetheless, in our study, GCD did not increase with the use of lubricants, probably because of the short duration of treatment.

Finally, as an ancillary part of this study, we also evaluated whether IVCM could be useful in providing cellular predictive biomarkers of surgical outcome in patients receiving pre-operative management with steroids.

As expected, because of their importance in bleb functionality, the discriminant analysis found that DCD and SMR, only when considered together, were highly significant confocal variables which correctly distinguished groups in 90% of cases. In this way, CDA further confirmed the impact of steroids on FS outcomes, since the analysis showed that patients presenting a higher reduction of pre-operative DCD and SMR were part of Groups 1 and 2.

The present study presents some limitations. First, we did not consider patients treated with topical non-steroidal anti-inflammatory drugs (NSAIDs). However, previous studies documented that the effects of steroids and NSAIDs on FS outcomes are similar, although a significantly higher efficacy of steroids over NSAIDs was described [14,27,28]. Second, since SMR is an arbitrary index and an indirect indicator of the tissue density, this parameter could not clearly indicate the collagen amount of the conjunctival stroma. Third, because we did not consider intermediate follow-up time points between pre-operative and 12 months, we are unable to describe how conjunctival features progressively changed during the first year after surgery. Fourth, we did not investigate the relations between IVCM variables and post-operative bleb features. This may be an additional important factor that could further clarify the impact of pre-operative steroids on surgical outcomes. Finally, we did not repeat IVCM at last follow-up to evaluate whether confocal parameters and 12-month follow up were correlated. However, based on a previous confocal study which found that the bleb-wall features were better when the ocular surface was less inflamed, we can hypothesize that steroid-treated patients may develop a more favorable bleb morphology after surgery [30]. Further studies aimed at investigating whether GCD, DCD, SMR, and surgical success rate correlate are warranted to clarify this aspect.

Furthermore, considering the potential effects of sodium hyaluronate on AH resorption through the bleb-wall, a prospective study aimed at investigating the impact of this treatment on FS outcomes is warranted.

5. Conclusions

In conclusion, the present study confirmed the positive effects of topical, low-potency steroids in promoting less intensive post-operative management after FS, rather than in increasing the success rate of surgery. At the same time, this study unraveled, in vivo, the cellular modifications underlying the mechanism of action of steroids, and preliminarily found IVCM to be a potentially useful system to predict surgical outcomes.

Author Contributions: Conceptualization, L.M. and L.A.; methodology, L.B.; software, M.T.; validation, G.D. and F.P.; formal analysis, G.D.; investigation, M.T.; resources, R.A.; data curation, F.D.; writing—original draft preparation, L.A.; writing—review and editing, L.B.; visualization, L.A.; supervision, L.M.; project administration, M.N. All authors have read and agreed to the published version of the manuscript.

Funding: This research received no external funding.

Institutional Review Board Statement: All procedures performed in studies involving human participants were in accordance with the ethical standards of the Ophthalmic Clinic, University G. d'Annunzio of Chieti-Pescara, Italy, and with the 1964 Helsinki Declaration and its later amendments or comparable ethical standards. We obtained an IRB approval from our Institutional Board Department (n.123/2021). This article does not contain any studies with animals performed by any of the authors.

Informed Consent Statement: Informed consent was obtained from all subjects involved in the study.

Data Availability Statement: Not applicable.

Acknowledgments: The author F.D. passed away during the manuscript preparation.

Conflicts of Interest: The authors declare no conflict of interest.

References

1. Parc, C.E.; Johnson, D.H.; Oliver, J.E.; Hattenhauer, M.G.; Hodge, D.O. The long-term outcome of glaucoma filtration surgery. *Am. J. Ophthalmol.* **2001**, *132*, 27–35. [CrossRef]
2. Molteno, A.C.; Bosma, N.J.; Kittelson, J.M. Otago glaucoma surgery outcome study: Long-term results of trabeculectomy-1976 to 1995. *Ophthalmology* **1999**, *106*, 1742–1750. [CrossRef]
3. Galin, M.A.; Baras, I.; McLean, J.M. The mechanism of external filtration. *Am. J. Ophthalmol.* **1966**, *61*, 3–68. [CrossRef]
4. Yu, D.Y.; Morgan, W.H.; Sun, X.; Su, E.N.; Cringle, S.J.; Yu, P.K.; House, P.; Guo, W.; Yu, X. The critical role of the conjunctiva in glaucoma filtration surgery. *Prog. Retin. Eye Res.* **2009**, *28*, 303–328. [CrossRef]
5. Johnson, D.H.; Yoshikawa, K.; Brubaker, R.F.; Hodge, D.O. The effect of long-term medical therapy on the outcome of filtration surgery. *Am. J. Ophthalmol* **1994**, *117*, 139–148. [CrossRef]
6. Baudouin, C. Ocular surface and external filtration surgery: Mutual relationships. *Dev. Ophthalmol.* **2012**, *50*, 64–78. [CrossRef] [PubMed]
7. Mastropasqua, L.; Agnifili, L.; Mastropasqua, R.; Fasanella, V. Conjunctival modifications induced by medical and surgical therapies in patients with glaucoma. *Curr. Opin. Pharmacol.* **2013**, *13*, 56–64. [CrossRef]
8. Agnifili, L.; Fasanella, V.; Mastropasqua, R.; Frezzotti, P.; Curcio, C.; Brescia, L.; Marchini, G. In vivo goblet cell density as a potential indicator of glaucoma filtration surgery outcome. *Investig. Ophthalmol. Vis. Sci.* **2016**, *57*, 2928–2935. [CrossRef]
9. Mastropasqua, R.; Fasanella, V.; Brescia, L.; Oddone, F.; Mariotti, C.; Di Staso, S.; Agnifili, L. In vivo confocal imaging of the conjunctiva as a predictive tool for the glaucoma filtration surgery outcome. *Investig. Ophthalmol. Vis. Sci.* **2017**, *58*, BIO114–BIO120. [CrossRef]
10. Kronfeld, P.C. The chemical demonstration of trans-conjunctival passage of aqueous after antiglaucomatous operations. *Am. J. Ophthalmol.* **1952**, *35*, 38–45. [CrossRef]
11. Amar, N.; Labbè, A.; Hamard, P.; Dupas, B.; Baudouin, C. Filtering blebs and aqueous pathway: An immunocytological and in vivo confocal microscopy study. *Ophthalmology* **2008**, *115*, 1154–1161. [CrossRef] [PubMed]
12. Boimer, C.; Birt, C.M. Preservative exposure and surgical outcomes in glaucoma patients: The PESO study. *J. Glaucoma* **2013**, *22*, 730–735. [CrossRef] [PubMed]
13. Tailor, R.; Batra, R.; Mohamed, S. A National Survey of Glaucoma Specialists on the Preoperative (Trabeculectomy) Management of the Ocular Surface. *Semin. Ophthalmol.* **2016**, *31*, 519–525. [CrossRef] [PubMed]
14. Agnifili, L.; Sacchi, M.; Figus, M.; Posarelli, C.; Lizzio, R.A.U.; Nucci, P.; Mastropasqua, L. Preparing the ocular surface for glaucoma filtration surgery: An unmet clinical need. *Acta Ophthalmol.* **2022**, 15098. [CrossRef]
15. Breusegem, C.; Spielberg, L.; Van Ginderdeuren, R.; Vandewalle, E.; Renier, C.; Van de Veire, S.; Fieuws, S.; Zeyen, T.; Stalmans, I. Preoperative nonsteroidal anti-inflammatory drug or steroid and outcomes after trabeculectomy: A randomized controlled trial. *Ophthalmology* **2010**, *117*, 1324–1330. [CrossRef] [PubMed]
16. Lorenz, K.; Wasielica-Poslednik, J.; Bell, K.; Renieri, G.; Keicher, A.; Ruckes, C.; Pfeiffer, N.; Thieme, H. Efficacy and safety of preoperative IOP reduction using a preservative-free fixed combination of dorzolamide/timolol eye drops versus oral acetazolamide and dexamethasone eye drops and assessment of the clinical outcome of trabeculectomy in glaucoma. *PLoS ONE* **2017**, *12*, e0171636. [CrossRef]
17. Law, S.K.; Shih, K.; Tran, D.H.; Coleman, A.L.; Caprioli, J. Long-term outcomes of repeat vs initial trabeculectomy in open-angle glaucoma. *Am. J. Ophthalmol.* **2009**, *148*, 685–695.e1. [CrossRef]
18. Hoffmann, E.M.; Herzog, D.; Wasielica-Poslednik, J.; Butsch, C.; Schuster, A.K. Bleb grading by photographs versus bleb grading by slit-lamp examination. *Acta Ophthalmol.* **2019**, *98*, e607–e610. [CrossRef]
19. Lakhani, B.K.; Giannouladis, K.; Leighton, P.; King, A.J. Seeking a practical definition of stable glaucoma: A Delphi consensus survey of UK glaucoma consultants. *Eye* **2020**, *34*, 335–343. [CrossRef]
20. Mastropasqua, R.; Agnifili, L.; Fasanella, V.; Lappa, A.; Brescia, L.; Lanzini, M.; Oddone, F.; Perri, P.; Mastropasqua, L. In vivo distribution of corneal epithelial dendritic cells in patients with glaucoma. *Investig. Ophthalmol. Vis. Sci.* **2016**, *57*, 5996–6002. [CrossRef]
21. Dale, S.B.; Saban, D.R. Linking immune responses with fibrosis in allergic eye disease. *Curr. Opin. Allergy Clin. Immunol.* **2015**, *15*, 467–475. [CrossRef] [PubMed]
22. Efron, N.; Al-Dossari, M.; Pritchard, N. In vivo confocal microscopy of the bulbar conjunctiva. *Clin. Exp. Ophthalmol.* **2009**, *37*, 335–344. [CrossRef] [PubMed]
23. Messmer, E.M.; Zapp, D.M.; Mackert, M.J.; Thiel, M.; Kampik, A. In vivo confocal microscopy of filtering blebs after trabeculectomy. *Arch. Ophthalmol.* **2006**, *124*, 1095–1103. [CrossRef] [PubMed]
24. Messmer, E.M.; Mackert, M.J.; Zapp, D.M.; Kampik, A. In vivo confocal microscopy of normal conjunctiva and conjunctivitis. *Cornea* **2006**, *25*, 781–788. [CrossRef]
25. Seo, J.H.; Kim, Y.A.; Park, K.H.; Lee, Y. Evaluation of Functional Filtering Bleb Using Optical Coherence Tomography Angiography. *Transl. Vis. Sci. Technol.* **2019**, *8*, 14. [CrossRef]
26. Baudouin, C. Ocular Surface and External Filtration Surgery: Mutual Relationships. *Dev. Ophthalmol.* **2017**, *59*, 67–79. [CrossRef]
27. Baudouin, C.; Nordmann, J.P.; Denis, P.; Creuzot-Garcher, C.; Allaire, C.; Trinquand, C. Efficacy of indomethacin 0.1% and fluorometholone 0.1% on conjunctival inflammation following chronic application of antiglaucomatous drugs. *Graefes Arch. Clin. Exp. Ophthalmol.* **2002**, *240*, 929–935. [CrossRef]

28. Nguyen, K.D.; Lee, D.A. Effect of steroids and nonsteroidal antiinflammatory agents on human ocular fibroblast. *Investig. Ophthalmol. Vis. Sci.* **1992**, *33*, 2693–2701.
29. Broadway, D.C.; Grierson, I.; Sturmer, J.; Hitchings, R.A. Reversal of topical antiglaucoma medication effects on the conjunctiva. *Arch. Ophthalmol.* **1966**, *114*, 262–267. [CrossRef]
30. Agnifili, L.; Brescia, L.; Oddone, F.; Sacchi, M.; D'Ugo, E.; Di Marzio, G.; Perna, F.; Costagliola, C.; Mastropasqua, R. The ocular surface after successful glaucoma filtration surgery: A clinical, in vivo confocal microscopy, and immune-cytology study. *Sci. Rep.* **2019**, *9*, 11299. [CrossRef]

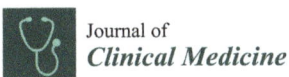

Article

Steroid Response after Trabeculectomy—A Randomized Controlled Trial Comparing Dexamethasone to Diclofenac Eye Drops

Afrouz Ahmadzadeh [1,*], Line Kessel [1,2], Bo Simmendefeldt Schmidt [3] and Daniella Bach-Holm [1,2]

1. Department of Ophthalmology, Copenhagen University Hospital—Rigshospitalet, 2600 Copenhagen, Denmark
2. Department of Clinical Medicine, University of Copenhagen, 2100 Copenhagen, Denmark
3. Department of Physics, Technical University of Denmark, 2800 Kongens Lyngby, Denmark
* Correspondence: afrouz.ahmadzadeh.01@regionh.dk

Abstract: This prospective randomized controlled trial aimed to compare changes in intraocular pressure in three different anti-inflammatory regimens following trabeculectomy. Sixty-nine patients were randomized to receive either postoperative prophylaxis with topical preservative-free dexamethasone (DEX), diclofenac (DICLO), or their combination (DEX+DICLO). Our main outcome measure was an intraocular pressure (IOP) change of a minimum 4 mmHg following the withdrawal of anti-inflammatory prophylaxis 9 weeks after trabeculectomy. We found that the IOP decreased $\geq$ 4 mmHg in 18.6% of eyes after cessation of the topical steroid DEX (n = 3/22) and DEX+DICLO (n = 5/21), whereas a decrease in IOP was not observed in the DICLO group. In conclusion, IOP decreased in nearly 1/5 of patients after cessation of topical steroidal anti-inflammatory prophylaxis after trabeculectomy. This points toward a steroid-induced increase in IOP even after trabeculectomy. Thus, increased postoperative IOP may be related to steroid use, and the success or failure of a trabeculectomy cannot be fully evaluated before anti-inflammatory prophylaxis with steroids is stopped or changed to non-steroidal eye drops.

Keywords: glaucoma; NSAID; steroid; trabeculectomy

1. Introduction

Increased intraocular pressure (IOP) is a well-documented adverse effect of steroids [1]. Steroid responders are individuals who are susceptible to increased IOP during systemic or topical steroid therapy. This side effect of corticosteroids is more prevalent in glaucoma patients and children than in the general population [2–5]. The mechanism by which steroids cause elevated IOP is not fully known, but morphological changes in the trabecular meshwork associated with increased resistance of aqueous outflow are considered a possible site of action [6].

The treatment of choice for medically uncontrolled glaucoma is trabeculectomy, as elevated IOP remains the major modifiable risk factor for preserving visual function [7]. To control the inflammation, postoperative topical anti-inflammatory medication is used, most commonly steroids [8,9]. In a successful trabeculectomy, the aqueous humour leaves the eye through the bleb; therefore, steroid-induced changes in the trabecular meshwork should have minimal or no influence on IOP. However, it has been observed that some patients have elevated IOP during topical treatment with steroids after a trabeculectomy despite a functional filtering bleb [10,11]. This may lead to reoperations, such as needling or a revision of the trabeculectomy, due to the impression that the primary surgery was ineffective.

Non-steroidal anti-inflammatory drugs (NSAID) are attractive alternatives as postoperative treatment after a trabeculectomy, as they have not been associated with IOP increase.

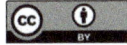

Additionally, previous studies have shown that NSAIDs are comparable with topical steroids in controlling early inflammation after trabeculectomy and cataract surgery [12–14].

In this randomized controlled clinical trial, we sought to identify if corticosteroid use is associated with a rise in IOP following trabeculectomy.

2. Materials and Methods

The Steroids and/or Non-steroidal Anti-inflammatory Drugs in the Postoperative Regime After Trabeculectomy Study (SNAP) is a prospective randomized controlled clinical trial conducted at the Department of Ophthalmology at Rigshospitalet-Glostrup, Denmark. Three topical and preservative-free anti-inflammatory regimens, dexamethasone (DEX) (Monopex 1 mg/mL, Théa), diclofenac (DICLO) (Voltaren Ophta 1 mg/mL, GSK Consumer Healthcare) or a combination of dexamethasone (Monopex 1 mg/mL, Théa) and diclofenac (Voltaren Ophta 1 mg/mL, GSK Consumer Healthcare) (DEX+DICLO) following trabeculectomy were compared.

A topical antibiotic (Chloramphenicol 5 mg/mL) was prescribed four times daily for the first week. Anti-inflammatory prophylaxis was planned to last a minimum nine weeks. For the first two weeks, the drops were used six times daily, followed by four drops daily for four weeks. After six weeks, the topical anti-inflammatory medication was reduced by one daily drop per week, depending on the clinical status of the eye. Preservative-free topical DEX was used if topical therapy was required for more than 15 weeks following the filtration operation.

The study was approved by the Danish Committee on Health Research Ethics (Journal nr.: H-18056701), the Danish Medicines Agency (Journal nr.: 2018082465) and the Danish Data Protection Agency (VD-2018-477, I-Suite nr.: 6736). The study was registered at www.clinicaltrials.gov (accessed on 7 December 2022) (NCT04054830) and the European Union Drug Regulating Authorities Clinical Trials Database (EudraCT, 2018-001855-10), was conducted in accordance with Good Clinical Practice guidelines, and adhered to the tenets of the Declaration of Helsinki [15]. All participants provided written informed consent and received no incentives or compensation for participation. The Consolidated Standards of Reporting Trials (CONSORT) reporting guideline was followed.

2.1. Study Participants

Participants were recruited from 1 August 2019 to 11 July 2021, from patients scheduled for trabeculectomy at the Department of Ophthalmology, Rigshospitalet-Glostrup, Denmark. Participants had to be older than 50 years, and women had to be postmenopausal. We included participants with either primary open-angle glaucoma (POAG), pseudoexfoliation syndrome (PEX), pigment dispersion syndrome (PDS) or ocular hypertension (OH). Participants had to be able to comply with study procedures and consent to participation.

Exclusion criteria were known allergy to any content of the pharmaceuticals used in the study, previous history of steroid response mentioned in the medical charts (using the definition of the treating physician or confirmed by questioning study participants), systemic treatment with NSAIDs or steroids, prior intraocular surgery (except for cataract surgery), medical history of anterior segment dysgenesis, inflammatory/uveitic glaucoma, angle closure glaucoma, neovascular glaucoma or traumatic glaucoma.

2.2. Randomization and Blinding

Participants were randomized to one of the three interventional groups (Figure 1). A computerized algorithm determined which eye to include in the study if both eyes were eligible. An independent researcher generated a block-randomized list in Sealed Envelope (https://www.sealedenvelope.com/simple-randomiser/v1/lists (accessed on 7 December 2022)) and uploaded it to Research Electronic Data Capture (REDCap) [16,17], a randomization instrument hosted at Capital Region, Denmark. The list length was 123, with block sizes 6 and 9 in random order. The study was designed as single blinded, with primary outcome assessors masked to the randomization status. All statistical calculations were performed in a blinded manner.

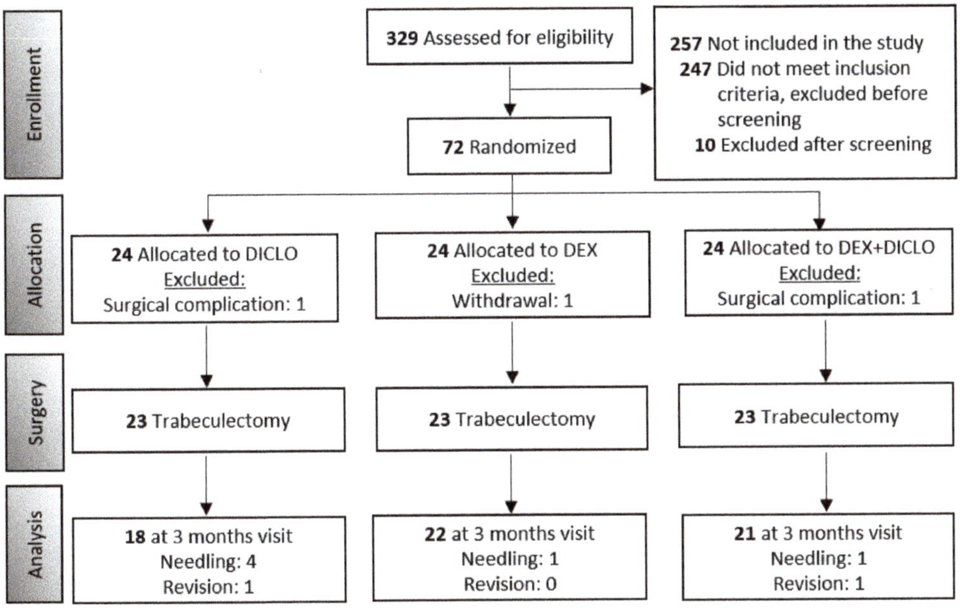

```
Enrollment:
  329 Assessed for eligibility
  257 Not included in the study
    247 Did not meet inclusion criteria, excluded before screening
    10 Excluded after screening
  72 Randomized

Allocation:
  24 Allocated to DICLO
    Excluded:
    Surgical complication: 1
  24 Allocated to DEX
    Excluded:
    Withdrawal: 1
  24 Allocated to DEX+DICLO
    Excluded:
    Surgical complication: 1

Surgery:
  23 Trabeculectomy
  23 Trabeculectomy
  23 Trabeculectomy

Analysis:
  18 at 3 months visit
    Needling: 4
    Revision: 1
  22 at 3 months visit
    Needling: 1
    Revision: 0
  21 at 3 months visit
    Needling: 1
    Revision: 1
```

Figure 1. Consort Diagram for IOP analysis.

2.3. Surgical Technique

The trabeculectomies were performed by three experienced surgeons with a standard limbus-based scleral technique using 0.2 mg/mL Mitomycin (MMC) on sponges subconjunctivally for 3 min. The surgery was concluded by injecting 1 mL cefuroxime 2.5 mg/mL into the anterior chamber and applying 0.5 mL of 4 mg/mL dexamethasone 180° away from the trabeculectomy subconjunctivally. One operation was performed using general anesthesia, and all other surgical procedures were performed using peribulbar or topical anesthesia according to the surgeon's preference.

2.4. Follow-Up Examinations and Outcome

The primary outcome in the present study was the IOP change from 6 weeks to 3 months postoperatively. IOP was measured using Goldmann applanation tonometry. Two measurements were taken and averaged to the mean IOP if the two values were within 2 mmHg. A third measurement was taken if the first two deviated ≥ 3 mmHg. If so, the median value was used [18]. Participants were identified as steroid responders if they experienced a pressure decrease ≥ 4 mmHg at 3 months (off topical anti-inflammatory eye drops) compared to 6 weeks after surgery (on anti-inflammatory eye drops). At 6 weeks, patients received 4 or 8 anti-inflammatory eye drops a day (according to the randomization), whereas participants had been free of anti-inflammatory eye drops for 4 weeks at the 3 month visit. If a participant required surgical intervention, e.g., needling or revision, in the first 3 postoperative months, the patient was excluded from the analysis due to the incomparable postoperative medical prophylaxis with steroids.

2.5. Statistical Analysis

A one-way ANOVA was used to calculate *p*-values for the baseline characteristics of the participants, including gender, age, pre-operative IOP, MD and the number of glaucoma medications; see Table 1. The dependent variables were tested for normality using Shapiro–Wilk's test and for homogeneity of variances using Levene's test. From the IOP changes from 6 to 12 weeks, participants who experienced a drop in IOP (steroid responders) were analyzed using descriptive statistics for inter-group differences.

Table 1. Baseline characteristics.

	All Participants	DICLO	DEX	DEX + DICLO	*p*-Value
Participants, n	61	18	22	21	
F/M, n (%)	27/34 (44/56)	5/13 (27.8/72.2)	12/10 (54.5/45.5)	10/11 (47.6/52.4)	0.40
Age (yrs), mean (SD)	71.5 (8.8)	70.1 (7.3)	73.2 (8.0)	71.0 (10.8)	0.53
Pre-operative IOP (mm Hg), mean (SD)	18.8 (5.8)	18.2 (6.8)	18.4 (5.7)	19.8 (5.2)	0.62
Visual field MD (dB), mean (SD)	15.3 (5.7)	16.0 (5.4)	15.1 (6.6)	15.0 (5.1)	0.86
No. of glaucoma medications, mean (SD)	3.4 (0.8)	3.5 (0.8)	3.3 (0.8)	3.5 (0.7)	0.64
Prostaglandin, n (%)	61 (100)	18 (100)	22 (100)	21 (100)	
Beta-blocker, n (%)	56 (91.8)	16 (88.9)	20 (90.9)	20 (95.2)	
Topical Carbonic Anhydrase Inhibitor, n (%)	56 (91.8)	17 (94.4)	19 (86.4)	20 (95.2)	
Alpha agonist, n (%)	37 (60.7)	12 (66.7)	12 (54.5)	13 (61.9)	
Systemic Carbonic Anhydrase Inhibitor, n (%)	7 (11.5)	2 (11.1)	2 (9.1)	3 (14.3)	

F/M = female/male; SD = standard deviation; IOP = intraocular pressure; MD = mean deviation; HTG = high tension glaucoma; NTG = normal tension glaucoma; PXG = pseudoexfoliative glaucoma; PG = pigmentary glaucoma; OH = ocular hypertension.

3. Results

Between August 2019 and June 2021, 72 participants were randomized and scheduled for trabeculectomy. One participant withdrew consent, two experienced complications during surgery, six required needling, and two required revision. A total of 61 eyes (27 women (44%) and 34 men (56%)) were included in the analyses with a mean age of 71.5 ± 8.8 years (range, 51 to 88 years). Figure 1 and Table 1 summarize the demographics of the study sample.

A reduction ≥4 mmHg was observed in 18.6% of eyes that received steroids (n = 8/43). None of the participants in the DICLO group had a reduction ≥4 mmHg following cessation of anti-inflammatory prophylaxis. After discontinuation of anti-inflammatory prophylaxis, 8.2% (n = 5/61) of study participants had unchanged IOP, whereas IOP increased in 32.8% (n = 20/61). For those participants who experienced an increase after prophylactic treatment stopped, the mean IOP reached 11.3 mmHg (6.8 to 15.7 mmHg, 95% CI) in the DICLO group, compared to 9.5 mmHg (8.2 to 10.8 mmHg, 95% CI, DEX group) and 12.4 mmHg (10.5 to 14.3 mmHg, 95% CI, DEX+DICLO group) in the steroid groups. The mean IOP at 3 months was 8.8 mmHg for all participants with no significant difference between groups; see Table 2.

Table 2. Change in IOP from 6 weeks to 3 months.

	All Participants	DICLO	DEX	DEX+DICLO	STEROID (DEX, DEX + DICLO)
Participants, n	61	18	22	21	43
IOP at 6 w, (mmHg), mean (SD)	9.4 (3.7)	8.6 (3.3)	9.1 (4.0)	10.3 (3.7)	9.7 (3.8)
IOP at 3 m, (mmHg), mean (SD)	8.8 (2.61)	8.6 (2.6)	9.0 (3.3)	8.9 (2.0)	8.9 (2.7)
Increased IOP, n (%)	20 (32.8)	7 (38.9)	6 (27.3)	7 (33.3)	13 (30.2)
Increased IOP, (mmHg), mean (SD) *	11.1 (2.9)	11.3 (4.2)	9.5 (1.2)	12.4 (2.1)	11.1 (2.3)
Unchanged IOP, n (%)	5 (8.2)	2 (11.1)	1 (4.5)	2 (9.5)	3 (7.0)
Decreased IOP, n (%)					
0 to < −2 mmHg	14 (23.0)	3 (16.7)	8 (36.4)	3 (14.3)	11 (25.6)
−2 to < −4 mmHg	14 (23.0)	6 (33.3)	4 (18.2)	4 (19.0)	8 (18.6)
−4 to < −6 mmHg	3 (4.9)	-	2 (9.1)	1 (4.8)	3 (7.0)
−6 to < −8 mmHg	4 (6.6)	-	1 † (4.5)	3 (14.3)	4 (9.3)
−8 to < −10 mmHg	1 (1.6)	-	-	1 † (4.8)	1 (2.3)

Table 2 shows changes in IOP from when patients were using topical eye drops (6 weeks) to when topical eye drops use stopped (3 months). Thus, higher pressure during eye drop treatment was seen as a drop in IOP at 3 months. IOP = intraocular pressure (mean value); w = week; m = month; * IOP indicates participants who experienced increased pressure after discontinuation of anti-inflammatory prophylaxis; † indicates two participants who were suspected to be anti-inflammatory responders and received topical anti-glaucomatous treatment.

4. Discussion

We investigated if an anti-inflammatory regime after trabeculectomy affects IOP by evaluating the change in IOP after cessation of anti-inflammatory prophylaxis. We used a cut-off of a 4 mmHg decrease in IOP from 6 weeks (during anti-inflammatory prophylaxis) to 3 months (4 weeks after withdrawal of anti-inflammatory prophylaxis). We found that nearly one in five subjects receiving topical dexamethasone (18.6 %, n = 8/43) experienced a decrease in IOP after cessation of anti-inflammatory prophylaxis, whereas such a reduction was not observed among those who received non-steroidal anti-inflammatory prophylaxis alone (n = 0/18). This observation indicates that there is a risk of a steroid-induced increase in intraocular pressure after trabeculectomy. Notably, patients who were known to be steroid responders were excluded from the study. Topical steroids (compared to no anti-inflammatory prophylaxis) generally improves outcomes after trabeculectomy [19,20]; however, our results suggest that apparent surgical failure (increased IOP) during steroid therapy may be related to steroid use and that a steroid-free period may be warranted before deciding if needling or a revision of the trabeculectomy should be performed.

The definition of steroid responders in the general population varies among studies. Yamamoto et al. [21] and Abtahi et al. [22] define steroid responders as individuals with an IOP rise of 5 mmHg from baseline, whereas Chang et al. describe steroid responsiveness as an IOP increase of at least 25% when on topical prednisolone, and up to 28 mmHg, followed by a drop of at least 25%, when the medication is withdrawn [23]. Steroid response may be divided into three categories: approximately 2/3 are low responders, with a pressure increase <6 mmHg and an IOP < 20 mmHg; approximately 1/3 are intermediate responders, with IOPs between 20 and 31 mmHg or a pressure increase of 6–15 mmHg; and 4–6% are high responders, with an IOP above 31 mm Hg or an increase of more than 15 mm Hg above baseline [24]. Typically, these steroid responders are young, or have a family history of glaucoma, myopia or diabetes [2–5].

When using topical steroids, IOP increases three to six weeks after initiation and usually returns to normal within two weeks after discontinuation [25]. Considering that our participants had undergone a trabeculectomy (and there should have been no aqueous outflow resistance at the trabecular meshwork), we set our steroid response cut-off at

4 mmHg. Although we excluded known steroid responders, we found that 18.6% of participants experienced a decrease in IOP of ≥4 mmHg after cessation of topical steroids, whereas this was not observed in the group that did not receive steroids.

Reports describing the occurrence of steroid response after trabeculectomy are limited. Thomas et al. studied 87 eyes of 52 participants with POAG and found a significant steroid-induced increase in 23% of the eyes with a mean pressure of 25.1 mmHg; Wilensky et al. reported an IOP between 25 to 42 mmHg following trabeculectomy during postoperative steroid prophylaxis [10,11]. The incidence of steroid response after combined phacoemulsification with either Trabectome or iStent is reported to be 12.7% [22]. Several studies have assessed the efficacy of steroids and NSAIDs in controlling early postoperative inflammation. Regarding anterior chamber flare, no significant difference was found among the different anti-inflammatory treatments [26–28]. Taking the inflammation parameter into account, no participant in the DICLO group had an IOP decrease ≥ 4 mmHg, compared to eight participants in the DEX and DEX+DICLO groups following their sessions of anti-inflammatory treatment. Surgical manipulation leading to increased inflammation may have contributed to this transient postoperative increase in IOP. To ascertain this, histological testing of the trabecular meshwork would be necessary.

NSAID eye drops may be a good alternative to topical steroids after filtering surgery as they have an anti-inflammatory effect without an IOP increase during treatment. The most common complications associated with topical NSAID are irritation when the eye drop is applied, impaired vision shortly after application, redness and corneal melts that usually occur in individuals with a cornea weakened due to diabetes, ocular surgery or systemic immunological disorders, and have only been documented in rare cases [29,30].

The key strengths of our trial were its randomized design, large sample size and a control group that did not receive steroids. As one group had combination therapy, the study could not be fully masked. However, the primary outcome assessors and all statistical analyses were conducted in a blinded manner. Increased IOP was observed in 1/3 of participants between the three-month and six-week visits, likely due to bleb fibrosis. It would have been informative to compare bleb appearance between treatment groups to ascertain the effect of the previously administered anti-inflammatory prophylaxis.

5. Conclusions

Nearly 1/5 of individuals undergoing trabeculectomy experienced increased intraocular pressure during postoperative treatment with topical steroids—an increase that was not seen after NSAID treatment. It is important to recognize a steroid response following trabeculectomy since erroneous decisions may be taken, such as initiating a prolonged pressure lowering treatment or intervening surgically. Steroid treatment should be discontinued before determining if a trabeculectomy is unsuccessful and further measures should be taken.

Author Contributions: Concept and design, A.A., D.B.-H. and L.K.; acquisition or interpretation of data, all authors; statistical analysis, A.A. and B.S.S.; writing—original draft preparation, A.A.; writing—critical revision and editing, all authors; funding acquisition, A.A., D.B.-H. and L.K. All authors have read and agreed to the published version of the manuscript.

Funding: This research was funded by Fight for Sight Denmark, the Danish Eye Research Foundation, the Synoptik Foundation, the Gangsted Fond, the Fabrikant Einar Willumsens Fond, the Aase og Ejnar Danielsens Fond and the Henry og Astrid Møllers Fond. Funding organizations had no role in the design or conduct of this research.

Institutional Review Board Statement: The study was approved by the Committee on Health Research Ethics (Journal nr.: H-18056701), the Danish Medicines Agency (Journal nr.: 2018082465), and The Danish Data Protection Agency (VD- 2018-477, I-Suite nr.: 6736). The study was registered in the European Union Drug Regulating Authorities Clinical Trials Database (EudraCT, 2018-001855-10) and at www.clinicaltrials.gov (accessed on 7 December 2022) (NCT04054830) before initiation. The study was conducted following the tenets of the Declaration of Helsinki of 1964 and its later amendments.

Informed Consent Statement: Written informed consent was obtained from participants before the screening visit.

Data Availability Statement: The datasets generated and/or analyzed during this study are available from the corresponding author upon reasonable request.

Acknowledgments: The authors thank all the participants for participating in this clinical trial.

Conflicts of Interest: The authors declare no conflict of interest.

References

1. Phulke, S.; Kaushik, S.; Kaur, S.; Pandav, S.S. Steroid-induced Glaucoma: An Avoidable Irreversible Blindness. *J. Curr. Glaucoma Pract.* **2017**, *11*, 67. [CrossRef] [PubMed]
2. Fini, M.E.; Schwartz, S.G.; Gao, X.; Jeong, S.; Patel, N.; Itakura, T.; Price, M.O.; Price, F.W.; Varma, R.; Stamer, W.D. Steroid-Induced Ocular Hypertension/Glaucoma: Focus on Pharmacogenomics and Implications for Precision Medicine. *Prog. Retin. Eye Res.* **2017**, *56*, 58. [CrossRef] [PubMed]
3. Becker, B.; Mills, D.W. Corticosteroids and Intraocular Pressure. *Arch. Ophthalmol.* **1963**, *70*, 500–507. [CrossRef] [PubMed]
4. Armaly, M.F. Effect of Corticosteroids on Intraocular Pressure and Fluid Dynamics: II. The Effect of Dexamethasone in the Glaucomatous Eye. *Arch. Ophthalmol.* **1963**, *70*, 492–499. [CrossRef] [PubMed]
5. Armaly, M.F. Effect of Corticosteroids on Intraocular Pressure and Fluid Dynamics: I. The Effect of Dexamethasone in the Normal Eye. *Arch. Ophthalmol.* **1963**, *70*, 482–491. [CrossRef] [PubMed]
6. Clark, A.F.; Wordinger, R.J. The role of steroids in outflow resistance. *Exp. Eye Res.* **2009**, *88*, 752–759. [CrossRef]
7. Cordeiro, M.F.; Siriwardena, D.; Chang, L.; Khaw, P.T. Wound healing modulation after glaucoma surgery. *Curr. Opin. Ophthalmol.* **2000**, *11*, 121–126. [CrossRef]
8. Panarelli, J.F.; Nayak, N.V.; Sidoti, P.A. Postoperative management of trabeculectomy and glaucoma drainage implant surgery. *Curr. Opin. Ophthalmol.* **2016**, *27*, 170–176. [CrossRef]
9. Lama, P.J.; Fechtner, R.D. Antifibrotics and wound healing in glaucoma surgery. *Surv. Ophthalmol.* **2003**, *48*, 314–346. [CrossRef]
10. Thomas, R.; Jay, J.L. Raised intraocular pressure with topical steroids after trabeculectomy. *Graefes Arch. Clin. Exp. Ophthalmol.* **1988**, *226*, 337–340. [CrossRef]
11. Wilensky, J.T.; Snyder, D.; Gieser, D. Steroid-induced ocular hypertension in patients with filtering blebs. *Ophthalmology* **1980**, *87*, 240–244. [CrossRef] [PubMed]
12. Kessel, L.; Tendal, B.; Jørgensen, K.J.; Erngaard, D.; Flesner, P.; Andresen, J.L.; Hjortdal, J.; Jorgensen, K.J.; Erngaard, D.; Flesner, P.; et al. Post-cataract Prevention of Inflammation and Macular Edema by Steroid and Nonsteroidal Anti-inflammatory Eye Drops A Systematic Review. *Ophthalmology* **2014**, *121*, 1915–1924. [CrossRef] [PubMed]
13. Wielders, L.H.P.P.; Schouten, J.J.S.A.G.; Nuijts, R.M.M.A.R. Prevention of macular edema after cataract surgery. *Curr. Opin. Ophthalmol.* **2018**, *29*, 48–53. [CrossRef] [PubMed]
14. Kent, A.R.; Dubiner, H.B.; Whitaker, R.; Mundorf, T.K.; Stewart, J.A.; Cate, E.A.; Stewart, W.C. The efficacy and safety of diclofenac 0.1% versus prednisolone acetate 1% following trabeculectomy with adjunctive mitomycin-C. *Ophthalmic Surg. Lasers* **1998**, *29*, 562–569. [CrossRef] [PubMed]
15. Association, W.M. World Medical Association Declaration of Helsinki: Ethical Principles for Medical Research Involving Human Subjects. *JAMA* **2013**, *310*, 2191–2194. [CrossRef]
16. Harris, P.A.; Taylor, R.; Thielke, R.; Payne, J.; Gonzalez, N.; Conde, J.G. Research Electronic Data Capture (REDCap)—A metadata-driven methodology and workflow process for providing translational research informatics support. *J. Biomed. Inform.* **2009**, *42*, 377. [CrossRef]
17. Harris, P.A.; Taylor, R.; Minor, B.L.; Elliott, V.; Fernandez, M.; O'Neal, L.; McLeod, L.; Delacqua, G.; Delacqua, F.; Kirby, J.; et al. The REDCap Consortium: Building an International Community of Software Platform Partners. *J. Biomed. Inform.* **2019**, *95*, 103208. [CrossRef]
18. Shaarawy, T.; Sherwood, M.; Grehn, F. World Glaucoma Association Guidelines on Design & Reporting of Glaucoma Surgical Trials. 2009. Available online: https://wga.one/wga/guidelines-on-design-reporting-glaucoma-trials/ (accessed on 7 March 2022).
19. Almatlouh, A.; Bach-Holm, D.; Kessel, L. Steroids and nonsteroidal anti-inflammatory drugs in the postoperative regime after trabeculectomy—Which provides the better outcome? A systematic review and meta-analysis. *Acta Ophthalmol.* **2018**, *97*, 146–157. [CrossRef]
20. Khaw, P.T.; Bouremel, Y.; Brocchini, S.; Henein, C. The control of conjunctival fibrosis as a paradigm for the prevention of ocular fibrosis-related blindness. "Fibrosis has many friends.". *Eye* **2020**, *34*, 2163. [CrossRef]

21. Yamamoto, Y.; Komatsu, T.; Koura, Y.; Nishino, K.; Fukushima, A.; Ueno, H. Intraocular pressure elevation after intravitreal or posterior sub-Tenon triamcinolone acetonide injection. *Can. J. Ophthalmol.* **2008**, *43*, 42–47. [CrossRef]
22. Abtahi, M.; Rudnisky, C.J.; Nazarali, S.; Damji, K.F. Incidence of steroid response in microinvasive glaucoma surgery with trabecular microbypass stent and ab interno trabeculectomy. *Can. J. Ophthalmol.* **2022**, *57*, 167–174. [CrossRef] [PubMed]
23. Chang, D.F.; Tan, J.J.; Tripodis, Y. Risk factors for steroid response among cataract patients. *J. Cartaract Refract. Surg.* **2011**, *37*, 675–681. [CrossRef] [PubMed]
24. Armaly, M.F. Statistical attributes of the steroid hypertensive response in the clinically normal eye. I. The demonstration of three levels of response. *Investig. Ophthalmol.* **1965**, *4*, 187–197.
25. Weinreb, R.N.; Polansky, J.R.; Kramer, S.G.; Baxter, J.D. Acute effects of dexamethasone on intraocular pressure in glaucoma. *Investig. Ophthalmol. Vis. Sci.* **1985**, *26*, 170–175.
26. Erichsen, J.H.; Forman, J.L.; Holm, L.M.; Kessel, L. Effect of anti-inflammatory regimen on early postoperative inflammation after cataract surgery. *J. Cataract Refract. Surg.* **2021**, *47*, 323–330. [CrossRef]
27. Ylinen, P.; Holmström, E.; Laine, I.; Lindholm, J.-M.; Tuuminen, R. Anti-inflammatory medication following cataract surgery: A randomized trial between preservative-free dexamethasone, diclofenac and their combination. *Acta Ophthalmol. (Cph.)* **2018**, *96*, 486–493. [CrossRef]
28. Laurell, C.G.; Zetterström, C. Effects of dexamethasone, diclofenac, or placebo on the inflammatory response after cataract surgery. *Br. J. Ophthalmol.* **2002**, *86*, 1380. [CrossRef]
29. Flach, A.J. Corneal melts associated with topically applied nonsteroidal anti-inflammatory drugs. *Trans. Am. Ophthalmol. Soc.* **2001**, *99*, 202–205.
30. Rigas, B.; Huang, W.; Honkanen, R. NSAID-induced corneal melt: Clinical importance, pathogenesis, and risk mitigation. *Surv. Ophthalmol.* **2020**, *65*, 1–11. [CrossRef]

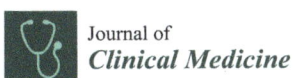

Article

Effect of Combined Surgery in Patients with Complex Nanophthalmos

Yantao Wei [1,†], Yihua Su [1,2,†], Lei Fang [1,†], Xinxing Guo [3], Stephanie Chen [4], Ying Han [4], Yingting Zhu [1], Bing Cheng [1], Shufen Lin [1], Yimin Zhong [1] and Xing Liu [1,*]

1. State Key Laboratory of Ophthalmology, Zhongshan Ophthalmic Center, Sun Yat-sen University, Guangdong Provincial Key Laboratory of Ophthalmology and Visual Science, Guangdong Provincial Clinical Research Center for Ocular Diseases, Guangzhou 510060, China
2. The Ophthalmology Department, The First Affiliated Hospital of Sun Yat-sen University, Guangzhou 510060, China
3. Wilmer Eye Institute, Johns Hopkins University, Baltimore, MD 21287, USA
4. Department of Ophthalmology, San Francisco School of Medicine, University of California, San Francisco, CA 94143, USA
* Correspondence: liuxing@mail.sysu.edu.cn; Tel.: +86-20-66678990; Fax: +86-20-66686996
† These authors contributed equally to this work.

Abstract: (1) Background: To evaluate the efficacy and safety of combined surgery (limited pars plana vitrectomy, anterior-chamber stabilized phacoemulsification, IOL implantation and posterior capsulotomy, LPPV + ACSP + IOL + PC) in complex nanophthalmos. (2) Methods: Patients with complex nanophthalmos were recruited to undergo LPPV + ACSP + IOL + PC from January 2017 to February 2021. Preoperative and post-operative intraocular pressure (IOP), best corrected visual acuity (BCVA), anterior chamber depth (ACD), and number of glaucoma medications were compared using the paired t-test or Wilcoxon signed rank sum tests. Surgical success rate was evaluated. Surgery-associated complications were documented. (3) Results: Forty-five eyes of 37 patients with complex nanophthalmos were enrolled. The mean follow-up period was 21.7 ± 10.6 months after surgery. Mean IOP decreased from 32.7 ± 8.7 mmHg before surgery to 16.9 ± 4.5 mmHg ($p < 0.001$) at the final follow-up visit, mean logMAR BCVA improved from 1.28 ± 0.64 to 0.96 ± 0.44 ($p < 0.001$), mean ACD significantly increased from 1.14 ± 0.51 mm to 3.07 ± 0.66 mm ($p < 0.001$), and the median number of glaucoma medications dropped from 3 (1, 4) to 2 (0, 4) ($p < 0.001$). The success rate was 88.9% (40 eyes) at the final follow-up visit. Two eyes had localized choroidal detachments which resolved with medical treatment. (4) Conclusions: LPPV + ACSP + IOL + PC is a safe and effective surgical procedure, which can decrease IOP, improve BCVA, deepen the anterior chamber, and reduce the number of glaucoma medications in patients with complex nanophthalmos. It can be considered as one of the first treatment in nanophthalmic eyes with complex conditions.

Keywords: nanophthalmos; glaucoma; vitrectomy; phacoemulsification; posterior capsulotomy

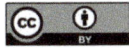

1. Introduction

Nanophthalmos is a relatively rare disease characterized by a short axial length (AL, <20.0 mm), crowded anterior chamber, high lens/eye volume ratio, and axial hypermetropia [1–4]. Angle-closure glaucoma (ACG) is a common complication in eyes with nanophthalmos, mainly due to pupillary block, displacement of the peripheral iris, and development of peripheral anterior synechia (PAS) [5,6]. The treatment in nanophthalmic eyes, especially in complex nanophthalmos with acute angle-closure glaucoma (AACG) or with failed glaucoma surgery, is difficult and challenging. Usually, the response to medical treatment is poor in such patients. Prior studies supported performing laser or surgical peripheral iridectomy to control intraocular pressure (IOP) in the early stages of nanophthalmos-induced ACG [7–11]. However, surgical intervention is usually required in more severe disease with uncontrolled IOP or progressive shallowing of the anterior chamber. Due to the multiple anatomic abnormalities in nanophthalmos eyes, routine operations become quite challenging and associated with high incidences of significant intra- and postoperative complications, such as malignant glaucoma, uveal effusion, and uveal hemorrhage, as previously reported [12,13].

Phacoemulsification surgery has been shown to be a feasible option for patients who are diagnosed with microphthalmos or nanophthalmos and cataracts and desire to improve vision and are willing to accept the risks of surgical complications [14–16]. For nanophthalmic eyes with glaucoma, disproportionately large lenses are thought to contribute to pupillary or ciliolenticular block in the pathogenesis of glaucoma [5]. Theoretically, phacoemulsification alone can help to eliminate lens-associated block and reconstruct the aqueous outflow pathway, thereby treating complex nanophthalmos. Nevertheless, previous assessments of intraocular surgery in nanophthalmic eyes, such as phacoemulsification alone, documented high incidences of uveal effusion or intraocular hemorrhage, primarily due to intraoperative rapid IOP fluctuations and sudden shallows in anterior chamber depth (ACD) when removing the intraocular instruments (phaco or irrigation-aspiration (I/A) tips) during an operation [17–19]. Thus, maintenance of IOP and ACD were considered critical throughout the entire operation. In this study, we describe a combined surgical technique for stabilizing IOP and anterior chamber during cataract surgery for complex nanophthalmos. This technique involves limited pars plana vitrectomy, anterior-chamber stabilized phacoemulsification, IOL implantation and posterior capsulotomy (LPPV + ACSP + IOL + PC). Moreover, the efficacy and safety profile of this combined procedure are evaluated.

2. Materials and Methods

This retrospective case series was performed in accordance with the World Medical Association's Declaration of Helsinki and was approved by the Ethics Committee of the Zhongshan Ophthalmic Center, Sun Yat-sen University (2021KYPJ181). Informed consent was obtained from each subject or their guardians.

2.1. Patients

This study included patients with complex nanophthalmos between January 2017 to February 2021. The inclusion criteria for our study were as follows: (1) diagnoses of nanophthalmos; (2) at least 12 months of follow-up after surgery; (3) combined with complex conditions, as evaluated by the attending physician meeting, including at least one of the following clinical criteria: (i) secondary AACG; (ii) with uncontrolled IOP or had complications (such as malignant glaucoma and extremely shallow ACD (<1 mm)) following a previous failed glaucoma surgery. The previous failed glaucoma surgeries included laser or surgical peripheral iridectomy (LPI, SPI), trabeculectomy, or ultrasound cycloplasty (UCP). Patients with uncontrolled ocular infection and severe systemic diseases were excluded. Nanophthalmos was defined as having a shorter AL (<20.0 mm), a shallow anterior chamber, high lens/eye volume ratio, moderate to severe hyperopia, and choroidal-scleral thickening measured by B-scan ultrasonography (Quantel Medical, CF, Cournon d'Auvergne Cedex, France) and optical coherence tomography (OCT, Heidelberg Engineering, Heidelberg, Germany) [20–22]. The medical records of the enrolled patients were recorded.

2.2. Examinations

All patients underwent ophthalmic examinations, involving best-corrected visual acuity (BCVA) testing with Snellen charts, IOP measurements with Goldmann applanation tonometry, refraction, slit-lamp biomicroscopy, and ophthalmoscopy. For subjects with clear cornea, gonioscopy was performed by an experienced glaucoma specialist (X.L.) to evaluate the degree of angle closure. The ACD was measured by anterior segment of optical coherence tomography (AS-OCT, CASIA SS-1000TM, Tomey, Aichi, Japan). Ciliary body and zonule was evaluated by ultrasound biomicroscopy (UBM, model SW-3200L; Tianjin Sower Electronic Technology Co., Ltd., Tianjin, China). Axial length (AL) and lens thickness (LT) were measured by A-scan ultrasound biometry (Quantel Medical, CF, France). B-scan ultrasonography was performed to assess for retinal detachment or uveal effusion. The horizontal corneal diameter (HCD) was measured by a keratometer (WAM-5500 Grand Seiko, Hiroshima, Japan). Visual field (VF) testing was performed by standard automated perimetry with the SITA standard 30–2 program (Zeiss Humphrey visual field 750i, Carl Zeiss Meditec Inc., Dublin, CA, USA). Patients with BCVA <20/200 or poor fixation did not undergo VF testing. Color fundus photography (TRC-NW6S; Topcon, Tokyo, Japan), scanning laser ophthalmoscopy (Optos PLC, Dunfermline, UK), and OCT were performed if permissible based on media clarity.

2.3. Surgical Procedure

One hour before surgery, 20% mannitol was intravenously administered to reduce intraoperative vitreous pressure in all cases. All surgeries were performed under general anesthesia by two experienced ophthalmologists (X.L, Y.W).

2.3.1. Limited Pars Plana Vitrectomy (LPPV)

A 25-gauge trocar was placed in a transconjunctival and transscleral fashion in the inferotemporal quadrant 2 mm posterior to the limbus in order to account for the extremely short AL (Figure 1A,B). With the 25-gauge Constellation system (Alcon Laboratories, Fort Worth, TX, USA), a limited pars plana vitrectomy was performed via this trocar to moderately reduce posterior pressure and deepen the anterior chamber. The vitrectomy cut rate was set at 5000 cpm to minimize vitreous traction.

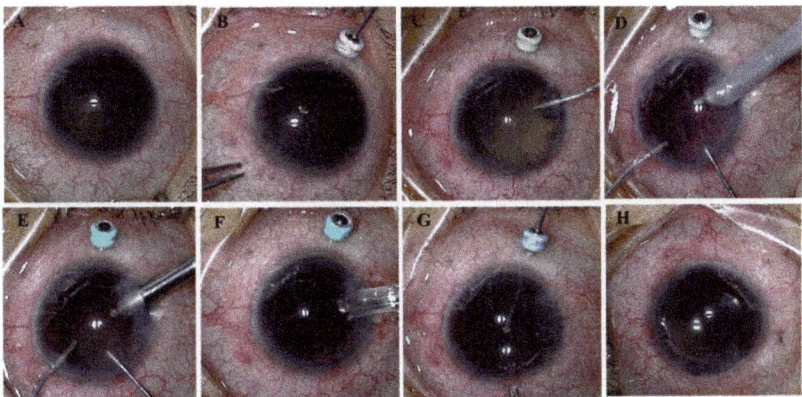

Figure 1. Surgical view of phacoemulsification combined with pars plana vitrectomy and posterior capsulotomy. (**A**) Preoperative view of the anterior segment. (**B**) Limited pars plana vitrectomy. A 25-gauge trocar was inserted in a transconjunctival and transscleral fashion 2 mm posterior to the limbus in the inferotemporal quadrant. (**C**) Deepening of the anterior chamber with a viscoelastic agent through a temporal clear corneal incision. (**D,E**) Prior to removal of the intraocular instruments (phaco or I/A tips), viscoelastic was injected into the anterior chamber from one paracentesis to prevent sudden change in IOP and ACD. (**F**) Implantation of a foldable single-piece IOL. (**G**) Posterior capsulotomy; (**H**) Removal of trocar.

2.3.2. Anterior-Chamber Stabilized Phacoemulsification and IOL Implantation (ACSP + IOL)

A 3.2 mm temporal clear corneal incision was created, followed by injection of a viscoelastic agent (Healon 5, Abbott Medical Optics, AMO, Santa Ana, CA, USA) to sufficiently flatten the iris and deepen the anterior chamber (Figure 1C). Two paracenteses were made at 12 and 6 o'clock in the left eye and 11 and 1 o'clock in the right eye. Posterior synechiolysis or sphincterotomies were performed as needed to facilitate pupillary dilation and maximize visualization. A 5.5 mm continuous curvilinear capsulotomy was completed with Utrata forceps. Phacoemulsification of the nucleus and I/A of the cortex were performed. To help prevent IOP fluctuations and stabilize the anterior chamber, prior to removal of the intraocular instruments (phaco or I/A tips), the viscoelastic agent was injected into the anterior chamber from one of the paracenteses (Figure 1D,E). In all patients, a foldable, single-piece intraocular lens (IOL) (Acrysof SA60AT; Alcon) was implanted in the capsular bag (Figure 1F).

2.3.3. Posterior Capsulotomy (PC)

A 4–5 mm posterior capsulectomy (capsulotomy) was performed with the 25-gauge vitrector (Figure 1G). Once completed, the trocar was removed. The incision site was sealed without suturing (Figure 1H). The remaining viscoelastic agent in the anterior chamber was then carefully exchanged with balanced salt solution.

Postoperatively, prednisolone acetate 1% (Allergan, Parsippany-Troy Hills, NJ, USA) and topical antibiotics (Ofloxacin, Santen Pharmaceutical Co., Ltd. Noto Plant, Osaka, Japan) were administered four times daily for 4 weeks. All patients were followed at postoperative day 1, week 1, month 1, month 3, and every 3 months thereafter. Glaucoma eye drops or oral medications were administered for IOP > 21 mmHg.

The occurrence of intraoperative complications, including dropped nucleus, iris prolapse, anterior chamber hemorrhage, choroidal detachment, uveal effusion, or suprachoroidal hemorrhage, were noted. Postoperative complications were also documented, including uveal effusion, choroid detachment, vitreous hemorrhage, malignant glaucoma, rhegmatogenous or serous retinal detachment, and persistent iritis, as was the need for additional surgeries during the entire follow-up period.

Surgical success was defined as: (1) postoperative IOP (≥ 5 mmHg and ≤ 21 mmHg) with or without use of glaucoma medications; (2) the absence of severe, vision-threatening complications, such as suprachoroidal hemorrhage, retinal detachment, endophthalmitis, or loss of light perception; and (3) not requiring additional glaucoma surgery.

2.4. Statistical Analysis

For statistical analyses, BCVA was converted to logarithm of the minimum angle of resolution (logMAR) visual acuity. Counting fingers, hand motion, light perception, or no light perception vision were noted as logMAR values of 2.1, 2.4, 2.7, and 3.0, respectively [23]. Descriptive statistics were reported as means and standard deviations (SD), medians and interquartile ranges, or numbers and percentages as appropriated. The normality of continuous variable distributions was examined using the Kolmogorov–Smirnov test. Paired t-tests and Wilcoxon signed rank sum tests were used to assess differences between preoperative and postoperative values according to whether variables conformed to a normal distribution. Statistical significance was defined as $p < 0.05$. All statistical analyses were performed using SPSS software, version 22.0 (SPSS, Inc., Chicago, IL, USA).

3. Results

3.1. Patient Characteristics

LPPV + ACSP + IOL + PC surgery was performed on 45 eyes of 37 patients with complex nanophthalmos. There were 12 (32.4%) male and 25 (67.6%) female patients. The mean age was 46.6 ± 12.2 years (range 17–78 years). Thirteen eyes (28.9%) presented secondary AACG with uncontrolled IOP despite maximum tolerated medical therapy. Thirty-two eyes (71.1%) had undergone prior glaucoma procedures, including LPI in 12 eyes, SPI in 13 eyes, trabeculectomy in 5 eyes, and UCP in 2 eyes. Of the 32 eyes, 28 eyes had uncontrolled IOP following previous surgery. Among them, 11 eyes developed malignant glaucoma. The remaining four eyes had extremely shallow ACD (<1 mm) after surgery. The clinical parameters at baseline are summarized in Table 1. The mean duration of follow-up after surgery was 21.7± 10.6 months (range 15–72 months).

Table 1. Baseline characteristics of 37 patients with complex nanophthalmos (n = 45).

Characteristics	Mean ± SD/Median (Q1, Q3)	Range
IOP (mmHg)	32.7 ± 8.7	22.0–52.0
BCVA, logMAR	1.28 ± 0.64	0.2–2.6
HCD (mm)	10.7 ± 0.6	9.1–11.8
ACD (mm)	1.14 ± 0.51	0–2.22
LT (mm)	5.03 ± 0.75	3.08–5.99
AL (mm)	16.68 ± 1.18	14.67–19.50
LT/AL ratio (%)	30.4 ± 5.1	17.7–38.0
Degrees of angle closure [&]	330 (210, 360)	0–360
RNFL thickness (μm) *	115.1 ± 52.8	24–237
SFCT (μm) *	472.3 ± 104.5	243.0–676.0
FRT (μm) *	350.7 ± 130.7	150.0–617.5
Number of medications	3 (2, 3)	1–4

IOP: intraocular pressure, BCVA: best-corrected visual acuity, HCD: horizontal corneal diameter, ACD: anterior angle chamber depth, LT: lens thickness, AL: axial length, RNFL: retinal nerve fiber layer, SFCT: subfoveal choroidal thickness, FRT: foveal retinal the thickness. Q1: 25th percentile, Q3: 75th percentile. [&]: Ten eyes did not have gonioscopic exam due to corneal edema. * Three eyes were not able to obtain macular scan.

3.2. Intraocular Pressure (IOP) and Surgical Success Rate

Preoperatively, the mean IOP was 32.7 ± 8.7 mmHg in our case series. Mean IOPs with or without glaucoma medications decreased to 17.2 ± 6.5 mmHg at 1 week, 18.6 ± 7.2 mmHg at 1 month, 18.4 ± 7.7 mmHg at 3 months, 19.5 ± 8.0 mmHg at 6 months, 19.1 ± 6.9 mmHg at 12 months and 16.9 ± 4.5 mmHg at the final follow-up visit postoperatively (Figure 2). The difference in IOP before and after surgery was statistically significant at all visits (all $p < 0.001$).

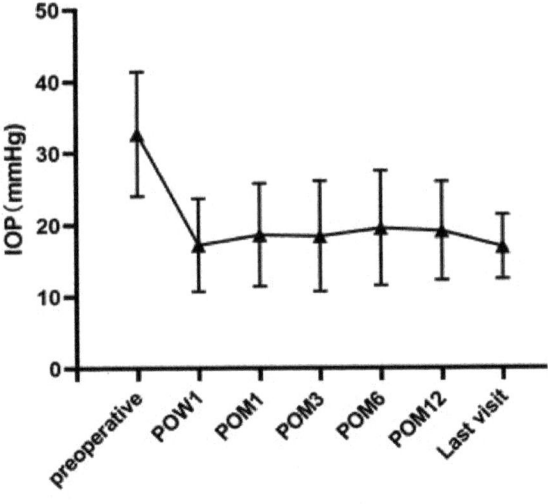

Figure 2. Pre- and postoperative intraocular pressure (IOP) changes at week 1 (POW1), month 1 (POM1), month 3 (POM3), month 6 (POM6), month 12 (POM12) and the final visit. The mean postoperative IOP was significantly reduced at all postoperative follow-up visits compared with preoperative measurements.

Surgical success was found in 40 of 45 eyes (88.9%) at the last documented follow-up visit. Among these, 17 eyes (42.5%) did not require glaucoma medications. Five eyes (11.1%) were classified as failures because of the need for additional glaucoma procedures to adequately control IOP. Cyclophotocoagulation was performed in 2 of the 5 eyes, while the remaining 3 eyes underwent uncomplicated Ahmed glaucoma valve implantation. All 5 eyes achieved IOP control during the postoperative follow-up period (7.0 ± 4.6 months), with a mean final IOP of 11.4 ± 3.2 mmHg.

3.3. Best-Corrected Visual Acuity (BCVA)

At the final follow-up visit, the mean logMAR BCVA (0.96 ± 0.44) was significantly improved from baseline (1.28 ± 0.64) ($p < 0.001$). Of the 45 eyes, the BCVA of 33 eyes (73.3%) showed improvement, 10 eyes (22.3%) remained unchanged from baseline, and 2 (4.4%) eyes decreased (one eye lost 3 Snellen lines and 1 Snellen line in the other) but no eye lost vision. The two eyes had a decrease in visual acuity because of perioperative choroidal detachment.

3.4. Anterior Chamber Depth (ACD) and Degrees of Angle Closure

Preoperatively, the mean ACD was 1.14 ± 0.51 mm. At the final visit after surgery, the mean ACD was significantly deeper at 3.07 ± 0.66 mm ($p < 0.001$). Gonioscopy was performed in 21 patients (25 eyes) before surgery. The median postoperative degree of angle closure reduced from 330° (range 0–360°) at baseline to 240° (0–360)° at the final visit; however, the difference was not statistically significant ($p = 0.172$).

3.5. Number of Glaucoma Medications

The median number of glaucoma medications was 3 (range 1–4) before surgery and significantly decreased to 2 (range 0–4, $p < 0.001$) at the final postoperative visit. A total of 17 eyes (17/40, 42.5%) did not require any glaucoma medication at the final follow-up.

3.6. Surgical Complications

Intra- and postoperative complications were observed in 2 eyes (4.4%). A localized choroidal detachment was noted intraoperatively in one eye and on the first postoperative day in the other eye. In both, the choroidal detachment resolved with conservative treatment within 2 weeks. During the postoperative follow-up period, there was no sight-threatening postoperative complication, such as retinal detachment, uveal hemorrhage, hypotony, or endophthalmitis.

3.7. Typical Case

A 39-year-old male was referred to the glaucoma division in July 2019 with complaints of poor vision in both eyes since childhood and aggravation of the right eye (RE) associated with headaches for the past 6 months. He was subsequently diagnosed with nanophthalmos and secondary glaucoma in both eyes. Although LPIs had been performed in both eyes, the IOP in the RE could not be controlled with glaucoma medications.

At his examination in January 2020, BCVA was 20/100 with +12.75 diopters of hyperopia RE and 20/125 with +13.00 diopters of hyperopia in the left eye (LE). IOP was 38 mmHg RE and 21 mmHg LE with brinzolamide (S. A. ALCON-COUVREURN. V, UK) and brimonidine tartrate eye drops (Allergan Pharmaceuticals, Ireland). Slit-lamp biomicroscopy showed shallow anterior chambers and mild nuclear sclerotic cataracts in both eyes (Figure 3A,B). The vertical C/D ratio was 0.5 RE and 0.2 LE (Figure 3C). A-scan ultrasonography revealed an AL of 16.19 mm RE and 16.48 mm LE. OCT demonstrated that the average retinal nerve fiber layer thickness was 87 μm RE and 95 μm LE, and the subfoveal choroidal thickness was 524 μm RE and 576 μm LE (Figure 3D). AS-OCT showed a central ACD of 0.75 mm RE and 0.76 mm LE.

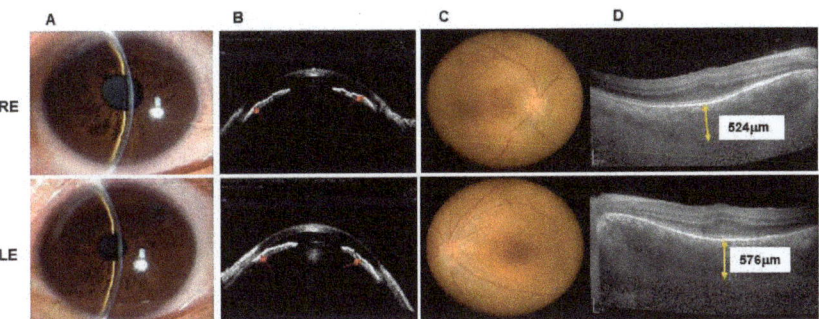

Figure 3. Preoperative images of 39-year-old man with nanophthalmos. (**A,B**) the preoperative anterior segment of both eyes showed a shallow anterior chamber (RE: 0.75 mm, LE: 0.76 mm) with angle closure (red arrow). (**C**) The fundus photographs of both eyes showed disappearance of macular fovea reflection. (**D**) Linear horizontal macular OCT scan revealed absence of a foveal depression, persistence of inner nuclear layers and thickened choroid. RE: right eye, LE: left eye.

The patient subsequently underwent bilateral LPPV + ACSP + IOL + PC successively. On the first day after surgery, his uncorrected visual acuity was 20/200 RE and 20/500 LE. The central ACD significantly increased (RE: 3.71 mm, LE: 3.33 mm) compared to the preoperative ACD (Figure 4A,B). B-scan ultrasonography and SLO showed flat and attached retinas in both eyes (Figure 4C,D). At the last visit (RE: 6 months after surgery, LE: 3 months after surgery), BCVAs of both eyes were 20/100. IOP was 21 mmHg RE with glaucoma medications (brinzolamide and brimonidine tartrate eye drops) and 20 mmHg LE without medication.

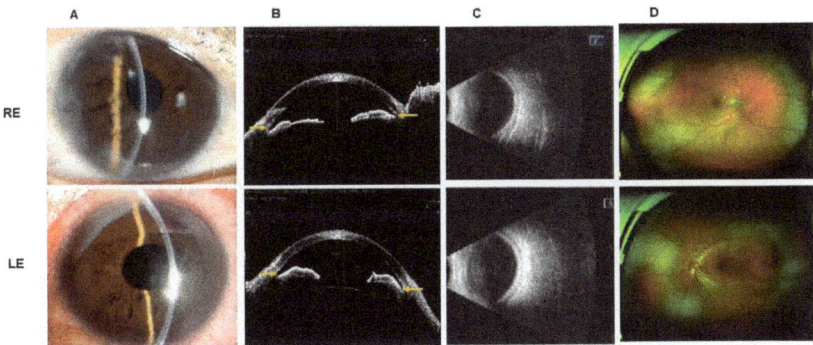

Figure 4. One-day postoperative images of the patient in Figure 1. (**A,B**) Postsurgical anterior segment of both eyes showed significantly increased center ACD (RE: 3.71 mm, LE: 3.33 mm) and open angle (yellow arrow). (**C,D**) B-scan ultrasonography and scanning laser ophthalmoscope showed flat retina in both eyes. RE: right eye, LE: left eye.

4. Discussion

This study showed that limited pars plana vitrectomy, anterior-chamber stabilized phacoemulsification, IOL implantation, and posterior capsulotomy (LPPV + ACSP + IOL + PC) can effectively decrease IOP, deepen the anterior chamber, reduce the number of IOP-lowering medications, and improve BCVA with few complications in patients with complex nanophthalmos.

Cataract surgery in nanophthalmic patients has always been technically challenging due to the limited space in the anterior chamber [14–16]. Previous studies showed that shorter AL and smaller ACD were associated with higher risks of complications [24,25].

In our enrolled subjects, the mean ACD was extremely shallow, and the mean AL was extremely short, even more so than those reported by Day [24] and Ye et al. [25]. Moreover, eyes with nanophthalmic glaucoma are usually associated with elevated vitreous pressure, which makes cataract surgery complicated and may lead to several secondary complications [26]. Therefore, limited PPV combined with phacoemulsification is a reasonable approach to such a high-risk situation. Sharma et al. [27] described combining PPV with phacoemulsification to successfully manage malignant glaucoma in phakic eyes. Using a 25-gauge system, Chalam et al. [26] also reported the advantages of limited vitrectomy to deepen the anterior chamber and facilitate phacoemulsification in eyes with positive vitreous pressure and shallow anterior chambers. However, combined PPV and phacoemulsification, as was previously performed for nanophthalmic glaucoma, has a few challenges. First, severe vision-threatening complications such as uveal effusion and uveal hemorrhage have been reported because of rapid IOP fluctuations and a sudden shallower anterior chamber during surgery [17–19]. Second, nanophthalmic patients at baseline have a high incidence of postoperative aqueous misdirection [28].

In this study, we described a combined procedure to manage eyes with complex nanophthalmos. In our surgical procedure, LPPV was considered the first step to reduce vitreous pressure and deepen the anterior chamber. A viscoelastic agent was used to strictly control the IOP and stabilize the anterior chamber throughout the entire surgery. Finally, a posterior capsulotomy was performed to reduce the risk of postoperative aqueous misdirection. Our results show that LPPV + ACSP + IOL + PC is effective and safe in the management of patients with complex nanophthalmos with minimal intra- and postoperative complications.

A significant reduction of IOP and deepening of ACD in eyes with complex nanophthalmos treated with LPPV + ACSP + IOL + PC was detected in the follow-up period, with an 88.9% success rate. The success rate of antiglaucoma surgery for nanophthalmic glaucoma varies in previous studies [1,11,29]. Singh et al. [1] reported that of 15 patients with nanophthalmic glaucoma undergoing filtration surgery, 60.0% failed treatment, and 86.6% suffered a visual loss. Yalvac et al. [11] reported that the total success rate was 85.0, 78.5, and 47.0% at 1, 2, and 5 years after trabeculectomy for patients with nanophthalmic glaucoma. Zhang et al. [29] reported results of 23-G vitrectomy combined with lensectomy in 21 eyes with nanophthalmic glaucoma. The total success rates were 85.7%, 81.0%, and 85.7% at the 6-month, 12-month, and final follow-up visits, respectively, consistent with our results. However, all the eyes in their study underwent lensectomy without IOL implantation, which resulted in the limited visual outcomes.

Generally, visual impairment in nanophthalmic patients is associated with amblyopia, macular abnormalities, or other ocular disorders [1]. In our cohort, poor vision before surgery was further exacerbated by glaucoma-related damage. The preoperative mean logMAR BCVA noted here (1.28 ± 0.64) was worse than that previously seen [11,30]. Yalvac et al. [11] reported a mean preoperative BCVA of 0.24 ± 0.15 in 20 patients (28 eyes) with nanophthalmic glaucoma, while Steijins et al. [30] described a median preoperative BCVA of 20/60 (HM to 20/25) or approximately 0.48 logMAR equivalent. Nevertheless, despite worse vision preoperatively, our results also showed that the mean postoperative BCVA was significantly better compared to baseline, with 73.3% of eyes exhibiting an improvement in visual acuity after surgery. This percentage is higher than what has been found in the literature, where only 40–66% of nanophthalmic eyes without glaucoma demonstrated improved visual acuity after routine cataract surgery [30,31]. Given the visual acuity benefit as well as refractive compensation for postoperative hyperopia, we would recommend primary implantation of IOLs in nanophthalmic glaucoma eyes at the time of surgery.

Not only does LPPV + ACSP + IOL + PC appear to be effective in lowering IOP and improving vision, but it is also safe for nanophthalmic glaucoma. Cataract surgery of nanophthalmic eyes is usually associated with a high risk of severe perioperative complications, such as choroidal effusions. Uveal effusions often occur following intraocular surgery because of sudden change in IOP and ACD and are a major cause of severe vision loss in nanophthalmic eyes. Yalvac et al. [11] evaluated the surgical results of trabeculectomy in patients with nanophthalmic glaucoma and found that choroidal detachments occurred in 50% and 25% of patients in the early and late postoperative periods, respectively. However, in our study, only 2 eyes developed localized choroidal detachments perioperatively, both of which resolved with conservative therapy. Neither early nor later uveal effusion, suprachoroidal hemorrhage, retinal detachment, or endophthalmitis was observed in the follow-up period. One of the most important reasons for the low incidence of complications was the surgical technique. Control of IOP fluctuations and stabilization of the anterior chamber were considered critical throughout the entire operation. To achieve this, LPPV was performed early to moderately decrease vitreous pressure, preventing acute IOP drops. Moreover, to avoid the dramatic pressure and ACD changes that occur from the sudden cessation of irrigation, viscoelastic agents were injected into the anterior chamber each time before the removal of the phacoemulsification or irrigation-aspiration tips from the eye. This step ensures the maintenance of IOP and ACD and prevents the development of severe uveal effusions or even expulsive choroidal hemorrhages. Chalam et al. [26] also demonstrated that anterior chamber maintainer may be another option to achieve anterior chamber stability during the phacoemulsification phase.

Day et al. [24] found that the occurrence of malignant glaucoma was 9.5% in nanophthalmic patients after cataract surgery; however, there were no cases of malignant glaucoma in our case series. This is likely because a posterior capsulotomy was performed during surgery, which is known to be effective for preventing aqueous misdirection [32]. While some anterior segment surgeons will create a posterior capsulotomy from an anterior approach through a corneal incision [32,33], we describe here and recommend using the 25-G vitrector through a scleral incision to form the posterior capsulotomy. The advantages of a posterior approach are manifold: first, the IOL can be kept in its original position without disturbing any zonules or the capsular bag; second, the surgeon is better able to control the size of the capsulotomy using the vitrector; and finally, the anterior vitreous attached to the posterior capsule can be simultaneously removed, decreasing the risk of postoperative aqueous misdirection.

Studies have reported that the risk for complications after incisional surgery is greater in eyes with nanophthalmic glaucoma [8,12]. However, in our study, no intra- or postoperative complications were observed in the 3 eyes that required Ahmed glaucoma valve implantation for additional IOP control. We suspect this is attributable to the effective decrease of positive vitreous pressure and increase of ACD achieved as a result of the modified procedure.

This study has several limitations. First, the retrospective nature may result in potential bias in our conclusions. Second, because this is a descriptive case series, the study did not include a control group. Finally, because of the short follow-up period, there may be long-term complications that are not captured in this study.

In summary, our study showed that altogether, LPPV + ACSP + IOL + PC is an effective and safe option for patients with complex nanophthalmos with successful IOP control, deepening of the ACD, improvement in visual acuity, and reduction of glaucoma medications required. Thus, this procedure may be considered for the treatment of eyes with complex nanophthalmos.

Author Contributions: Conceptualization, X.L.; methodology, Y.S. and L.F.; software, Y.S. and L.F.; validation, X.L. and Y.W.; formal analysis, Y.S.; investigation, Y.S., S.L., Y.Z. (Yimin Zhong) and B.C.; resources, X.L.; data curation, Y.S.; writing—original draft preparation, Y.W., Y.S. and L.F.; writing—review and editing, X.L., X.G., S.C., Y.H. and Y.Z. (Yingting Zhu); visualization, X.G.; supervision, X.L.; project administration, X.L.; funding acquisition, X.L. All authors have read and agreed to the published version of the manuscript.

Funding: This work was supported by the Sun Yat-Sen University Clinical Research 5010 Program (2014016), and the Fundamental Research Funds of the State Key Laboratory of Ophthalmology. The sponsor or funding organization had no role in the design or conduct of this research.

Institutional Review Board Statement: The study was conducted in accordance with the Declaration of Helsinki and approved by the Ethics Committee of the Zhongshan Ophthalmic Center, Sun Yat-sen University (2021KYPJ181).

Informed Consent Statement: Informed consent was obtained from all subjects involved in the study.

Data Availability Statement: Not applicable.

Acknowledgments: We thank all the study subjects and their guardians for participating in this clinical trial. The authors would like to thank Minbin Yu, Mingkai Lin, Jingjing Huang, Shaochong Zhang, Yunlan Ling and Yangfan Yang from Zhongshan Ophthalmic Center, Sun Yat-Sen University, China for their support on patient assessment.

Conflicts of Interest: The authors declare no conflict of interest.

References

1. Singh, O.S.; Simmons, R.J.; Brockhurst, R.J.; Trempe, C.L. Nanophthalmos: A perspective on identification and therapy. *Ophthalmology* **1982**, *89*, 1006–1012. [CrossRef]
2. Auffarth, G.U.; Blum, M.; Faller, U.; Tetz, M.R.; Völcker, H.E. Relative anterior microphthalmos: Morphometric analysis and its implications for cataract surgery. *Ophthalmology* **2000**, *107*, 1555–1560. [CrossRef]
3. Khairallah, M.; Messaoud, R.; Zaouali, S.; Ben, Y.S.; Ladjimi, A.; Jenzri, S. Posterior segment changes associated with posterior microphthalmos. *Ophthalmology* **2002**, *109*, 569–574. [CrossRef]
4. Nowilaty, S.R.; Khan, A.O.; Aldahmesh, M.A.; Tabbara, K.F.; Al-Amri, A.; Alkuraya, F.S. Biometric and molecular characterization of clinically diagnosed posterior microphthalmos. *Am. J. Ophthalmol.* **2013**, *155*, 361–372. [CrossRef] [PubMed]
5. Kimbrough, R.L.; Trempe, C.S.; Brockhurst, R.J.; Simmons, R.J. Angle-closure glaucoma in nanophthalmos. *Am. J. Ophthalmol.* **1979**, *88*, 572–579. [CrossRef]
6. Burgoyne, C.; Tello, C.; Katz, L.J. Nanophthalmia and chronic angle-closure glaucoma. *J. Glaucoma* **2002**, *11*, 525–528. [CrossRef]
7. Calhoun, F.J. The management of glaucoma in nanophthalmos. *Trans. Am. Ophthalmol. Soc.* **1975**, *73*, 97–122.
8. Singh, O.S.; Belcher, C.D.; Simmons, R.J. Nanophthalmic eyes and neodymium-YAG laser iridectomies. *Arch. Ophthalmol.* **1987**, *105*, 455–456. [CrossRef]
9. Jin, J.C.; Anderson, D.R. Laser and unsutured sclerotomy in nanophthalmos. *Am. J. Ophthalmol.* **1990**, *109*, 575–580. [CrossRef]
10. Kocak, I.; Altintas, A.G.; Yalvac, I.S.; Nurozler, A.; Kasim, R.; Duman, S. Treatment of glaucoma in young nanophthalmic patients. *Int. Ophthalmol.* **1996**, *20*, 107–111. [CrossRef]
11. Yalvac, I.S.; Satana, B.; Ozkan, G.; Eksioglu, U.; Duman, S. Management of glaucoma in patients with nanophthalmos. *Eye* **2008**, *22*, 838–843. [CrossRef] [PubMed]
12. Schmoll, C.; Devlin, H.; Foster, P. Uveal effusion syndrome as a complication of cyclodiode therapy in nanophthalmos glaucoma. *Eye* **2011**, *25*, 963–964. [CrossRef] [PubMed]
13. Krohn, J.; Seland, J.H. Exudative retinal detachment in nanophthalmos. *Acta Ophthalmol. Scand.* **1998**, *76*, 499–502. [CrossRef] [PubMed]
14. Wu, W.; Dawson, D.G.; Sugar, A.; Elner, S.G.; Meyer, K.A.; McKey, J.B.; Moroi, S.E. Cataract surgery in patients with nanophthalmos: Results and complications. *J. Cataract Refract. Surg.* **2004**, *30*, 584–590. [CrossRef]
15. Carifi, G.; Safa, F.; Aiello, F.; Baumann, C.; Maurino, V. Cataract surgery in small adult eyes. *Br. J. Ophthalmol.* **2014**, *98*, 1261–1265. [CrossRef]
16. Zheng, T.; Chen, Z.; Xu, J.; Tang, Y.; Fan, Q.; Lu, Y. Outcomes and Prognostic Factors of cataract surgery in adult extreme microphthalmos with axial length <18 mm or corneal diameter <8 mm. *Am. J. Ophthalmol.* **2017**, *184*, 84–96. [CrossRef]
17. Brockhurst, R.J. Nanophthalmos with uveal effusion. A new clinical entity. *Arch. Ophthalmol.* **1975**, *93*, 1989–1999. [CrossRef]
18. Uyama, M.; Takahashi, K.; Kozaki, J.; Tagami, N.; Takada, Y.; Ohkuma, H.; Matsunaga, H.; Kimoto, T.; Nishimura, T. Uveal effusion syndrome: Clinical features, surgical treatment, histologic examination of the sclera, and pathophysiology. *Ophthalmology* **2000**, *107*, 441–449. [CrossRef]
19. Brockhurst, R.J. Vortex vein decompression for nanophthalmic uveal effusion. *Arch. Ophthalmol.* **1980**, *98*, 1987–1990. [CrossRef]
20. Awadalla, M.S.; Burdon, K.P.; Souzeau, E.; Landers, J.; Hewitt, A.W.; Sharma, S.; Craig, J.E. Mutation in TMEM98 in a large white kindred with autosomal dominant nanophthalmos linked to 17p12-q12. *JAMA Ophthalmol.* **2014**, *132*, 970–977. [CrossRef]
21. Utman, S.A.K. Small eyes big problems: Is cataract surgery the best option for the nanophthalmic eyes? *J. Coll. Physicians Surg. Pak.* **2013**, *23*, 653–656. [PubMed]
22. Seki, M.; Fukuchi, T.; Ueda, J.; Suda, K.; Nakatsue, T.; Tanaka, Y.; Togano, T.; Yamamoto, S.; Hara, H.; Abe, H. Nanophthalmos: Quantitative analysis of anterior chamber angle configuration before and after cataract surgery. *Br. J. Ophthalmol.* **2012**, *96*, 1108–1116. [CrossRef] [PubMed]
23. Gothwal, V.K.; Sharma, S.; Mandal, A.K. Beyond Intraocular Pressure: Visual Functioning and Quality of Life in Primary Congenital Glaucoma and Secondary Childhood Glaucoma. *Am. J. Ophthalmol.* **2020**, *209*, 62–70. [CrossRef] [PubMed]
24. Day, A.C.; Maclaren, R.E.; Bunce, C.; Stevens, J.D.; Foster, P.J. Outcomes of phacoemulsification and intraocular lens implantation in microphthalmos and nanophthalmos. *J. Cataract Refract. Surg.* **2013**, *39*, 87–96. [CrossRef]

25. Ye, Z.; Li, Z.; He, S.; Chen, B.; Xing, X.; Ren, C. Outcomes of Coaxial Micro-incision Phacoemulsification in Nanophthalmic Eyes: Report of Retrospective Case Series. *Eye Sci.* **2015**, *30*, 94–100.
26. Chalam, K.V.; Gupta, S.K.; Agarwal, S.; Shah, V.A. Sutureless limited vitrectomy for positive vitreous pressure in cataract surgery. *Ophthalmic Surg. Lasers Imaging* **2005**, *36*, 518–522. [CrossRef]
27. Sharma, A.; Sii, F.; Shah, P.; Kirkby, G.R. Vitrectomy-phacoemulsification-vitrectomy for the management of aqueous misdirection syndromes in phakic eyes. *Ophthalmology* **2006**, *113*, 1968–1973. [CrossRef]
28. Singh, H.; Wang, J.C.; Desjardins, D.C.; Baig, K.; Gagné, S.; Ahmed, I.I. Refractive outcomes in nanophthalmic eyes after phacoemulsification and implantation of a high-refractivepower foldable intraocular lens. *J. Cataract Refract. Surg.* **2015**, *41*, 2394–2402. [CrossRef]
29. Zhang, Z.; Zhang, S.; Jiang, X.; Wei, Y. Combined 23-G Pars Plana Vitrectomy and Lensectomy in the Management of Glaucoma Associated with Nanophthalmos. *Ophthalmic Res.* **2018**, *59*, 37–44. [CrossRef]
30. Steijns, D.; Van Der Lelij, A. Cataract surgery in patients with nanophthalmos. Author reply. *Ophthalmology* **2013**, *120*, e77–e78. [CrossRef]
31. Jung, K.I.; Yang, J.W.; Lee, Y.C.; Kim, S.Y. Cataract surgery in eyes with nanophthalmos and relative anterior microphthalmos. *Am. J. Ophthalmol.* **2012**, *153*, 1161–1168.e1. [CrossRef] [PubMed]
32. Liu, X.; Li, M.; Cheng, B.; Mao, Z.; Zhong, Y.; Wang, D.; Cao, D.; Yu, F.; Congdon, N.G. Phacoemulsification combined with posterior capsulorhexis and anterior vitrectomy in the management of malignant glaucoma in phakic eyes. *Acta. Ophthalmol.* **2013**, *91*, 660–665. [CrossRef] [PubMed]
33. Lois, N.; Wong, D.; Groenewald, C. New surgical approach in the management of pseudophakic malignant glaucoma. *Ophthalmology* **2001**, *108*, 780–783. [CrossRef]

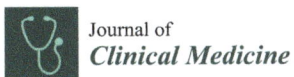

Article

Outcomes of Deep Sclerectomy for Glaucoma Secondary to Sturge–Weber Syndrome

Faisal A. Almobarak [1,2,*], Abdullah S. Alobaidan [1] and Mansour A. Alobrah [1]

1. Department of Ophthalmology, College of Medicine, King Saud University, Riyadh 11411, Saudi Arabia
2. Glaucoma Research Chair, King Saud University, Riyadh 11411, Saudi Arabia
* Correspondence: falmobarak@ksu.edu.sa; Tel.: +966-11-4786100 (ext. 1426); Fax: +966-11-4775731

Abstract: *Aims:* To report the outcomes and complications of deep sclerectomy in glaucoma secondary to Sturge–Weber syndrome (SWS). *Methods:* The retrospective case series included patients with SWS and secondary glaucoma who underwent deep sclerectomy at King Abdul Aziz University Hospital, Riyadh, Saudi Arabia between 2000 and 2021. The main outcome measures included intraocular pressure (IOP), the number of antiglaucoma medications, the presence of vision-threatening complications, and the need for further glaucoma surgery to control the IOP. The surgical outcome of each eye was based on the main outcome measures. *Results:* Twelve eyes of eleven patients were included in the study. The mean follow-up period was 83.00 months (±74.2) (range 1 to 251 months). The IOP and number of antiglaucoma medications decreased significantly from a mean of 28.75 mm Hg (±7.4) and 3.17 (±0.8) to 15.30 mm Hg (±3.5) and 0.3 (±0.7), and 18.83 (±9.3) and 1.67 (±1.7) on the 24th month and the last follow-up visit postoperatively, respectively ($p < 0.01$ for both). The success rate was 66.6% (8/12), while the failure rate was 33.3% (4/12) because of the uncontrolled IOP where a single repeat glaucoma surgery achieved controlled IOP. One procedure was complicated by choroidal detachment and one by choroidal effusion; both complications were resolved by medical treatments. *Conclusions:* Deep sclerectomy seems to be an effective treatment modality for controlling IOP and for decreasing the burden of antiglaucoma medications in patients with SWS and secondary glaucoma. Further studies are needed to confirm such a conclusion on larger number of patients with longer follow-up periods.

Keywords: glaucoma; Sturge–Weber syndrome; deep sclerectomy; intraocular pressure; filtering surgery; glaucoma surgery

Citation: Almobarak, F.A.; Alobaidan, A.S.; Alobrah, M.A. Outcomes of Deep Sclerectomy for Glaucoma Secondary to Sturge–Weber Syndrome. *J. Clin. Med.* 2023, 12, 516. https://doi.org/10.3390/jcm12020516

Academic Editors: Michele Figus and Karl Mercieca

Received: 22 December 2022
Revised: 6 January 2023
Accepted: 6 January 2023
Published: 8 January 2023

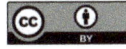

Copyright: © 2023 by the authors. Licensee MDPI, Basel, Switzerland. This article is an open access article distributed under the terms and conditions of the Creative Commons Attribution (CC BY) license (https://creativecommons.org/licenses/by/4.0/).

1. Introduction

Sturge–Weber syndrome (SWS) is a rare, sporadic, congenital neurocutaneous disorder that affects the brain, skin, and eyes. It is considered one of the phacomatoses that develop because of neural crest anomalies, such as neurofibromatosis, Klippel–Trenaunay syndrome, tuberous sclerosis, and von Hippel–Lindau syndrome. SWS is characterized by leptomeningeal hemangioma, facial angiomatosis, or nevus flammeus (port-wine stain) in the ophthalmic division of the trigeminal nerve, and ocular changes, such as glaucoma and choroidal hemangioma. The estimated incidence is between 1:20,000 and 1:50,000 infants, with no significant difference between the sexes [1]. Recently, somatic mosaic mutations in the *GNAQ* gene located on the long arm of chromosome 9 have been reported as a part of the genetic basis of SWS resulting in capillary malformations [2].

The incidence of glaucoma in patients with SWS varies between 30% and 70% [3]. The presentation and pathogenesis of glaucoma can be divided into two main categories: childhood and adulthood presentation. The early childhood or infancy presentation mainly develops because of outflow obstructions associated with angle malformations such as those observed in congenital glaucoma, while the adulthood presentation develops because of elevated episcleral venous pressure arising from vascular malformations that impede outflow and accelerated aging of the angle structures [4,5]. The conventional aqueous outflow faces the highest resistance in the juxtacanalicular trabecular meshwork. However, in SWS, the dilated episcleral vessels show a further, abnormal pressure gradient in the conventional pathway caused by vascular malformation [6]. Medical management seems to be less effective in SWS, and it cannot guarantee a good long-term control of glaucoma, especially for the childhood type [7,8]. When medical treatment fails to halt glaucoma progression, surgical intervention is needed. However, owing to the rare nature of the disease, few studies are available on the outcome of different surgical modalities; therefore, there is inconsistency in such interventions. Generally, the decision is based on the angle's status: with respect to whether it is open or closed. Trabeculectomy with or without trabeculotomy has been proposed as a choice for creating a new outflow tract for the aqueous humor, but it carries a significant risk of vision-threatening complications in patients with SWS which include massive choroidal detachment and expulsive hemorrhage [9,10]. Deep sclerectomy is a non-penetrating glaucoma surgery that allows a gradual egress of aqueous through the trabeculo-descemet's window (TDW) and, therefore, avoids hypotony and other choroidal-related complications in trabeculectomy. The efficacy and safety of deep sclerectomy have been previously described, even in patients with congenital glaucoma [11]. Nevertheless, there is insufficient evidence regarding the efficacy of deep sclerectomy in treating SWS. To our knowledge, only one study has reported the outcome of deep sclerectomy in patients with SWS [12]. Therefore, this study aimed to report the outcomes of deep sclerectomy in eyes with glaucoma secondary to SWS.

2. Materials and Methods

2.1. Patients

We reviewed the medical records of patients with SWS and secondary glaucoma who underwent deep sclerectomy at King Abdul Aziz University Hospital, Riyadh, Saudi Arabia. The study was approved by the Institutional Review Board (E-20-4996) of King Saud University as a part of a larger study on the outcomes of deep sclerectomy, and all procedures adhered to the tenets of the Declaration of Helsinki. In early childhood glaucoma, examinations under general anesthesia were performed, and the following observations were documented: the intraocular pressure (IOP) (measured using the Perkins applanation tonometer), horizontal corneal diameter, corneal edema, central corneal thickness, and cup-to-disc ratio, and dilated fundus examination. Surgery was performed when the patient was confirmed to have glaucoma. In patients with later presentation adulthood glaucoma, surgery was performed when the patient had the following: (i) medically uncontrolled IOP of ≥ 21 mmHg (measured using the Goldmann applanation tonometer) despite the maximum number of tolerated antiglaucoma medications and (ii) the presence of progressive glaucomatous optic nerve head damage.

2.2. Surgical Methods

One of several staff glaucoma specialists credentialed for the procedure performed the surgeries in accordance with standard documented techniques under general anesthesia. First, a fornix-based conjunctival peritomy was performed, and hemostasis of the episclera was achieved. A 4×5 mm superficial scleral flap was dissected toward the cornea, and 0.2 mg/mL of mitomycin C (MMC) soaked in a sponge was applied under the flap and conjunctiva for 2 min followed by balanced salt solution irrigation. A deeper scleral flap was dissected approximately 0.5 mm internal to the edges of the superficial flap right above the choroid, and a TDW was created, followed by deroofing of Schlemm's canal. When micro-perforations occurred in the TDW but with a normal depth anterior chamber, the procedure was completed as planned. When the TDW was perforated along with iris prolapse, peripheral iridectomy was performed, and the surgery was converted to a trabeculectomy. Thereafter, the deep flap was excised, and the superficial flap was closed using two 10.0 monofilament nylon sutures. The conjunctiva was closed using 9.0 vicryl sutures, and the wound was checked for the presence of leakage. Finally, antibiotics and steroids were subconjunctivally injected. After surgery, all patients were treated with topical ofloxacin and prednisolone acetate 1% drops.

2.3. Data Analysis

Postoperative visits were defined as those made on the first postoperative day; at 2–4 weeks, 3 months, 6 months, and 12 months postoperatively; and yearly thereafter. Pre and postoperative data were collected whenever available and applicable for the following variables: age at diagnosis and the time of surgery, sex, IOP, number of antiglaucoma medications, best-corrected visual acuity converted into logarithm of minimal angle of resolution format when available, time to failure, postoperative complications, and need for subsequent pressure-lowering procedures to control the IOP.

The variables were evaluated using Student's t-test and the Wilcoxon rank test and presented as means and standard deviations (SD). p values of <0.05 were considered significant. Surgical success was classified as follows: (i) complete success (IOP reduction of ≥20% from the baseline level or IOP between 6 and 21 mmHg without antiglaucoma medications, no loss of vision due to glaucoma progression, no postoperative vision-threatening complications, and no need for further glaucoma procedures to control the IOP); (ii) qualified success (IOP reduction of ≥20% from the baseline level or IOP between 6 and 21 mmHg with antiglaucoma medications, no loss of vision due to glaucoma progression, no postoperative vision-threatening complications, and no need for further glaucoma procedures to control the IOP); and (iii) failure (IOP reduction of <20% from the baseline level or IOP of >21 mmHg despite a maximum number of tolerated antiglaucoma medications on two visits, persistent hypotony [IOP of ≤5 mmHg] on two visits causing hypotony maculopathy, loss of vision due to glaucoma progression, postoperative vision-threatening complications, or the need for further glaucoma procedures to control the IOP). The cumulative probabilities of overall success, presented as percentages ± standard errors, were determined via a Kaplan–Meier life table analyses. Statistical analyses were carried out using SPSS version 23 (SPSS Inc., Chicago, IL, USA).

3. Results

3.1. Patient Characteristics

Eleven patients, including six boys and five girls (12 eyes), underwent deep sclerectomy as the first procedure for glaucoma secondary to SWS. One patient underwent a bilateral surgery, while the remaining patients underwent a unilateral surgery. The mean age at the time of surgery was 5.58 (±68.3) years (range, 2 months to 14 years). Three eyes (25%) had associated choroidal hemangioma. In all patients, there was no history of any ophthalmic surgery other than deep sclerectomy. The mean follow-up time was 83.00 (±74.2) months (range, 1–251 months). Most eyes had advanced glaucomatous disc damage (75%) (Table 1).

Table 1. Patient characteristics, complications, and success.

Patient	Eye	Age at Surgery	Preoperative IOP	No. of Preoperative Medications	Intraoperative Complications	Postoperative Complications	Follow-Up Duration	Status	Final IOP	No. of Final Medications
1	OD	2 months	43	4			7.8 years	Complete success	13	0
	OS	2 months	39	4			7.8 years	Complete success	13	0
2	OS	10 months	30	2	TDW perforation with iris prolapse		15.6 years	Failed	22	3
3	OD	8.5 years	28	4			1 month	Failed	37	2
4	OS	9.5 years	33	4	TDW perforation with iris prolapse	Choroidal detachment	7.8 years	Qualified success	16	4

Table 1. Cont.

Patient	Eye	Age at Surgery	Preoperative IOP	No. of Preoperative Medications	Intraoperative Complications	Postoperative Complications	Follow-Up Duration	Status	Final IOP	No. of Final Medications
5	OD	3 months	32	2	TDW perforation	Choroidal effusion	5.1 years	Failed	30	3
6	OS	1.3 years	25	3			4.1 years	Failed	32	3
7	OS	2 years	26	2	TDW perforation with iris prolapse		20.9 years	Qualified success	14	4
8	OD	8.3 years	20	3			8.8 years	Qualified success	18	1
9	OD	12.4 years	30	3			3.7 years	Complete success	12	0
10	OD	13.3 years	20	3			1 year	Complete success	10	0
11	OS	14.2 years	19	4			1 year	Complete success	9	0

OS: left eye; OD: right eye; IOP: intraocular pressure; TDW: trabeculo-descemet window.

3.2. Efficacy

The IOP decreased from a preoperative baseline of 28.75 (±7.4) mmHg to 14.90 (±3.9), 15.30 (±3.5), 15.57 (±4.3), 20.00 (±7.6), and 18.83 (±9.3) mmHg, while the number of antiglaucoma medications decreased from a preoperative baseline of 3.17 (±0.8) to 0.13 (±0.4), 0.30 (±0.7), 0.71 (±1.3), 1.00 (±1.3), and 1.67 (±1.7) on the 12th month, 24th month, 36th month, 48th month, and the last follow-up visit postoperatively, respectively (all $p < 0.05$). The cumulative probabilities of overall success were 75.0% (±12.5%) on the 12th month and 24th month, 66.7% (±13.6%) on the 36th month and 48th month, and 58.3% (±14.2%) on the 60th month postoperatively (Figure 1). Over the entire follow-up period, controlled IOP was achieved in eight eyes (66.6%) after deep sclerectomy: complete success in five eyes (41.7%) and qualified success in three eyes (25.0%). Meanwhile, the treatment failed in four eyes (33.3%) because of uncontrolled IOP, despite the maximum number of tolerated antiglaucoma medications and required additional glaucoma surgery to control the IOP: Ahmed implantation in two eyes and deep sclerectomy in two eyes. The mean failure time was 75.0 (±78.9) months (range, 2–187 months). One eye failed within the first 3 months after deep sclerectomy, while the remaining eyes failed after 50 months. All four eyes achieved IOP control after a single repeat glaucoma surgery.

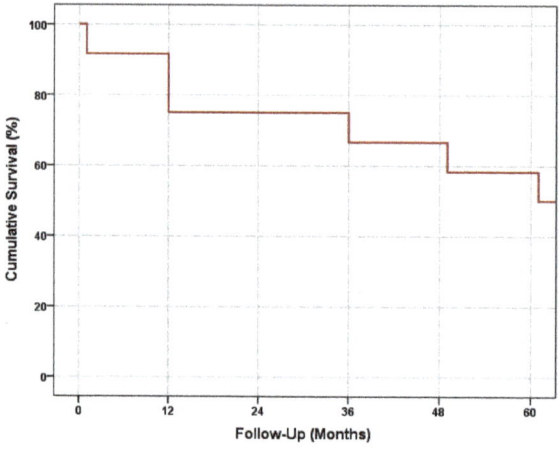

Figure 1. Kaplan–Meier survival curves showing the cumulative probability of success.

3.3. Safety

Intraoperative complications occurred in four eyes: two eyes had TDW perforations, but without iris prolapse, wherein the procedure was continued while maintaining a formed anterior chamber; two eyes had TDW perforation with iris prolapse, wherein peripheral iridectomy and iris repositioning were performed without sclerotomy. The deep flap was excised, and the procedure was continued. Postoperative choroidal effusions occurred in one eye with existing choroidal hemangioma, while isolated choroidal detachments occurred in one eye with no choroidal hemangioma. Both conditions resolved within 1 month after medical treatment including topical steroids and cycloplegic agents.

4. Discussion

Glaucoma that is secondary to SWS is a complex disease. The etiology has been attributed to trabecular meshwork anomalies for early-onset glaucoma and elevated episcleral venous pressure due to arteriovenous shunts and the premature aging of the trabeculae for juvenile/adult-onset glaucoma [13,14]. Medical therapy usually fails to achieve long-term IOP control; therefore, surgery is required to avoid visual loss. The type of surgical intervention usually depends on the pathophysiology of the disease. In SWS, deep sclerectomy is a preferred option, as it creates a new outflow tract, therefore avoiding episcleral venous pressure elevation. Furthermore, deep sclerectomy has been reported to be successful in treating primary congenital glaucoma (PCG). Eyes with PCG and glaucoma secondary to SWS have been shown to have trabecular meshwork anomalies; however, such anomalies seem less severe in patients with SWS than in those with PCG [15]. To the best of our knowledge, only one study has evaluated the outcomes of deep sclerectomy for glaucoma secondary to SWS [12]. The current study showed that deep sclerectomy is effective as an initial procedure for glaucoma secondary to SWS.

Herein, the IOP and number of antiglaucoma medications decreased significantly during the first year and the years thereafter. Complete success was achieved in 41.7% of the eyes and qualified success in 25.0% of the eyes on the last follow-up visit. Audren et al. reported a complete success rate of 56%, 28%, and 0% at 6, 13, and 26 months after deep sclerectomy, respectively. Our study showed a comparable survival rate in the short-term among the eyes that received Ahmed implants, but the results show better long-term survival rates. In their study that included 11 eyes, Hamush et al. reported a 2-year success rate of 79% and a 5-year success rate of 30% after using Ahmed implants. Kaushik et al. reported a 24-month success rate of 75% in 24 eyes that received Ahmed implants with a mean follow-up period of 2.12 years [16]. However, long-term survival seems to be better in the current study compared with both studies. Herein, the IOP increased over the follow-up period, and some eyes needed more antiglaucoma medications over time to control the IOP; this case is well known in bleb-dependent filtering surgery, which carries a high risk for surgical failure. Furthermore, the effect of a higher concentration of MMC is not expected to contribute to the surgical success and IOP control [17,18]. Other studies have reported encouraging outcomes of trabeculotomy and goniotomy. Olsen et al. [19] reported a success rate of 66.7% in 14 patients with early-onset glaucoma secondary to SWS after a mean follow-up of 5.4 years after one or more procedures, while Wu et al. [15]. reported a 1-year success rate of 86.6% in 32 patients; both results are comparable to our report. Of the four failed eyes herein, one eye with juvenile-onset glaucoma failed within the first 3 months and achieved IOP control after Ahmed implants; meanwhile, three eyes with early-onset glaucoma failed after 50 months and achieved IOP control after repeat deep sclerectomy (two eyes) and Ahmed implant (one eye).

Postoperative choroidal detachment occurred in one eye with intraoperative TDW perforation; choroidal effusion occurred in one eye with intraoperative TDW perforation and iris prolapse and co-existing choroidal hemangioma, wherein iridectomy was performed. No expulsive choroidal hemorrhage occurred. Both complications were self-limiting and responded well to medical treatments in the form of topical atropine and prednisolone drops. In SWS, the presence of aberrant clusters of capillary–venule-like blood vessels, choroidal vessel's overgrowth and thickening, and overabundant vessels increases not only the risk of glaucoma but also that of choroidal effusion. Since the mitogen-activated kinase pathway does not show significantly increased signaling activities in cells with *GNAQ*, the β-blocker propranolol could not have a crucial role in such cases [20]. Nevertheless, in intractable choroidal effusion failing to respond to medical treatments, propranolol could still have a long-term role in resolving such complications [21]. Although bleb-dependent procedures for SWS are associated with high rates of complications, such as expulsive hemorrhage and prolonged hypotony, none of these complications were observed in the current study [6]. However, a major advantage of deep sclerectomy is the higher safety profile and fewer postoperative complications because of the progressive outflow of aqueous through an intact TDW, which precludes complications, such as sudden hypotony, aqueous misdirection, and expulsive hemorrhage [22]. Adding a control group that underwent other surgical modalities in the current study to compare the IOP control and complications would be ideal. However, this was not possible because of the rare nature of the disease.

5. Conclusions

Although the current retrospective study included a small number of eyes because of the rare nature of the disease, it showed the efficacy of deep sclerectomy in treating glaucoma secondary to SWS. All complications were self-limiting and responded to medical treatments. Further studies are needed to compare the outcomes of deep sclerectomy with those of other filtering procedures.

Author Contributions: All authors contributed to the study conception, design and data collection. F.A.A. wrote the initial draft and analyzed the data. All authors have read and agreed to the published version of the manuscript.

Funding: This research received no external funding.

Institutional Review Board Statement: The study was conducted according to the guidelines of the Declaration of Helsinki and approved by the Institutional Review Board of King Saud University (E-20-4996). All patients provided informed consent.

Informed Consent Statement: Informed consent was obtained from all subjects involved in the study.

Data Availability Statement: All data are available from the corresponding author upon request.

Conflicts of Interest: The authors declare no conflict of interest.

References

1. Comi, A.M. Update on Sturge-Weber syndrome: Diagnosis, treatment, quantitative measures, and controversies. *Lymphat. Res. Biol.* **2007**, *5*, 257–264. [CrossRef] [PubMed]
2. Shirley, M.D.; Tang, H.; Gallione, C.J.; Baugher, J.D.; Frelin, L.P.; Cohen, B.; Pevsner, J. Sturge-Weber syndrome and port-wine stains caused by somatic mutation in GNAQ. *N. Engl. J. Med.* **2013**, *368*, 1971–1979. [CrossRef] [PubMed]
3. Hassanpour, K.; Nourinia, R.; Gerami, E.; Mahmoudi, G.; Esfandiari, H. Ocular Manifestations of the Sturge-Weber Syndrome. *J. Ophthalmic. Vis. Res.* **2021**, *16*, 415–431. [CrossRef] [PubMed]
4. Sullivan, T.J.; Clarke, M.P.; Morin, J.D. The ocular manifestations of the Sturge-Weber syndrome. *J. Pediatr. Ophthalmol. Strabismus* **1992**, *29*, 349–356. [CrossRef] [PubMed]
5. Cibis, G.W.; Tripathi, R.C.; Tripathi, B.J. Glaucoma in Sturge-Weber syndrome. *Ophthalmology* **1984**, *91*, 1061–1071. [CrossRef] [PubMed]
6. Mantelli, F.; Bruscolini, A.; La Cava, M.; Abdolrahimzadeh, S.; Lambiase, A. Ocular manifestations of Sturge-Weber syndrome: Pathogenesis, diagnosis, and management. *Clin. Ophthalmol.* **2016**, *10*, 871–878. [PubMed]
7. Basler, L.; Sowka, J. Sturge-Weber syndrome and glaucoma. *Optometry* **2011**, *82*, 306–309. [CrossRef] [PubMed]
8. Board, R.J.; Shields, M.B. Combined trabeculotomy-trabeculectomy for the management of glaucoma associated wih Sturge-Weber syndrome. *Ophthalmic. Surg.* **1981**, *12*, 813–817.
9. Keverline, P.O.; Hiles, D.A. Trabeculectomy for adolescent onset glaucoma in the Sturge-Weber syndrome. *J. Pediatr. Ophthalmol.* **1976**, *13*, 144–148. [CrossRef]
10. Iwach, A.G.; Hoskins, H.D., Jr.; Hetherington, J., Jr.; Shaffer, R.N. Analysis of surgical and medical management of glaucoma in Sturge-Weber syndrome. *Ophthalmology* **1990**, *97*, 904–909. [CrossRef]

11. Al-Obeidan, S.A.; Osman Eel, D.; Dewedar, A.S.; Kestelyn, P.; Mousa, A. Efficacy and safety of deep sclerectomy in childhood glaucoma in Saudi Arabia. *Acta Ophthalmol.* **2014**, *92*, 65–70. [CrossRef]
12. Audren, F.; Abitbol, O.; Dureau, P.; Hakiki, S.; Orssaud, C.; Bourgeois, M.; Dufier, J.L. Non-penetrating deep sclerectomy for glaucoma associated with Sturge-Weber syndrome. *Acta Ophthalmol. Scand.* **2006**, *84*, 656–660. [CrossRef]
13. Phelps, C.D. The pathogenesis of glaucoma in Sturge-Weber syndrome. *Ophthalmology* **1978**, *85*, 276–286. [CrossRef] [PubMed]
14. Arora, K.S.; Quigley, H.A.; Comi, A.M.; Miller, R.B.; Jampel, H.D. Increased choroidal thickness in patients with Sturge-Weber syndrome. *JAMA Ophthalmol.* **2013**, *131*, 1216–1219. [CrossRef] [PubMed]
15. Wu, Y.; Peng, C.; Ding, X.; Zeng, C.; Cui, C.; Xu, L.; Guo, W. Episcleral hemangioma distribution patterns could be an indicator of trabeculotomy prognosis in young SWS patients. *Acta Ophthalmol.* **2020**, *98*, e685–e690. [CrossRef] [PubMed]
16. Kaushik, J.; Parihar, J.K.S.; Jain, V.K.; Mathur, V. Ahmed valve implantation in childhood glaucoma associated with Sturge-Weber syndrome: Our experience. *Eye* **2019**, *33*, 464–468. [CrossRef] [PubMed]
17. Almobarak, F.A.; Alharbi, A.H.; Morales, J.; Aljadaan, I. The influence of mitomycin C concentration on the outcome of trabeculectomy in uveitic glaucoma. *Int. Ophthalmol.* **2018**, *38*, 2371–2379. [CrossRef] [PubMed]
18. Almobarak, F.A.; Alharbi, A.H.; Morales, J.; Aljadaan, I. Intermediate and Long-term Outcomes of Mitomycin C-enhanced Trabeculectomy as a First Glaucoma Procedure in Uveitic Glaucoma. *J. Glaucoma* **2017**, *26*, 478–485. [CrossRef]
19. Olsen, K.E.; Huang, A.S.; Wright, M.M. The efficacy of goniotomy/trabeculotomy in early-onset glaucoma associated with the Sturge-Weber syndrome. *J. Aapos* **1998**, *2*, 365–368. [CrossRef] [PubMed]
20. Bichsel, C.A.; Goss, J.; Alomari, M.; Alexandrescu, S.; Robb, R.; Smith, L.E.; Bischoff, J. Association of Somatic GNAQ Mutation with Capillary Malformations in a Case of Choroidal Hemangioma. *JAMA Ophthalmol.* **2019**, *137*, 91–95. [CrossRef] [PubMed]
21. Kaushik, S.; Kaur, S.; Pandav, S.S.; Gupta, A. Intractable choroidal effusion with exudative retinal detachment in Sturge-Weber syndrome. *JAMA Ophthalmol.* **2014**, *132*, 1143–1144. [CrossRef] [PubMed]
22. Almobarak, F.A. Aqueous misdirection after Nd:YAG goniopuncture in deep sclerectomy treated with Nd:YAG irido-zonulo-hyaloidotomy. *Eur. J. Ophthalmol.* **2022**, *32*, NP28–NP31. [CrossRef] [PubMed]

Disclaimer/Publisher's Note: The statements, opinions and data contained in all publications are solely those of the individual author(s) and contributor(s) and not of MDPI and/or the editor(s). MDPI and/or the editor(s) disclaim responsibility for any injury to people or property resulting from any ideas, methods, instructions or products referred to in the content.

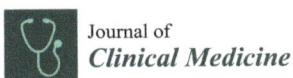

Article

Plasma Rich in Growth Factors as an Adjuvant Agent in Non-Penetrating Deep Sclerectomy

Pedro P. Rodríguez-Calvo [1,2], Ignacio Rodríguez-Uña [1,2,*], Andrés Fernández-Vega-Cueto [1,2], Ronald M. Sánchez-Ávila [3], Eduardo Anitua [3,4] and Jesús Merayo-Lloves [1,2]

1. Instituto Universitario Fernandez-Vega, Fundación de Investigación Oftalmológica, University of Oviedo, 33012 Oviedo, Spain
2. Instituto de Investigación Sanitaria del Principado de Asturias, 33011 Oviedo, Spain
3. Biotechnology Institute (BTI), 01007 Vitoria, Spain
4. Regenerative Medicine Laboratory, University Institute for Regenerative Medicine and Oral Implantology (UIRMI), 01007 Vitoria, Spain
* Correspondence: irodriguezu@fernandez-vega.com; Tel.: +34-985-240-141

Abstract: Background: The purpose of this study is to evaluate the utility and safety of plasma rich in growth factors immunosafe eye drops (is-ePRGF) in the postoperative treatment of non-penetrating deep sclerectomy (NPDS). Methods: This is a case–control study in patients with open-angle glaucoma. Group one (control) was not treated with is-ePRGF, while group two (is-ePRGF) was treated (four times a day for four months). Postoperative evaluations were performed at one day, one month, three months and six months. The main outcomes were: intraocular pressure (IOP), microcysts in blebs with AS-OCT and the number of hypotensive eye drops. Results: Preoperatively, group one (n = 48 eyes) and group two (n = 47 eyes) were similar in age (71.5 ± 10.7 vs. 70.9 ± 10.0 years; p = 0.68), IOP (20.6 ± 10.2 vs. 23.0 ± 9.0 mmHg; p = 0.26) and number of hypotensive drugs (2.7 ± 0.8 vs. 2.8 ± 0.9; p = 0.40). The IOP at six months dropped to 15.0 ± 8.0 mmHg (IOP reduction: −27.2%) and 10.9 ± 4.3 mmHg (IOP reduction: −52.6%) for group one and group two, respectively (p < 0.01). At six months, blebs with microcysts were 62.5% (group one) and 76.7% (group two). Postoperative complications were observed in 12 eyes (25%) for group one and in 5 eyes (11%) for group two (p = 0.06). No specific complications related to the use of is-ePRGF were identified. Conclusions: Topical is-ePRGF seems to reduce IOP and the rate of complications in the medium term after NPDS, so it can be considered as a possible safe adjuvant to achieve surgical success.

Keywords: glaucoma filtration surgery; non-perforating deep sclerectomy; open-angle glaucoma; plasma rich in growth factors; PRGF; surgery outcome; plasma rich in growth factors; immunosafe eye drops; is-ePRGF

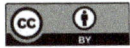

1. Introduction

Non-penetrating deep sclerectomy (NPDS) is a safe and effective option for intraocular pressure (IOP) reduction in glaucoma patients with a rapid disease progression, high IOP values or poor response to medical therapy [1–3]. The long-term success of this filtering surgery depends, in part, on maintaining adequate bleb morphology. Indeed, one of the leading causes of failure in this surgical technique is excessive scarring in the subconjunctival area or the intra-scleral space, causing fibrotic adhesions which compromise aqueous humor drainage and, consequently, increase IOP [1,4,5]. Therefore, prevention and postoperative management of fibrosis would determine postoperative outcomes, in terms of IOP and surgical success rate.

Intraoperative mitomycin C (MMC) and postoperative topical corticosteroids are widely used to prevent bleb fibrosis. Guedes et al. [4] reported that the use of MMC increased the success rate by 2.4-fold compared with not using it. Despite applying intraoperative MMC, postoperative bleb manipulations are often required to maintain IOP control [1]. Therefore, it is of interest to explore adjuvant therapeutic approaches to MMC to preserve bleb morphology and reduce the postoperative scarring response, aiming to promote long-term IOP control and decrease the incidence of postoperative bleb manipulations.

Plasma rich in growth factors (PRGF) is a blood derivative product of autologous origin with important biological features such as antimicrobial, anti-inflammatory and anti-fibrotic properties. PRGF, in its different therapeutic formulations (eye drops, clot and membrane), has been effectively used to treat several ocular surface and corneal diseases [6,7] and even in macular-hole surgery [8,9], demonstrating its role in tissular regeneration, inflammation control and fibrosis modulation [10,11]. The biological properties of PRGF would theoretically be of great help in reducing fibrosis after NPDS. Rodriguez-Agirretxe et al. [12], in a pilot study, evaluated a case series of 10 eyes that underwent NPDS with a PRGF clot inserted in the subconjunctival space. The authors concluded that PRGF might enhance surgery success rates and reduce the need for postoperative medications. Furthermore, they also pointed out that postoperative treatment with PRGF eye drops could improve the results.

The present study aimed to evaluate the potential benefits of the coadjuvant postoperative treatment with PRGF eye drops in patients who underwent NPDS with MMC.

2. Materials and Methods

This study included patients diagnosed with primary open-angle glaucoma (POAG) with uncontrolled IOP ($\geq$22 mm Hg), even with maximal tolerated medical therapy or laser trabeculoplasty, who underwent NPDS. Exclusion criteria were: age < 18 years, treatment with PRGF over the 12 months previous to NPDS surgery, previous glaucoma surgery, severe ocular surface disease, infectious illness (HIV, HBV, HDV, syphilis) and pregnancy or lactation. The study was approved by the Ethics Committee of the 'Principado de Asturias' (Oviedo, Spain) and adhered to the tenets of the Declaration of Helsinki. All the patients signed a consent form providing their approval for glaucoma surgery and blood extraction for PRGF elaboration.

The patients were divided into two groups: group 1 (control) corresponded to patients operated with NPDS who received standard postoperative treatment and did not receive PRGF eye drops as adjuvant treatment after surgery; these patients were selected retrospectively and sequentially immediately before the inclusion of the patients in group 2. Group 2 corresponded to the prospective cohort of patients who received standard postoperative treatment associated with PRGF eye drops as adjuvant therapy. Fifty eyes were included in each treatment group, which had to be followed up to 6 months after surgery.

2.1. Surgical Technique

All procedures were performed under peribulbar anesthesia by the same surgeon (P.P.R.-C.). A fornix-based peritomy was performed using a 7-0 silk corneal traction suture with conjunctival pocket dissection, followed by gentle cautery to achieve hemostasis. A 5 × 5 mm partial thickness superficial scleral flap was dissected (extended 1–2 mm into clear cornea) and 0.02% mitomycin C (MMC) was applied for 2 min between the sclera and conjunctiva. Then, the area was irrigated thoroughly with a balanced salt solution. Resection of a 4 × 4 mm deep scleral flap was performed, followed by trabecular-Descemet membrane (TDM) dissection and resection of the Schlemm's canal using Mermoud forceps. A supraciliary pocket was made with a 45° blade for the incision and a blunt spatula, 2 mm behind the scleral spur, following the technique first described by Muñoz (2009) [13], and a hema implant (either Esnoper® V-2000 or Esnoper® Clip, AJL Ophthalmic S.A., Miñano, Alava, Spain) was placed inside [14]. The superficial scleral flap was reflected back without sutures and conjunctiva was closed with interrupted 10-0 nylon sutures. In the postoperative follow-up, a goniopuncture with Nd-Yag laser was performed when insufficient filtration was observed through the TDM [15].

2.2. PRGF Preparation

The PRGF elaboration was developed following the steps already published by our group elsewhere [16]. Before surgery, during the anesthetic process, blood from patients was collected into 9 mL tubes. Samples were centrifuged at $580\times g$ for 8 min at room temperature in an Endoret System centrifuge (BTI Biotechnology Institute, S.L., Miñano, Alava, Spain). The whole column of PRGF was collected after centrifugation, avoiding the buffy coat that contains the leukocytes, using an Endoret ophthalmology kit (BTI Biotechnology Institute, S.L., Miñano, Spain). The obtained supernatant was incubated at 37 °C for 1 h and then heat treated at 56 °C for 60 min. The plasma supernatants were filtered, aliquoted and stored at -20 °C until use.

Highly sterile conditions were followed for all procedures, operating inside a laminar flow hood. In order to inactivate the complement, the PRGF eye drops were heated to 57 °C; the resulting product is called immunosafe eye drops (is-ePRGF). Patients were instructed to keep the PRGF eye-drop dispensers at -20 °C; each dispenser was used for 3 consecutive days (the eye drops could be at 8 °C or ambient temperature).

2.3. Postoperative Treatment

Standard postoperative treatment consisted of moxifloxacin eye drops 4 times a day for one week, and dexamethasone eye drops every 2 h for one week and then in tapering frequency over the following 10 weeks after surgery: 5 times a day for 2 weeks, 4 times a day for 2 weeks, 3 times a day for 2 weeks, twice a day for 2 weeks and once a day for 2 weeks. Group 1 and group 2 patients received standard postoperative treatment. Patients in group 2 were additionally treated with is-ePRGF 4 times a day for 4 months (uninterruptedly). The is-ePRGF were prescribed to be used 4 times a day distributed throughout the day, approximately every 6 h, leaving a 5 min interval among the other drops. In the hypothetical case of loss or completion, a new blood test was performed at one of the routine follow-up visits to prevent the patient from running out of treatment.

2.4. Study Variables

Follow-up visits were at 1 day and 1-, 3- and 6 months after NPDS. The variables analyzed included IOP measurement, bleb height and presence of microcysts in bleb (Anterior Segment Optical Coherence Tomography; AS-OCT, CASIA2, Tomey, Japan), the incidence of complications and frequency of bleb manipulations. The measurements and assessment of AS-OCT parameters were carried out by one observer (P.P.R.-C.) masked to the IOP level and surgical outcome.

Furthermore, the surgical outcomes were stratified into three levels: (1) complete success, defined as having an IOP $\leq$ 21 mmHg without antiglaucoma medications; (2) qualified success, defined as having an IOP $\leq$ 21 mmHg with antiglaucoma medications; (3) failure, defined as having IOP $\leq$ 6 mmHg in two consecutive visits, additional glaucoma surgeries (needling was not considered as secondary glaucoma surgery), or not achieving the qualification of complete or qualified success.

2.5. Statistical Analisys

Data analysis was performed using SPSS for Windows, version 25.0 (SPSS Inc., Chicago, IL, USA). Normality was checked by means of the Kolmogorov–Smirnov test. A descriptive analysis of the sociodemographic variables expresses the mean values with their standard deviation. The absolute and relative frequencies were determined for categorical variables, and for continuous variables, the mean, standard deviation, minimum and maximum were calculated. For comparisons between pre-and post-treatment values, parametric (Student's t or ANOVA) or non-parametric (Mann–Whitney or Kruskal–Wallis) tests are used in the case of continuous variables, and for categorical variables, the chi-square test was used. Continuous variables were analyzed using repeated-measures analysis of variance (ANOVA). Bonferroni test was performed to analyze significant differences for the variables throughout the time within a group, while differences between two groups at each visit were analyzed with the independent-sample *t*-test. Fisher exact test was used to compare categorical data between both studied groups. Differences were considered statistically significant when the *p* value was <0.05.

3. Results

Forty-eight eyes were included in group one (control) and forty-seven in group two (is-ePRGF). The detailed characteristics of the patients before surgery are shown in Table 1. Among the 50 selected controls (group one), there were two losses: one died during follow-up, and one did not attend scheduled appointments. In group two, three withdrawals of the fifty selected cases that had signed the informed consent were reported: one patient requested to leave the study by their own decision, and in the other two cases the sample was not valid to prepare the is-ePRGF. No differences were found in the demographic data or the preoperative clinical characteristics between the two groups studied (Table 1).

Table 1. Baseline demographics and preoperative clinical characteristics by subgroups.

Parameter	Group 1 (Control) n = 48		Group 2 (Is-ePRGF) n = 47		*p* Value
	NPDS	NPDS + Phaco	NPDS	NPDS + Phaco	
Eyes (*n*)	19	29	31	16	
Age (years)	72.7 ± 8.4	70.7 ± 12.0	69.7 ± 11.1	69.6 ± 7.5	0.73
	(58–91)	(34–88)	(51–91)	(52–80)	
Sex (Female/Male)	10/9	12/17	18/13	6/10	0.46
	(52.6%/47.4%)	(41.4%/58.6%)	(58.1%/41.9%)	(37.5%/62.5%)	
CDVA (logMAR)	0.39 ± 0.38	0.25 ± 0.44	0.27 ± 0.27	0.10 ± 0.14	0.01 *
	(1.00–0.00)	(1.70–0.00)	(1.30–0.00)	(0.40–0.00)	
IOP (mmHg)	21.9 ± 12.6	17.9 ± 7.3	18.3 ± 6.8	19.6 ± 7.1	0.79
	(9.0–50.0)	(10.0–44.0)	(8.0–37.0)	(11.0–35.0)	
Eyes with glaucoma eyedrop treatment	19 (100%)	29 (100%)	31 (100%)	16 (100%)	
No. of hypotensive medications	2.6 ± 0.6	2.9 ± 0.8	2.9 ± 0.9	2.8 ± 0.8	0.44
Visual field mean deviation (dB)	−18.7 ± 7.2	−13.5 ± 7.7	−16.1 ± 9.2	−15.0 ± 7.7	0.21
Glaucoma severity					
Early	1 (5.3%)	6 (20.7%)	5 (16.1%)	2 (12.5%)	0.42
Moderate	3 (15.8%)	8 (27.6%)	6 (19.4%)	7 (43.8%)	
Advanced	14 (73.7%)	12 (41.4%)	15 (48.4%)	7 (43.8%)	
Terminal	1 (5.3%)	3 (10.3%)	5 (16.1%)	−	
Type of glaucoma, *n* (%)					
POAG	4 (21.1)	12 (41.4)	8 (25.8)	5 (31.3)	0.50
Glaucoma and high myopia	6 (31.6)	3 (10.3)	11 (35.5)	−	
PXFG	5 (26.3)	11 (37.9)	9 (29.0)	7 (43.8)	
UG	1 (5.3)	1 (3.4)	−	1 (3.2)	
NTG	2 (10.5)	1 (3.4)	1 (3.2)	1 (3.2)	
TG	1 (5.3)	−	1 (3.2)	1 (3.2)	
PG	−	1 (3.4)	1 (3.2)	1 (3.2)	

Data presented as mean ± SD (range) or No. (%). * NPDS group 1 vs. NPDS + Phaco group 2. is-ePRGF: immunosafe eye drops plasma rich in growth factors; CDVA: corrected distance visual acuity; IOP: intraocular pressure; NPDS: non-penetrating deep sclerectomy; NTG: normal-tension glaucoma; PG: pigmentary glaucoma; Phaco: Phacoemulsification and intraocular lens implantation; POAG: primary open angle glaucoma; PXFG: pseudoexfoliative glaucoma; TG: secondary open angle glaucoma due to ocular trauma; UG: uveitic glaucoma.

NPDS showed a significant reduction in IOP at each postoperative follow-up visit concerning preoperative values in both groups. In group one (control), there was a significant IOP increase between 3- and 6-month follow-up visits ($p = 0.01$). In group two (is-ePRGF), IOP was maintained from the first month throughout the follow-up period ($p = 0.15$). At the last follow-up visit, the IOP was significantly lower in group two than that in group one ($p < 0.01$) (Figure 1). The IOP reduction at 6 months compared with that preoperatively was 27.2% and 52.6% in group one and group two, respectively. In a further analysis, each patient's IOP reduction was calculated, showing mean values of 11.0 ± 51.5% in group one and 34.5 ± 30.9%

in group two ($p < 0.01$). The number of hypotensive medications significantly decreased to 0.3 ± 0.9 and 0.2 ± 0.6 in group one and group two, respectively ($p < 0.01$).

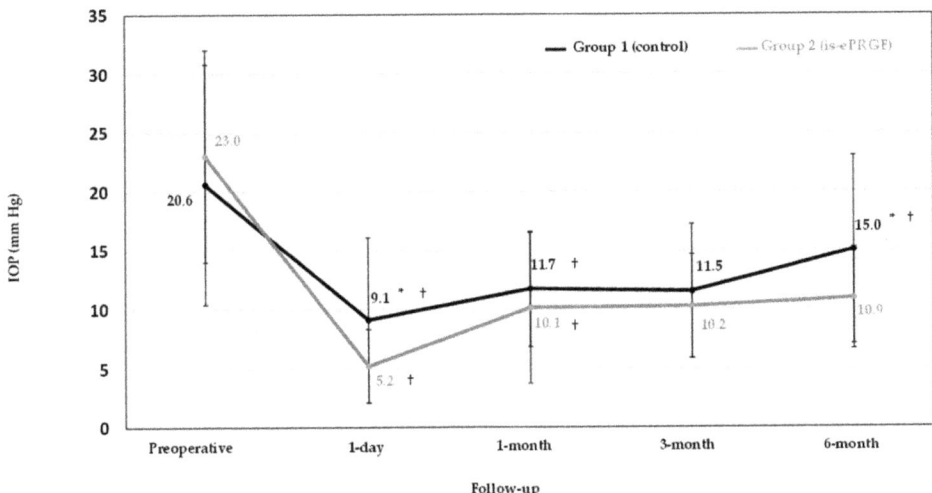

Figure 1. Measurement of intraocular pressure after surgery. *: Differences between groups at the follow-up visit. †: Differences with previous visit within the group. is-ePRGF: immunosafe eye drops plasma rich in growth factors; IOP: intraocular pressure.

Further comparisons according to the surgical technique (Figure 2) showed statistically significant differences at 6 months between controls that underwent NPDS + Phaco and NPDS + Phaco in the is-ePRGF group ($p = 0.01$). IOP was also lower in NPDS with is-ePRGF compared with that in NPDS in controls ($p = 0.26$).

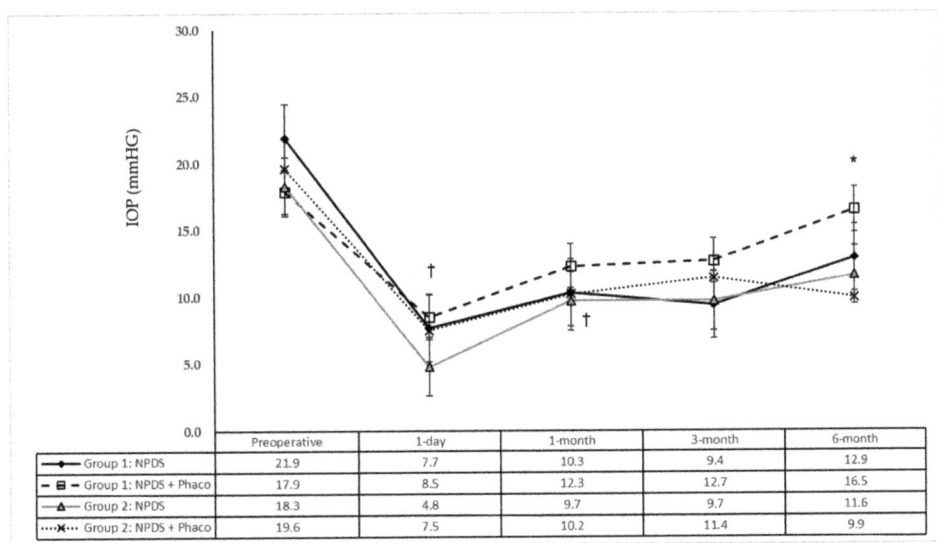

Figure 2. Measurement of intraocular pressure after surgery. *: Differences between groups at the follow-up visit. †: Differences with previous visit within the group. IOP: intraocular pressure; NPDS: non-penetrating deep sclerectomy; Phaco: phacoemulsification and intraocular lens implantation.

The percentages of complete and qualified success at the end of the follow-up were 66.7% and 83.3%, respectively, in group one, and 72.3% and 93.6% in group two. A further analysis by subgroups is shown in Table 2: the subgroup of NPDS + phaco treated with is-ePRGF presented the lowest failure rate (6.3%), followed by the subgroup of NPDS with is-ePRGF (6.5%).

Table 2. Success rates at 6 months (intraocular pressure ≤ 21 mm Hg) by subgroups.

	Group 1 (Control)		Group 2 (Is-ePRGF)	
	NPDS	NPDS + Phaco	NPDS	NPDS + Phaco
	(n = 19)	(n = 29)	(n = 31)	(n = 16)
Complete success, n (%)	14 (73.7)	18 (62.1)	21 (67.7)	13 (81.3)
Qualified success (complete success + success with treatment), n (%)	16 (84.2)	24 (82.8)	29 (93.5)	15 (93.8)
Failure, n (%)	3 (15.8)	5 (17.2)	2 (6.5)	1 (6.3)

The bleb evaluation with AS-OCT revealed a higher bleb height at all follow-up visits in group two compared with that in group one. In group two, an increase in bleb height was observed between 1 day and 1 month, and then it remained stable (Figure 3A). At the final visit, the percentages of blebs presenting microcysts were 62.5% and 76.7% in group one and group two, respectively (Figure 3B).

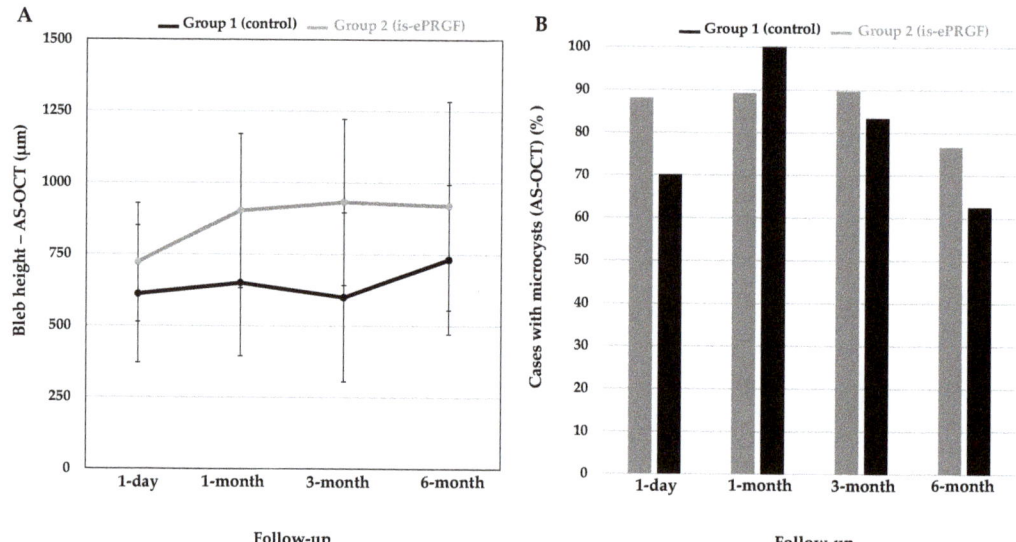

Figure 3. Measurement of bleb with AS-OCT. (**A**) Bleb height; (**B**) frequency of microcysts. is-ePRGF: immunosafe eye drops plasma rich in growth factors.

Table 3 shows the postoperative complications and frequency of bleb manipulations in each group. There were no complications related to the use of is-ePRGF. Bleb manipulations (laser goniopuncture or needling) were performed in 39.6% and 38.3% of the eyes in group one and group two, respectively. Hypotensive medication was required in 29.2% of the cases in group one and in 21.3% of group two. Postoperative complications were more frequent in group one. In group one, 6.3% of the eyes required a secondary glaucoma surgery, and this was 2.1% in group two.

Table 3. Comparison of bleb manipulations, hypotensive medication, postoperative complications and secondary glaucoma surgery between groups.

Parameter	Group 1 (Control)	Group 2 (Is-ePRGF)	p Value
Bleb manipulation	19 (39.6%)	18 (38.3%)	0.58
Laser goniopuncture	14 (29.2%)	10 (21.3%)	0.36
Needling	5 (10.4%)	8 (17.0%)	0.58
Hypotensive medications	14 (25.0%)	10 (21.3%)	0.42
Postoperative complications	12 (25.0%)	5 (10.6%)	0.06
Hyphema	4 (8.3%)	2 (4.3%)	
Atalamia	2 (4.2%)	0 (0.0%)	
Hypotony	3 (6.3%)	1 (2.1%)	
Iris incarceration	2 (4.2%)	0 (0.0%)	
TDM rupture	1 (2.1%)	2 (4.3%)	
Secondary glaucoma surgery	3 (6.3%)	1 (2.1%)	0.78
Bleb revision	2 (4.2%)	1 (2.1%)	
GDD implantation	1 (2.1%)	0 (0.0%)	

GDD: Glaucoma drainage device; TDM: Trabecular-Descemet membrane.

The requirement of hypotensive medications and further glaucoma surgery were both less frequent in group two, without reaching statistical significance ($p = 0.42$ and $p = 0.78$, respectively).

4. Discussion

NPDS is a filtering glaucoma surgery that emerged as an alternative to trabeculectomy in patients with open-angle glaucoma [2], providing satisfactory efficacy and a low rate of complications [3]. However, the surgical success rate (meaning a goal IOP within adequate limits) tends to decrease over the long-term [1,17]. Postoperative fibrosis is the leading cause of surgical failure [17,18]. Consequently, huge efforts are performed to find effective strategies to modulate the healing process. To this extent, the strategies may aim to act on the four wound-healing pathways, coagulative, inflammatory, proliferative and post-proliferative remodeling [19], and may be applied at three different stages: pre-, intra- and postoperatively. In the current study, we evaluated a strategy which consisted of reinforcing the conventional one (that is, intraoperative MMC [20,21] and postoperative steroids) with PRGF at the postoperative stage. PRGF has demonstrated its role in tissular regeneration, inflammation control and fibrosis modulation. Hence, it could act on the inflammatory, proliferative and post-proliferative remodeling of the wound-healing pathways.

Our results showed that reinforcing the conventional strategy with postoperative is-ePRGF yielded a higher IOP reduction at 6 months postoperatively (27.2% vs. 52.6% of IOP reduction in the control and PRGF groups, respectively) and a lower percentage of failed surgical outcomes (16.7% vs. 6.4%).

Furthermore, AS-OCT analysis of bleb morphologies showed a higher bleb height as well as a higher proportion of blebs presenting microcysts in the PRGF group than in the control group. AS-OCT has been widely used in the postoperative evaluation of conjunctival blebs of several glaucoma filtering techniques [22–25]. Several parameters, such as bleb thickness, bleb height, bleb wall reflectivity, the presence or absence of microcysts, etc., have been studied, looking for an association with better IOP control. In general, a tall bleb with a thick hypo-reflective wall is considered as a feature of a well-functioning bleb [26]. Hirooka et al. [27] studied trabeculectomy bleb images with time-domain OCT, looking for an association between morphological features and function. They found that the so-called cystoid-type blebs (characterized by the presence of multiple small cysts inside the bleb) were related to a higher probability of success compared with other filtering blebs presenting less cystic spaces. This is in accordance with other studies [28,29].

In addition, a higher proportion of blebs presenting microcysts as well as taller blebs were observed in the is-ePRGF group compared with the control group. These facts could be related with the lower IOP and the higher success rate in the is-ePRGF group at the final follow-up visit. Therefore, the better feature appearance of the bleb morphology in the is-ePRGF group would also support the benefits of using coadjuvant is-ePRGF eye drops in NPDS.

To the best of our knowledge, this is the first study that evaluated coadjuvant postoperative treatment with PRGF immunosafe eye drops in patients who underwent NPDS. However, it is worth noting the study by Rodriguez-Agirretxe et al. [12], who also evaluated PRFG, although in another therapeutic formulation (fibrin membrane), and in another stage (intraoperatively). The IOP reduction in our study at the 6-month follow-up visit was comparable to that reported by Rodriguez-Agirretxe et al. [12] (around 50%); they extended the follow-up for two years, finding that IOP was stabilized at levels of approximately 15 mmHg. Furthermore, their complete and qualified success percentages were 80 and 90%, respectively, two years after NPDS. These results support the hypothesis of the benefit of PRGF for enhancing the surgical success rate of NPDS.

The use of amniotic membrane (AM) has also been reported to be a safe and effective adjuvant treatment in glaucoma filtering surgery [30]. Similarly to the present study, Sheha et al. [31] reported that the use of single-layer AM under the scleral flap in trabeculectomy with MMC provided lower IOP, higher success rates and lower complication rates compared with trabeculectomy with MMC alone. However, the method of application of AM in filtering surgery (whether above or below the scleral flap) is yet to be standardized [32].

Despite the positive presented results in our study in terms of IOP control, surgical success rate and bleb features, it is interesting to note that there were no differences between groups in the rate of postoperative bleb manipulation, number of required hypotensive medications and necessity of secondary glaucoma surgery (Table 2). We hypothesized that depending on the formulation (eye drop or fibrin membrane), PRGF could have a different effect on NPDS surgery. In eye drops, the percentage of penetration reaching the bleb would be lower than the fibrin membrane. Consequently, its impact on modulating bleb fibrosis would be limited, and it would explain the absence of differences between the control and PRGF groups in postoperative management. By contrast, the use of postoperative PRGF eye drop formulation, beyond the moderate healing process in the bleb (which could depend on the degree of PRGF eye drop penetration), could contribute to other properties to improve IOP control after NPDS. Firstly, the PRGF eye drop itself could decrease the IOP by modulating the transforming growth factor-β (TGF-β) activity [16]. The increased activity of TGF-β may provide an accumulation of deposits in the extracellular matrix of the trabecular tissue, limiting the aqueous humor flow through the trabecular meshwork and causing an IOP rise [33,34]. Consequently, the capability of PRGF eye drops to modulate the TGF-β activity would act as hypotensive and could explain the lower postoperative IOP in the PRGF group. Secondly, for those patients who required postoperative hypotensive medication, the anti-inflammatory properties of the PRGF eye drop could contribute to higher treatment adherence, augmenting the hypotensive effect and increasing the rate of qualified success (defined as having an IOP $\leq$ 21 mmHg with antiglaucoma medications).

There were no PRGF-related complications over the follow-up. Of note that in this study, we evaluated the postoperative PRGF eye drop combined with intraoperative MMC and postoperative steroids. The absence of potential complications associated with PRGF eye drops is another crucial aspect owing to be combined with any of the strategies studied to modulate wound healing of filtering blebs, such as preoperative steroids, intraoperative antifibrotics, anti-VEGF, PRGF membrane, or amniotic membrane. Furthermore, we observe a decrease in the rate of postoperative complications in the PRGF group compared with the control group.

Despite these encouraging outcomes, it should be noted that our study has limitations, such as the retrospective analysis in the control group and a short follow-up. In addition, the postoperative AS-OCT evaluation did not include bleb wall reflectivity assessment, which might be related to bleb functionality [22,25,26]. Finally, the relatively small sample size within some subgroups might imply that some results need to be analyzed with caution.

Ideally, in the design of future prospective randomized clinical trials, a larger number of patients undergoing only one type of surgical technique may be selected in order to reduce the risk of bias.

5. Conclusions

The results of this study would suggest that PRGF immunosafe eye drops may be considered as a safe non-invasive adjuvant agent in the postoperative treatment of NPDS. Further prospective and randomized clinical trials should be performed to confirm the potential therapeutic efficacy of PRGF eye drops in glaucoma surgery.

Author Contributions: Conceptualization, P.P.R.-C., I.R.-U., A.F.-V.-C., R.M.S.-Á., E.A. and J.M.-L.; methodology, P.P.R.-C., I.R.-U., A.F.-V.-C. and J.M.-L.; software, I.R.-U. and R.M.S.-Á.; validation, P.P.R.-C., I.R.-U., A.F.-V.-C., R.M.S.-Á., E.A. and J.M.-L.; formal analysis, R.M.S.-Á.; investigation, P.P.R.-C., I.R.-U., A.F.-V.-C., R.M.S.-Á., E.A. and J.M.-L.; resources, A.F.-V.-C., E.A. and J.M.-L.; data curation, P.P.R.-C., I.R.-U. and R.M.S.-Á.; writing—original draft preparation, P.P.R.-C. and I.R.-U.; writing—review and editing, I.R.-U. and R.M.S.-Á.; supervision, I.R.-U., E.A. and J.M.-L.; project administration, E.A. and J.M.-L. All authors have read and agreed to the published version of the manuscript.

Funding: This research was funded by grant RD21/0002/0041 (Instituto de Salud Carlos III, Spain).

Institutional Review Board Statement: The study was approved by the regional clinical research ethics committee (Comité de Ética de la Investigación del Principado de Asturias, CEImPA n# 2019.84, 8 January 2020). The research adhered to the guidelines of the Declaration of Helsinki.

Informed Consent Statement: Informed consent was obtained from all subjects involved in this study.

Data Availability Statement: The data used to support this study's findings are available upon request to the corresponding author.

Acknowledgments: The authors would like to express their gratitude to David Madrid from Complutense University of Madrid for his scientific guidance and advice. P.P.R.-C., I.R.-U. and A.F.-V.-C. would also like to give special thanks to Montserrat García, Lydia Álvarez and Héctor Iglesias from Fundación de Investigación Oftalmológica for their continuous support from their laboratory to our clinical department.

Conflicts of Interest: The authors declare the following conflicts of interest: E.A. is the Scientific Director and R.M.S.-Á. is a scientist at BTI Biotechnology Institute, a company that investigates in the fields of oral implantology and PRGF-Endoret technology. The other authors declare no conflicts of interest in developing this study.

References

1. Shaarawy, T.; Mansouri, K.; Schnyder, C.; Ravinet, E.; Achache, F.; Mermoud, A. Long-term results of deep sclerectomy with collagen implant. *J. Cataract Refract. Surg.* **2004**, *30*, 1225–1231. [CrossRef] [PubMed]
2. Mendrinos, E.; Mermoud, A.; Shaarawy, T. Nonpenetrating glaucoma surgery. *Surv. Ophthalmol.* **2008**, *53*, 592–630. [CrossRef] [PubMed]
3. Eldaly, M.A.; Bunce, C.; Elsheikha, O.Z.; Wormald, R. Non-penetrating filtration surgery versus trabeculectomy for open-angle glaucoma. *Cochrane Database Syst. Rev.* **2014**, CD007059. [CrossRef] [PubMed]
4. Guedes, R.A.P.; Guedes, V.M.P.; Chaoubah, A. Factors associated with non-penetrating deep sclerectomy failure in controlling intraocular pressure. *Acta Ophthalmol.* **2011**, *89*, 58–61. [CrossRef] [PubMed]
5. Roy, S.; Mermoud, A. Complications of deep nonpenetrating sclerectomy. *J. Fr. Ophtalmol.* **2006**, *29*, 1180–1197. [CrossRef]
6. Sanchez-Avila, R.M.; Merayo-Lloves, J.; Fernandez, M.L.; Rodriguez-Gutierrez, L.A.; Jurado, N.; Muruzabal, F.; Orive, G.; Anitua, E. Plasma Rich in Growth Factors for the Treatment of Dry Eye after LASIK Surgery. *Ophthalmic Res.* **2018**, *60*, 80–86. [CrossRef]
7. Sanchez-Avila, R.M.; Merayo-Lloves, J.; Riestra, A.C.; Fernandez-Vega Cueto, L.; Anitua, E.; Begona, L.; Muruzabal, F.; Orive, G. Treatment of patients with neurotrophic keratitis stages 2 and 3 with plasma rich in growth factors (PRGF-Endoret) eye-drops. *Int. Ophthalmol.* **2017**, *38*, 1193–1204. [CrossRef]
8. Sánchez-Ávila, R.M.; Robayo-Esper, C.A.; Villota-Deleu, E.; Fernández-Vega Sanz, Á.; Fernández-Vega González, Á.; de la Sen-Corcuera, B.; Anitua, E.; Merayo-Lloves, J. Plasma Rich in Growth Factors in Macular Hole Surgery. *Clin. Pract.* **2022**, *12*, 57–69. [CrossRef]

9. Figueroa, M.S.; Mora Cantallops, A.; Virgili, G.; Govetto, A. Long-term results of autologous plasma as adjuvant to pars plana vitrectomy in the treatment of high myopic full-thickness macular holes. *Eur. J. Ophthalmol.* **2020**, *31*, 2612–2620. [CrossRef]
10. Sanchez-Avila, R.M.; Merayo-Lloves, J.; Riestra, A.C.; Berisa, S.; Lisa, C.; Sanchez, J.A.; Muruzabal, F.; Orive, G.; Anitua, E. Plasma rich in growth factors membrane as coadjuvant treatment in the surgery of ocular surface disorders. *Medicine* **2018**, *97*, e0242. [CrossRef]
11. Anitua, E.; de la Sen-Corcuera, B.; Orive, G.; Sánchez-Ávila, R.M.; Heredia, P.; Muruzabal, F.; Merayo-Lloves, J. Progress in the use of plasma rich in growth factors in ophthalmology: From ocular surface to ocular fundus. *Expert Opin. Biol. Ther.* **2021**, *22*, 31–45. [CrossRef] [PubMed]
12. Rodríguez-Agirretxe, I.; Freire, V.; Muruzabal, F.; Orive, G.; Anitua, E.; Díez-Feijóo, E.; Acera, A. Subconjunctival PRGF Fibrin Membrane as an Adjuvant to Nonpenetrating Deep Sclerectomy: A 2-Year Pilot Study. *Ophthalmic Res.* **2018**, *59*, 45–52. [CrossRef] [PubMed]
13. Muñoz, G. Nonstitch suprachoroidal technique for T-flux implantation in deep sclerectomy. *J. Glaucoma* **2009**, *18*, 262–264. [CrossRef] [PubMed]
14. Bonilla, R.; Loscos, J.; Valldeperas, X.; Parera, M.A.; Sabala, A. Supraciliary hema implant in combined deep sclerectomy and phacoemulsification: One year results. *Open Ophthalmol. J.* **2012**, *6*, 59–62. [CrossRef] [PubMed]
15. Belda, J.I.; Loscos-Arenas, J.; Mermoud, A.; Lozano, E.; D'Alessandro, E.; Rebolleda, G.; Rodriguez-Agirretxe, I.; Canut, M.; Rodriguez-Calvo, P.P. Supraciliary versus intrascleral implantation with hema implant (Esnoper V-2000) in deep sclerectomy: A multicenter randomized controlled trial. *Acta Ophthalmol.* **2018**, *96*, e852–e858. [CrossRef]
16. Sánchez-Avila, R.M.; Merayo-Lloves, J.; Fernández, M.L.; Rodríguez-Gutiérrez, L.A.; Rodríguez-Calvo, P.P.; Fernández-Vega Cueto, A.; Muruzabal, F.; Orive, G.; Anitua, E. Plasma rich in growth factors eye drops to treat secondary ocular surface disorders in patients with glaucoma. *Int. Med. Case Rep. J.* **2018**, *11*, 97–103. [CrossRef]
17. Bergin, C.; Petrovic, A.; Mermoud, A.; Ravinet, E.; Sharkawi, E. Baerveldt tube implantation following failed deep sclerectomy versus repeat deep sclerectomy. *Graefe's Arch. Clin. Exp. Ophthalmol.* **2016**, *254*, 161–168. [CrossRef]
18. Bissig, A.; Rivier, D.; Zaninetti, M.; Shaarawy, T.; Mermoud, A.; Roy, S. Ten years follow-up after deep sclerectomy with collagen implant. *J. Glaucoma* **2008**, *17*, 680–686. [CrossRef]
19. Fan Gaskin, J.C.; Nguyen, D.Q.; Soon Ang, G.; O'Connor, J.; Crowston, J.G. Wound Healing Modulation in Glaucoma Filtration Surgery-Conventional Practices and New Perspectives: The Role of Antifibrotic Agents (Part I). *J. Curr. glaucoma Pract.* **2014**, *8*, 37–45. [CrossRef]
20. Cheng, J.-W.; Cai, J.-P.; Li, Y.; Wei, R.-L. Intraoperative mitomycin C for nonpenetrating glaucoma surgery: A systematic review and meta-analysis. *J. Glaucoma* **2011**, *20*, 322–326. [CrossRef]
21. Kozobolis, V.P.; Christodoulakis, E.V.; Tzanakis, N.; Zacharopoulos, I.; Pallikaris, I.G. Primary deep sclerectomy versus primary deep sclerectomy with the use of mitomycin C in primary open-angle glaucoma. *J. Glaucoma* **2002**, *11*, 287–293. [CrossRef]
22. Mastropasqua, R.; Fasanella, V.; Agnifili, L.; Curcio, C.; Ciancaglini, M.; Mastropasqua, L. Anterior segment optical coherence tomography imaging of conjunctival filtering blebs after glaucoma surgery. *Biomed Res. Int.* **2014**, *2014*, 610623. [CrossRef] [PubMed]
23. Fernández-Buenaga, R.; Rebolleda, G.; Casas-Llera, P.; Muñoz-Negrete, F.J.; Pérez-López, M. A comparison of intrascleral bleb height by anterior segment OCT using three different implants in deep sclerectomy. *Eye* **2012**, *26*, 552–556. [CrossRef] [PubMed]
24. Aptel, F.; Dumas, S.; Denis, P. Ultrasound biomicroscopy and optical coherence tomography imaging of filtering blebs after deep sclerectomy with new collagen implant. *Eur. J. Ophthalmol.* **2009**, *19*, 223–230. [CrossRef]
25. Pérez-Rico, C.; Gutiérrez-Ortíz, C.; Moreno-Salgueiro, A.; González-Mesa, A.; Teus, M.A. Visante anterior segment optical coherence tomography analysis of morphologic changes after deep sclerectomy with intraoperative mitomycin-C and no implant use. *J. Glaucoma* **2014**, *23*, e86–e90. [CrossRef] [PubMed]
26. Narita, A.; Morizane, Y.; Miyake, T.; Seguchi, J.; Baba, T.; Shiraga, F. Characteristics of early filtering blebs that predict successful trabeculectomy identified via three-dimensional anterior segment optical coherence tomography. *Br. J. Ophthalmol.* **2018**, *102*, 796–801. [CrossRef]
27. Hirooka, K.; Takagishi, M.; Baba, T.; Takenaka, H.; Shiraga, F. Stratus optical coherence tomography study of filtering blebs after primary trabeculectomy with a fornix-based conjunctival flap. *Acta Ophthalmol.* **2010**, *88*, 60–64. [CrossRef]
28. Singh, M.; Chew, P.T.K.; Friedman, D.S.; Nolan, W.P.; See, J.L.; Smith, S.D.; Zheng, C.; Foster, P.J.; Aung, T. Imaging of trabeculectomy blebs using anterior segment optical coherence tomography. *Ophthalmology* **2007**, *114*, 47–53. [CrossRef]
29. Cerdà-Ibáñez, M.; Pérez-Torregrosa, V.T.; Olate-Pérez, A.; Almor Palacios, I.; Gargallo-Benedicto, A.; Osorio-Alayo, V.; Barreiro Rego, A.; Duch-Samper, A. Qualitative analysis of repaired filtering blebs with anterior segment-optical coherence tomography. *Arch. Soc. Esp. Oftalmol.* **2017**, *92*, 359–365. [CrossRef]
30. Shen, T.-Y.; Hu, W.-N.; Cai, W.-T.; Jin, H.-Z.; Yu, D.-H.; Sun, J.-H.; Yu, J. Effectiveness and Safety of Trabeculectomy along with Amniotic Membrane Transplantation on Glaucoma: A Systematic Review. *J. Ophthalmol.* **2020**, *2020*, 3949775. [CrossRef]
31. Sheha, H.; Kheirkhah, A.; Taha, H. Amniotic membrane transplantation in trabeculectomy with mitomycin C for refractory glaucoma. *J. Glaucoma* **2008**, *17*, 303–307. [CrossRef] [PubMed]
32. Sharma, R.; Nappi, V.; Empeslidis, T. The developments in amniotic membrane transplantation in glaucoma and vitreoretinal procedures. *Int. Ophthalmol.* **2023**, *43*, 1771–1783. [CrossRef] [PubMed]

33. Raychaudhuri, U.; Millar, J.C.; Clark, A.F. Knockout of tissue transglutaminase ameliorates TGFβ2-induced ocular hypertension: A novel therapeutic target for glaucoma? *Exp. Eye Res.* **2018**, *171*, 106–110. [CrossRef] [PubMed]
34. Agarwal, R.; Agarwal, P. Future target molecules in antiglaucoma therapy: Tgf-Beta may have a role to play. *Ophthalmic Res.* **2010**, *43*, 1–10. [CrossRef] [PubMed]

Disclaimer/Publisher's Note: The statements, opinions and data contained in all publications are solely those of the individual author(s) and contributor(s) and not of MDPI and/or the editor(s). MDPI and/or the editor(s) disclaim responsibility for any injury to people or property resulting from any ideas, methods, instructions or products referred to in the content.

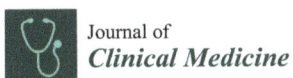

Article

Safety and Efficacy of Three Variants of Canaloplasty with Phacoemulsification to Treat Open-Angle Glaucoma and Cataract: 12-Month Follow-Up

Aleksandra K. Kicińska [1,*], Monika E. Danielewska [2] and Marek Rękas [1]

1 Department of Ophthalmology, Military Institute of Medicine, 04-141 Warsaw, Poland
2 Department of Biomedical Engineering, Faculty of Fundamental Problems of Technology, Wroclaw University of Science and Technology, 50-370 Wroclaw, Poland
* Correspondence: aleksandra.kicinska@gmail.com

Abstract: Background: A single-center prospective randomized observational study to compare three types of canaloplasty, i.e., ab externo (ABeC), minicanaloplasty (miniABeC) and ab interno, (ABiC) combined with cataract surgery in primary open-angle glaucoma (POAG) patients over 12 months. Methods: 48 POAG patients underwent one of three canaloplasty procedures: ABeC (16 eyes), miniABeC (16 eyes) or ABiC (16 eyes) or combined with phacoemulsification. Patients were assessed at baseline, at day 0–1–7 and at month 1–3–6–12. Successful treatment was defined as unmedicated IOP reduction ≥20%. Complete surgical success was defined as an IOP ≤ 15 mmHg without medications, and a qualified surgical success as IOP ≤ 15 mmHg with or without medications. Results: Pre-washout IOP median values (mmHg) were 17 (ABeC), 18 (miniABeC) and 17 (AbiC) and decreased at 12-month follow up postoperatively to 13 ($p = 0.005$), 13 ($p = 0.004$) and 14 ($p = 0.008$), respectively—successful treatment was achieved in approximately 100% of patients for ABeC and in 93.8% for both miniABeC and AbiC groups. Preoperatively, the median number of medications was 2.0 (range 1–3) (ABeC), 2.0 (1–3) (miniABeC) and 2.0 (0–4) (ABiC); 12-month post-operatively, all medications were withdrawn except in two patients (followed miniABeC and AbiC). Conclusions: The three variants of canaloplasty significantly reduced IOP and the number of medications in patients with mild to moderate POAG and gave no significant complications.

Keywords: MIGS; mini-invasive antiglaucoma surgery; POAG; canaloplasty; minicanaloplasty

Citation: Kicińska, A.K.; Danielewska, M.E.; Rękas, M. Safety and Efficacy of Three Variants of Canaloplasty with Phacoemulsification to Treat Open-Angle Glaucoma and Cataract: 12-Month Follow-Up. *J. Clin. Med.* **2022**, *11*, 6501. https://doi.org/10.3390/jcm11216501

Academic Editors: Michele Figus and Karl Mercieca

Received: 3 October 2022
Accepted: 29 October 2022
Published: 2 November 2022

Publisher's Note: MDPI stays neutral with regard to jurisdictional claims in published maps and institutional affiliations.

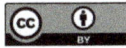

Copyright: © 2022 by the authors. Licensee MDPI, Basel, Switzerland. This article is an open access article distributed under the terms and conditions of the Creative Commons Attribution (CC BY) license (https://creativecommons.org/licenses/by/4.0/).

1. Introduction

In recent years, surgical methods to restore natural aqueous outflow systems to treat open angle glaucoma (OAG) have become an alternative to more invasive and risk-carrying penetrating surgeries. Among this group, canaloplasty and its various modifications have been of interest since 2005 when they were first introduced [1]. The concept of canaloplasty was born when adding a flexible microcannula to dilate 360° of Schlemm's canal by Kearney [2] during viscocanalostomy pioneered by Stegmann [3]. Since then, canaloplasty, performed as a single procedure or combined with phacoemulsification [4–8], has been shown to reduce IOP in patients with OAG in a safe and effective way. In terms of IOP-lowering potential canaloplasty was even described by some authors as comparable to trabeculectomy [9,10]. The surgical technique of canaloplasty is designed to address all aspects of outflow resistance—the trabecular meshwork (TM), Schlemm's canal and the distal outflow system beginning with the collector channels [2].

Over the years, canaloplasty has gained popularity and evolved into a group of procedures [1]. Various modifications of canaloplasty have been described, including catheterless suture placement [11], using various sutures [12], replacing suture with two Stegmann Canal Expander devices [13] or intubation without viscodilatation with Glaucolight [14].

In 2015, Sunman et al. described a variant of surgery with a deeper scleral excision facilitating the uveoscleral outflow pathway, and thus, intensifying the IOP reducing potential compared to the traditional method [15].

Growing demand for moving towards more sparing procedures caused a natural evolution into ab interno canaloplasty (ABiC) [16]. ABiC belongs to minimally invasive glaucoma surgery and as such requires neither peritomy nor sclerectomy and uses corneal incision to access the Schlemm's canal under the gonioscopic view. However, the ab interno variant makes the placement of a Prolene suture impossible, which imposes severe limitations on the use of this technique.

Minicanaloplasty, described by Rekas et al. [17], fills the gap between the traditional procedure, which originated from non-penetrating deep sclerectomy (NPDS), and viscocanalostomy, with its ab interno method. It allows for Schlemm's canal cannulation without meticulous dissection of the trabeculo-Descemet membrane (TDM)—in this procedure, scleral flaps are only needed for accessing the canal [17]. The initial results proved it to be as successful as traditional canaloplasty and ABiC in terms of IOP reduction with a similar safety profile [18]. Following these observations, the aim of this study was to compare three variants of canaloplasty, i.e., ab externo canaloplasty, minicanaloplasty and ab interno canaloplastyin, in terms of efficacy and safety after 12 months. The role of the scleral lake in canaloplasty and its effect on IOP reduction were also of interest to the investigation.

2. Materials and Methods

2.1. Study Design

This is a prospective randomized observational clinical study on canaloplasty. The study was performed in accordance with the principles of the Declaration of Helsinki and approved by the Bioethics Committee of the Military Institute of Medicine in Warsaw (decision no. 76/WIM/2015). All patients were over 18 years old and able to understand and provide informed consent. The study was registered at www.clinicaltrials.gov: NCT02908633.

A total of 48 eyes of 48 consecutive patients affected by primary open-angle glaucoma underwent one of three variants of canaloplasty, i.e., ab externo canaloplasty (ABeC), minicanaloplasty (miniC) or ab interno canaloplasty (ABiC), combined with phacoemulsification. Operations were performed at the Ophthalmology Department of the Military Institute of Medicine in Warsaw, Poland, by one surgeon, M.R., between February 2016 and July 2019. Patients were randomized into three groups of 16 by a random sorting algorithm using the maximum allowable 10% deviations in a 1:1 allocation ratio on the day of the surgery. Baseline examination, randomization and postoperative care were carried out by the first author (A.K.K.), who had no interest in selecting one procedure in favor of another. The surgeon was excluded from any evaluation to avoid bias. Study subjects remained blind to treatment assignment throughout the course of the study. Data from all of the patients were reviewed over an extended period of time to obtain a comparable sample size at the 12-month follow-up stage.

All enrollees underwent a full ophthalmic baseline assessment 30 days before surgery (pre-washout), including: history of glaucoma, medication use, IOP measurement using Goldmann applanation tonometry, corrected distance visual acuity (CDVA) converted to the logarithm of the minimum angle of resolution (logMAR), gonioscopy angle grading according to the Spaeth system, slit-lamp biomicroscopy of the anterior segment and fundus indirect ophthalmoscopy of the optic nerve head, including cup-to-disc ratio, presence of a notch or splinter hemorrhage and peripapillary atrophy. In addition, measurements of central corneal thickness (CCT), axial length (AXL) and keratometric parameters required for the intraocular lens (IOL) calculation were taken. All patients were washed out from antiglaucoma medications throughout a minimum 4-week period prior to surgery. On the day of surgery, IOP was measured and determined as post-washout IOP.

Postoperative follow-up examinations were at days 0, 1 and 7 and months 1, 3, 6 and 12. Postoperative evaluation included IOP measurements, CDVA, slit-lamp examination, gonioscopy and ophthalmic medication reporting. Each time, three IOP measurements were taken and the mean value of the IOP was used for the statistical analysis. Tonometry was always performed between 8 and 10 am.

All adverse events were reported; those within 90 days following surgery were considered early, whereas those after 90 days were counted as late.

Surgical success was analyzed in two categories. The definition of qualified success was based on IOP $\leq$ 15 mmHg with or without medications, while complete success was defined as IOP $\leq$ 15 mmHg with no antiglaucoma medications. Additionally, the proportion of eyes at 12 months with unmedicated IOP reduction $\geq$ 20% compared with post-washout was determined.

2.2. Patient Inclusion and Exclusion Criteria

Indications for surgery were: coexisting visually significant cataract and primary open-angle glaucoma (POAG) with progression in visual field (VF) loss despite the use of IOP-lowering medications (one to four active ingredients). Eligible patients presented with ophthalmoscopically detectable glaucomatous optic neuropathy and mild to moderate visual field (VF) loss according to Hodapp–Anderson–Parrish criteria [19] and were previously assigned to combined antiglaucoma and cataract surgery. The post-washout IOP value measured at the day of surgery was required to be 18 mmHg or higher.

Exclusion criteria were: secondary open-angle or narrow-angle glaucoma, history of ocular trauma or inflammation, previous ocular surgery or laser trabeculoplasty and clinically significant corneal dystrophy. Another excluding factor was a history of untreated IOP over 30 mmHg, based on the knowledge that the collector ostia are collapsed at this level of IOP [20].

Only subjects in whom a full procedure of canaloplasty with 360 degrees catheterization (in ABeC, miniABeC and AbiC) and suture placement (in the case of AbeC and miniABeC) could be performed were included in the study.

2.3. Surgical Technique

2.3.1. Canaloplasty

The surgeon followed the traditional ab externo canaloplasty technique, which has been extensively reported in the literature [5,7,8,12,21–26]. Scleral flaps were parabolic in shape and their size was 5.0 × 5.0 mm and 4.5 × 4 mm. Once the catheterization of the canal was completed and the distal tip exposed at the ostium, a double 10–0 polypropylene suture was tied to it. As the microcatheter was being withdrawn, a viscoelastic (Healon GV) was injected—once every two clock hours. The deep scleral flap was then excised and the superficial flap was sutured tightly with five 10–0 Nylon sutures in a watertight manner in order to avoid filtering bleb formation.

2.3.2. Minicanaloplasty

Minicanaloplasty is a method proposed by the co-author (M.R.), in which the sizes of both the scleral flaps are modified [17]. The superficial flap dimension was 4.0 × 1.5 mm and the deep flap was 1.0 × 1.0 mm. No TDM was dissected and the deep scleral flap remained unexcised. Sclerectomy was only performed to access Schlemm's canal. Catheterization and suture placement were performed in an identical fashion to that in ab externo canaloplasty.

2.3.3. Ab Interno Canaloplasty

Ab interno canaloplasty is a method belonging to mini-invasive antiglaucoma surgery (MIGS), and hence, it requires no sclerectomy [27]. This procedure was performed under gonioscopic view. The iTrack device was advanced through the canal's whole circumference and a viscoelastic was injected during its withdrawal as in ABeC. Prolene suture placement was not possible with this method.

All variants of canaloplasty were combined with cataract phacoemulsification.

2.4. Statistical Analysis

The mean values of IOP and CDVA in all patient groups did not follow a normal distribution at specific time stages before and after surgery (Kolmogorov–Smirnov test; $p < 0.05$). Hence, the Wilcoxon signed-rank test was used to test the temporal changes of values of these parameters in each group. Following Armstrong [28], no correction for multiple comparisons was applied.

To compare the median values of IOP, CDVA and glaucoma medications between the three considered groups of patients at each stage before and after surgery, the Kruskal–Wallis test was used. Additionally, Kaplan–Meier survival analysis and the log-rank test were used to compare the cumulative incidence of qualified and complete success between the considered groups. Fisher's exact independence test was used to compare dependence between the group factor and the proportion of patients who achieved a 20% reduction in IOP. Differences in complications between groups were determined using the Chi-square test.

In all tests, the significance level was set to an α of 0.05. Calculations were performed using SPSS 22.0 (SPSS, Inc., Chicago, IL, USA).

3. Results

All patients in each group met the study inclusion and exclusion criteria and completed the follow-ups over the period of 12 months. One patient was excluded from the study because the post-washout IOP value was below 18 mmHg and one because of incomplete catheterization of Schlemm's canal. Table 1 shows the patients' demographic data, and Table 2 presents the results of temporal changes in IOP values in all patient groups together with the results of the Wilcoxon signed-rank tests.

Table 1. Patients' demographics. Ab externo canaloplasty (ABeC), minicanaloplasty (miniABeC) and ab interno canaloplasty (ABiC).

Demographic.	ABeC	miniABeC	ABiC
General			
Patients, *n* (%)	16 (33)	16 (33)	16 (33)
Sex, *n* (%)			
Female	12 (75)	10 (62.5)	14 (87.5)
Male	4 (25)	6 (37.5)	2 (12.5)
Age (y)			
Mean ± SD	77 ± 7	74 ± 8	74 ± 7
Range	62–88	61–89	64–81
Eye			
Right, *n* (%)	6 (37.5)	6 (37.5)	7 (43.8)
Left, *n* (%)	10 (62.5)	10 (62.5)	9 (56.2)
Ethnicity, *n* (%)			
Caucasian	16 (100)	16 (100)	16 (100)
Glaucoma characteristics Glaucoma type			
POAG (primary open-angle glaucoma)	16 (100)	16 (100)	16 (100)
MD, Mean ± SD	4.0 ± 2.5	4.0 ± 2.5	4.0 ± 2.5
Drugs, median (range)	2.0 (1–3)	2.0 (1–3)	2.0 (1–3)

3.1. Intraocular Pressure Lowering

The washout procedure resulted in a statistically significant increase in the IOP median values by 5.0 mmHg, 4.0 mmHg and 4.0 mmHg in the ABeC, miniABeC and ABiC groups, respectively (Wilcoxon test, all $p \leq 0.001$). At 12 months after surgery, the IOP median values decreased statistically significantly, with respect to both pre- and post-washout stages, in all patient groups (see Table 2 and Figure 1). The same results were observed from 1 month postoperatively in the ABeC group as well as from 7 days postoperatively in the miniABeC and ABiC groups.

Table 2. First quartiles (Q1), medians, third quartiles (Q3) and interquartile ranges (IQRs) of IOP at each time stage before and after surgery in three groups of patients: ab externo canaloplasty (ABeC), minicanaloplasty (miniABeC) and ab interno canaloplasty (ABiC). *p* value * and *p* value ** correspond to the results of the Wilcoxon signed-rank tests between particular study stages and the pre-washout or post-washout stages, respectively. All patients in each group completed a 12-month follow-up. Italicized values indicate *p* < 0.05.

	ABeC			miniABeC			ABiC		
Time	IOP (intraocular pressure) (mmHg) Q1, Median, Q3, IQR	*p* Value *	*p* Value **	IOP (mmHg) Q1, Median, Q3, IQR	*p* Value *	*p* Value **	IOP (mmHg) Q1, Median, Q3, IQR	*p* Value *	*p* Value **
pre-washout	14.0, 17.0, 18.0, 4.0	-	*<0.001*	16.0, 18.0, 19.8, 3.8	-	*0.001*	16.3, 17.0, 19.8, 3.5	-	*0.001*
post-washout	20.0, 22.0, 24.0, 4.0	*<0.001*	-	20.3, 22.0, 23.8, 3.5	*0.001*	-	19.3, 21.0, 23.0, 3.7	*0.001*	-
1 d	12.0, 16.0, 19.0, 7.0	0.925	*0.008*	12.3, 16.5, 20.8, 8.5	0.795	*0.031*	12.0, 15.0, 18.0, 6.0	0.088	*0.003*
7 d	14.3, 16.5, 18.8, 4.5	0.705	*0.007*	12.3, 14.5, 17.0, 4.7	*0.007*	*<0.001*	13.3, 15.0, 18.8, 5.5	*0.030*	*<0.001*
1 m	10.3, 11.5, 13.8, 3.5	*0.004*	*<0.001*	11.0, 13.5, 16.0, 5.0	*0.002*	*<0.001*	12.3, 15.0, 17.0, 4.7	*0.003*	*<0.001*
3 m	11.3, 14.0, 16.8, 5.5	*0.016*	*<0.001*	12.0, 15.5, 16.8, 4.8	*0.006*	*0.001*	13.3, 15.0, 17.0, 3.7	*0.001*	*<0.001*
6 m	13.0, 13.0, 15.0, 2.0	*0.003*	*<0.001*	11.3, 14.0, 15.8, 4.5	*0.006*	*<0.001*	13.3, 16.5, 17.8, 4.5	*0.006*	*<0.001*
12 m	11.3, 13.0, 16.3, 5.0	*0.005*	*<0.001*	12.0, 13.0, 17.0, 5.0	*0.004*	*<0.001*	13.0, 14.0, 17.8, 4.8	*0.008*	*<0.001*

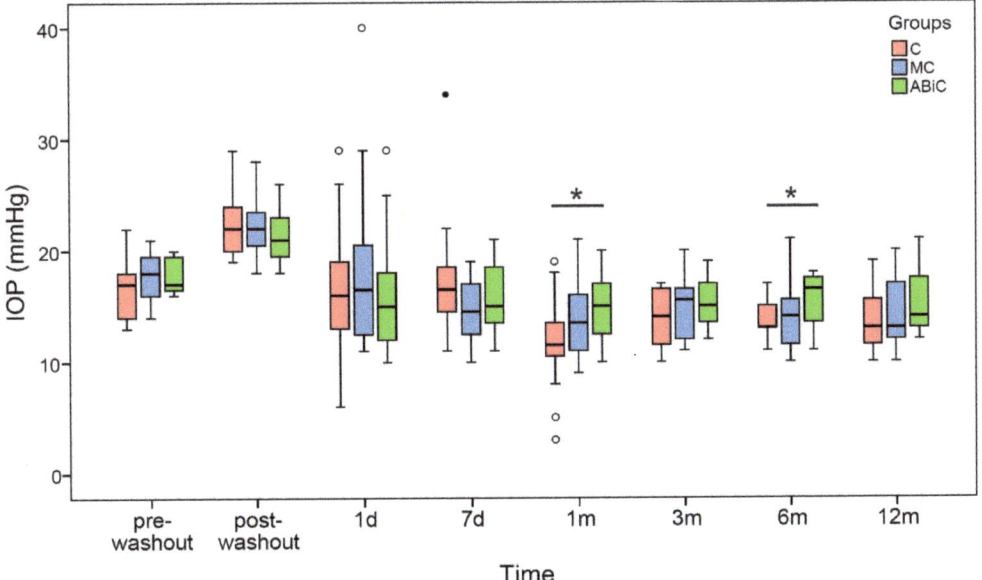

Figure 1. Boxplots of IOP median values at each time stage before and after surgery in three groups of patients: ab externo canaloplasty (ABeC), minicanaloplasty (miniABeC) and ab interno canaloplasty (ABiC). Asterisks denote statistically significant differences between particular groups ($p < 0.05$).

3.2. Comparison between Groups

There were statistically significant differences in the IOP median values between the ABeC and ABiC groups at the 1-month ($p = 0.022$) and 6-month ($p = 0.014$) follow-ups (Kruskal–Wallis test, all $p < 0.05$; see Figure 1). Based on the results of log-rank test examining the difference in the probability of surgical success between groups, there were no significant differences between the Kaplan–Meier curves of the individual groups ($p > 0.05$) for both complete and qualified success. Application of Fisher's exact independence test showed no significant dependence between the group factor and the proportion of patients who achieved a 20% reduction in intraocular pressure within one year ($df = 2$, $V = 0.17$, $p = 0.504$).

3.3. Change in Glaucoma Medication

The median numbers and ranges of medications at all time stages for all groups are presented in Table 3. At the 12-month follow up postoperatively, all medications were withdrawn in in all patients after ABeC and in 15 out of 16 patients in both after miniABeC and ABiC groups (~94%). One patient required addition of one topical medication after 1 month post miniABeC and further intensification of treatment ending with four topical medications at 12 months. A second patient following ABiC was using one medication at the 6-month and three medications at the 12-month follow-up.

Table 3. First quartiles (Q1), medians, third quartiles (Q3) and interquartile ranges (IQRs) of CDVA and number of medications (n) at each time stage before and after surgery in three groups of patients: ab externo canaloplasty (ABeC), minicanaloplasty (miniABeC) and ab interno canaloplasty (ABiC). *p* value * corresponds to the results of the Wilcoxon signed-rank tests for CDVA between particular study stages and the pre-washout stage. All patients in each group completed a 12-month follow-up. Italicized values indicate $p < 0.05$.

Time	ABeC Medications (n) Median (Range)	ABeC CDVA (logMAR) Q1, Median, Q3, IQR	*p* Value *	miniABeC Medications (n) Median (Range)	miniABeC CDVA (logMAR) Q1, Median, Q3, IQR	*p* Value *	ABiC Medications (n) Median (Range)	ABiC CDVA (logMAR) Q1, Median, Q3, IQR	*p* Value *
pre-washout	2.0 (1 to 3)	0.06, 0.26, 0.40, 0.34	-	2.0 (1 to 3)	0.10, 0.19, 0.28, 0.18	-	2.0 (0 to 4)	0.10, 0.22, 0.37, 0.27	-
post-washout	0	-	-	0	-	-	0	-	-
1 d	0	0.43, 0.81, 2.05, 1.62	*0.002*	0	0.11, 0.30, 0.88, 0.77	*0.038*	0	0.17, 0.35, 0.92, 0.75	0.069
7 d	0	0.19, 0.41, 0.66, 0.47	0.109	0	0.15, 0.26, 0.40, 0.25	0.272	0	0.10, 0.15, 0.30, 0.20	0.691
1 m	0	0.15, 0.22, 0.30, 0.15	0.637	0	0.00, 0.10, 0.22, 0.22	0.105	0	0.00, 0.00, 0.10, 0.10	*0.001*
3 m	0	0.00, 0.05, 0.10, 0.10	*0.001*	0 (0 to 1)	0.00, 0.02, 0.10, 0.10	*0.001*	0 (0 to 1)	0.00, 0.00, 0.10, 0.10	*0.001*
6 m	0	0.00, 0.10, 0.16, 0.16	*0.003*	0 (0 to 2)	0.00, 0.00, 0.10, 0.10	*0.002*	0 (0 to 1)	0.00, 0.00, 0.10, 0.10	*0.001*
12 m	0	0.00, 0.00, 0.10, 0.10	*0.004*	0 (0 to 4)	0.00, 0.00, 0.10, 0.10	*0.006*	0 (0 to 3)	0.00, 0.00, 0.00, 0.00	*0.001*

3.4. Surgical Success

Kaplan–Meier cumulative incidence of qualified success was 75.0% (ABeC), 65.6% (miniABeC) and 59.4% (ABiC) ($p = 0.398$) after 12 months, while cumulative incidence of complete success after 12 months of observation was 75.0% (ABeC), 65.6% (miniABeC) and 56.2% (ABiC) ($p = 0.269$; see Figure 2). At the 12-month follow-up, the unmedicated IOP reduction ≥ 20 mmHg was achieved in approximately 100% of patients for ABeC and in 93.8% for miniABeC and ABiC in relation to the post-washout stage.

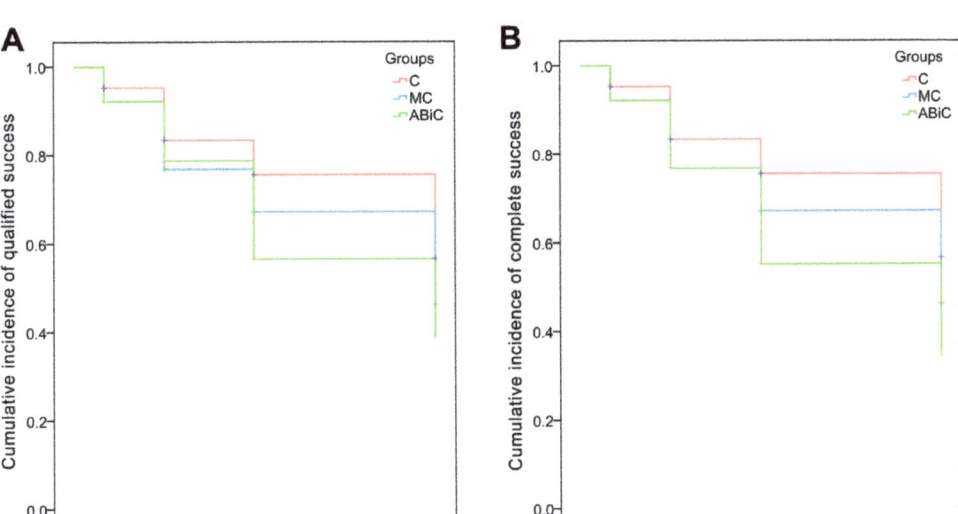

Figure 2. Kaplan–Meier survival analysis: (**A**) qualified success (IOP ≤ 15 mmHg with or without medications) and (**B**) complete success (IOP ≤ 15 mmHg without medications).

3.5. Visual Acuity Results

The median values for CDVA improved statistically significantly from 0.26 to 0.00 logMAR in the ABeC group, from 0.19 to 0.00 logMAR in the miniABeC group, and from 0.22 to 0.00 logMAR in the ABiC group, at 12 months after surgery compared to the pre-washout stage (Wilcoxon test, all $p \leq 0.006$). The CDVA differed statistically significantly between particular groups at 1 day and 1 month postoperatively (Kruskal–Wallis test, all $p < 0.05$; see Figure 3).

3.6. Incidence of Postsurgical Complications

The incidence of complications following all three procedures is shown in Table 4. No intraoperative adverse events were noted. In all variants requiring it, 360° dilation and insertion of a double suture into the Schlemm's canal was successful. The most common complications were microhyphema—defined as erythrocytes without a layer of blood (gonioscopically confirmed)—and hyphema—defined as layered blood in the anterior chamber. Only one patient required anterior chamber lavage for this reason, following ABeC. A raise in IOP of ≥30 mmHg was noted in all three variants of surgery, and in all cases, this was resolved within 2 weeks with topical antiglaucoma medications. One case of intravitreal hemorrhage occurred, following miniABeC; however, it resolved spontaneously. Two patients suffered from cystic macular edema: one after ABeC and one after miniABeC. Both were successfully treated with topical nepafenac 0.3% and dexamethasone 0.1% for 3 weeks. Interestingly, one patient undergoing ABeC developed a filtering bleb. Its morphology, however, did not resemble filtering blebs post sclerectomy. Additionally, this was the only case of transient hypotony (IOP of 3 mmHg) with a normal anterior chamber. Other complications included transient Descemet's membrane folds related to the phacoemulsification procedure and corneal erosion.

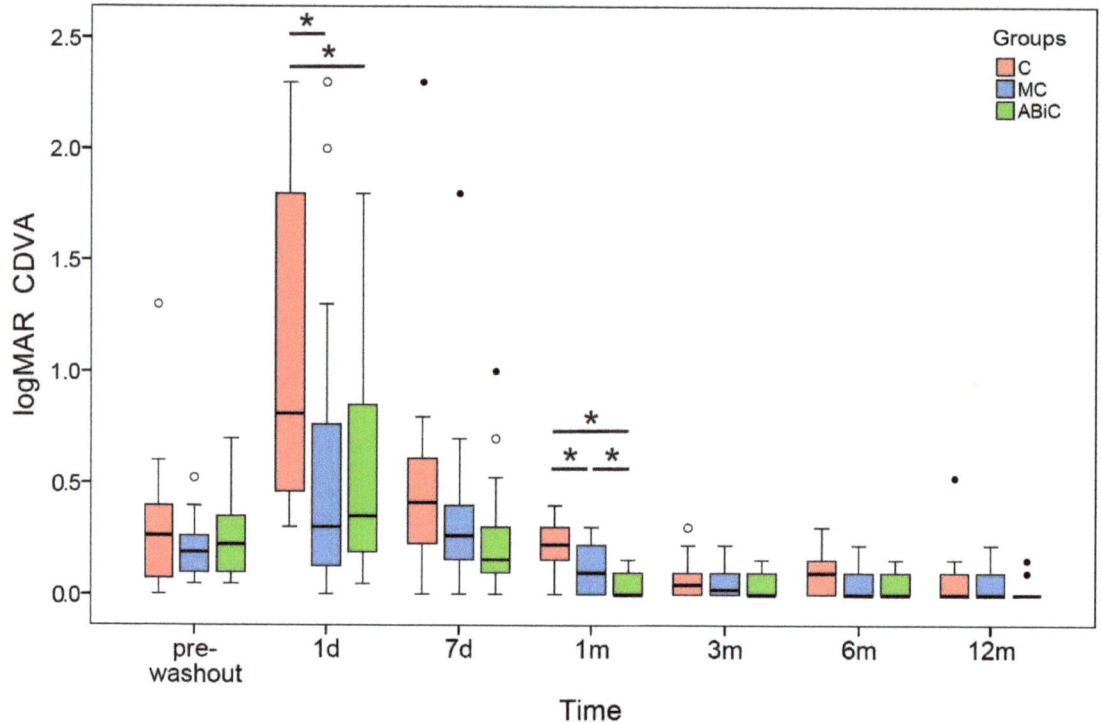

Figure 3. Boxplots of CDVA median values at each time stage before and after surgery in three groups of patients: ab externo canaloplasty (ABeC), minicanaloplasty (miniABeC) and ab interno canaloplasty (ABiC). Asterisks denote statistically significant differences between particular groups ($p < 0.05$).

Table 4. Evaluation of surgical and postsurgical complications with the aid of the Chi-square test. Italicized values indicate $p < 0.05$.

Complications	ABeC	miniABeC	ABiC	p Value
Early postoperative				
Elevated IOP (intraocular pressure) (≥30 mmHg)	2/16	1/16	2/16	0.800
Hyphema	8/16	3/16	1/16	*0.013*
Microhyphema	5/16	5/16	11/16	*0.047*
Fibrous strands	1/16	0/16	0/16	0.360
Cystic macular edema	1/16	1/16	0/16	0.593
Vitreous hemorrhage	0/16	1/16	0/16	0.360
Descemet folds	2/16	2/16	6/16	0.133
Corneal erosion	0/16	0/16	1/16	0.360
Bleb formation	0/16	1/16	0/16	0.360
Hypotony (IOP ≤ 5 mmHg)	0/0	1/16	0/0	0.360

4. Discussion

This prospective randomized trial was conducted to make a contribution to the existing literature on canaloplasty and its various modifications. The trial demonstrated that three variants of canaloplasty, i.e., ab externo, minicanaloplasty and ab interno, combined with cataract surgery provide effective reduction in IOP and medications in Caucasian patients with mild to moderate POAG in a safe way; however, the study was not powered to detect statistically significant changes in IOP. In that sense, our study has a pilot character. Twelve months postoperatively, there were no significant differences between the groups in terms of median IOP reduction and similar rates of effective treatment were observed in all groups, which suggests that all the procedures are effective and may be performed interchangeably. The results of this study are consistent with previously published data on phacocanaloplasty [5,6,10,29], and initial results of minicanaloplasty [17]. This study also shows promising results for ABiC, which was found to be as effective as other variants, and, to the authors' knowledge, this is the first trial to compare it to traditional canaloplasty in a prospective randomized manner. The amount of data on ABiC in the literature are still insufficient and a longer follow-up can show whether it will be a tissue-sparing alternative to ABeC or miniABeC. However, in our study, two patients following ABiC required readministration of antiglaucoma medication.

Restoring natural outflow pathways in canaloplasty is achieved in three ways. The trabecular tissues are stretched with the use of a tensioning suture in a so-called pilocarpine-like effect. Another way is viscodilating Schlemm's canal and keeping it open with a suture, which increases its diameter, thus lowering the resistance to flow. Finally, injecting viscoelastic material may open herniations and enable aqueous access to collector channel ostia throughout the whole circumference [21]. Canaloplasty evolved from viscocanalostomy where TDM functions as a site of controlled aqueous outflow [3]. In viscocanalostomy, however, viscodilatation was limited to sclerectomy margins only. This limits the IOP reducing potential of this procedure compared to canaloplasty, as shown by Koerber et al [30]. In NPDS, the inner wall of Schlemm's canal and the juxtacanalicular TM are peeled off the underlying trabeculum and the superficial flap is loosely attached in order to ease subconjunctival filtration. The aqueous humor that percolates through the TDM collects in the intrascleral space and acts as a reservoir. By contrast, the superficial flap in canaloplasty and viscocanalostomy is sutured tightly to avoid bleb formation and the internal wall of Schlemm's canal stays untouched. It remains unknown if and to what extent the intrascleral lake supports the IOP-lowering effect of canaloplasty; there are, however, alternate routes of aqueous humor percolation that are theoretically possible, such as transscleral into subconjunctival space. Grieshaber et al. have reported this type of outflow based on the migration of fluorescein dye from Schlemm's canal into episcleral veins. Mastropasqua et al. [31] supported this thesis by confirming the presence of epithelial microcysts in the bulbar conjunctiva after canaloplasty, similar to those found in filtering blebs after successful trabeculectomy [32–34]. These cysts were larger in number at the site of surgery. The authors explain this as occurring because of easier aqueous filtration through reduced scleral thickness after deep flap excision at the site of surgery. This was earlier postulated by Grieshaber et al. who noticed IOP drop caused by goniopuncture without bleb formation, suggesting that TDM plays a role in ABeC [7]. In a study by Byszewska et al., ABeC led to a more effective decrease in IOP than NPDS in a 24-month observation study [29], which, on the other hand, may suggest that restoring natural outflow pathways eventually wins over transscleral percolation. The main idea behind minicanaloplasty was to perform a minimal size sclerectomy only to access Schlemm's canal and to analyze whether it can compete with the traditional procedure. The 12-month follow-up period does not entitle us to make claims on the importance of the scleral lake; further observation might, however, indicate that its formation is necessary, which implies the need for more invasive procedures. Further observation is crucial in this matter, as one of the NPDS's long-term mechanisms of action–the presence of new aqueous vessels in the sclera adjacent to the dissection site and suprachoroidal drainage–could also possibly cause traditional canaloplasty to win over minicanaloplasty [35].

The tight closure of the scleral flaps in ABeC is intended to prevent filtering bleb formation. In our study, only one filtering bleb occurred following ABeC. It was more a bleb-like elevation of the conjunctiva similar to the ones described in previously published cases [36]. This was accompanied by IOP drop up to 3 mmHg persisting three months postoperatively. After this period IOP normalized and the bleb was not detectable in as-OCT. IOP measured in this individual at 12 months did not differ much from other patients following ABeC and reached 17 mmHg. The mechanism most probably responsible for bleb formation was TDM microperforation.

Canaloplasty has been of interest not only as an IOP-reducing procedure but also prospectively in antiglaucoma gene therapy. Schlemm's canal was suggested as a promising site of gene medication delivery which can be reached by catheterization or suture placement during surgery [37]. MiniABeC could be a faster method than the traditional procedure to gain access for TM-targeted gene therapeutics.

The safety profile of canaloplasty in the literature is very high [38]. In this study, none of the serious complications, such as choroidal detachment, retinal detachment, persistent hypotony or endophthalmitis, were observed. Postsurgical complications did not differ significantly between groups. None of the patients required additional glaucoma surgery within the first 12 months postoperatively; however, further observation will bring more information in this regard. The mean CDVA was significantly improved in the majority of cases and vision deterioration happened in only three individuals. This was mainly caused by simultaneous cataract phacoemulsification. The CDVA differed statistically significantly between particular groups at 1 day and 1 month postoperatively, which was probably due to differences in the amount of blood in the anterior chamber. The most frequent and only statistically significant complications in the early postoperative period were microhyphema/hyphema. Other common complications were Descemet folds, inflammation and transient IOP spikes. Presence of blood reflux is generally considered a good prognostic factor [39]; however, the fact that one of the patients after ABeC required surgical lavage is of note.

Another issue is the effect of phacoemulsification itself on post-surgical drop in IOP (in our study all eyes underwent a combined phacocanaloplasty procedure). According to different studies, it is on average: 1.4 mmHg, 1.9 mmHg, 1.55 mmHg, 1.88 mmHg, 2.9 mmHg, 3.1 mmHg and 4.9–5.3 mmHg [40–44]. Depending on the type of glaucoma, the largest decline in IOP is observed in eyes with angle-closure glaucoma, and in pseudoexfoliative glaucoma (this effect is transient and after a year IOP gradually increases). From an analysis of the published studies, it can be concluded that the largest decrease in intraocular pressure occurs between the third and sixth month after surgery [45,46]. From our previous studies, this effect remained at a similar level throughout the entire follow-up period which was 1 year, with the lowest values generally occurring after half a year of follow-up [47]. Hayashi et al. described an analogous IOP drop of 6.9 mmHg within 12 months after phacoemulsification, and even greater, as much as 7.2 mmHg, during 24 months after surgery. Generally, it can be concluded that this effect is most strongly expressed during the first year after surgery [48], although there are reports in the literature that a reduction in IOP was noted even 10 years postoperatively [49].

According to the data from the above-mentioned studies [40–50], the conclusion might be drawn that the decrease in IOP after surgery shows a strong inverse correlation with the preoperative depth of the anterior chamber, the width of the anterior chamber angle and the initial level of IOP.

Despite the promising outcome, the results of this study need to be interpreted with caution due to certain study limitations: a relatively small sample size and short follow-up period. Due to relatively small count of patients in the study, we performed a post-hoc estimation of statistical power. We have conducted our analysis according to Schoenfeld's formula for hazard ratio 0.7 at a statistical power of 80% a significance level of 5%. The required group sample should be n = 123. For the aforementioned reasons, it is stressed that data from this trial are of a preliminary nature. Furthermore, because the surgeon involved had many years of experience in non-penetrating and mini-invasive glaucoma surgery preparation in order to perform TDM in ABeC or mini-flaps in miniABeC did not require a long learning curve.

The main strength of the study is that it is the first to the authors' knowledge to compare different variants of canaloplasty as a treatment for POAG in a randomized prospective manner. The study demonstrates that all three variants of canaloplasty: ABeC, miniABeC and ABiC can be efficient in reducing IOP in mild to moderate POAG and are of a similar safety profile.

5. Conclusions

The aim of the study was to compare three variants of canaloplasty. All three variants occurred to result in effective IOP and medications' number reduction with mild complications. The results also did not differ significantly between groups. The authors conclude that canaloplasty combined with phacoemulsification is a procedure suitable for mild to moderate POAG patients with concomitant cataract, no previous damage to iridocorneal angle and assumed patent outflow system. Novel microsurgical variants of the procedure are unlikely to replace the conventional one; however, they provide alternatives for patients with early indication for surgical intervention.

6. Value Statement

What was known:
- ABeCy is a safe and effective technique to treat POAG with an IOP-reducing potential comparable with filtering surgeries.

What this paper adds:
- The study demonstrates that all three variants of canaloplasty, i.e., ABeC, miniABeC and AbiC, can be efficient in reducing IOP in mild to moderate POAG and are of a similar safety profile.
- Avoiding dissection of the TDM, as in miniABeC, may not affect IOP reduction, which questions the importance of the scleral lake in Schlemm's canal surgery.

Author Contributions: A.K.K. performed the research as well as analyzing and interpreting the data. M.R. performed the surgery. M.R and M.E.D. reviewed the whole manuscript. All authors contributed to data analysis, drafting or revising the article, agreeing to the journal to which the article would be submitted, gave final approval of the version to be published, and agreed to be accountable for all aspects of the work. All authors have read and agreed to the published version of the manuscript.

Funding: The work of two authors was funded by a Science Grant awarded by the Ministry of Science and Higher Education No 1/WMN/2017. The work of one author was funded by the National Centre for Research and Development, Poland, grant No LIDER/074/L-6/14/NCBR/2015.

Institutional Review Board Statement: The study was conducted according to the guidelines of the Declaration of Helsinki, and approved by the Ethics Committee of Military Institute of Medicine (decision no. 76/WIM/2015).

Informed Consent Statement: Informed consent was obtained from all subjects involved in the study.

Conflicts of Interest: The authors declare no conflict of interest.

References

1. Byszewska, A.; Konopińska, J.; Kicińska, A.K.; Mariak, Z.; Rękas, M. Canaloplasty in the Treatment of Primary Open-Angle Glaucoma: Patient Selection and Perspectives. *Clin. Ophthalmol.* **2019**, *13*, 2617–2629. [CrossRef]
2. Cameron, B.; Field, M.; Ball, J.K.S. Circumferential Viscodilation of Schlemm's Canal with a Flexible Microcannula during Non-penetrating Glaucoma Surgery. *Digit J. Ophthalmol.* **2006**, *12*. Available online: https://www.djo.harvard.edu/site.php?url=/physicians/oa/929 (accessed on 12 March 2022).

3. Stegmann, R.; Pienaar, A.; Miller, D. Viscocanalostomy for open-angle glaucoma in black African patients. *J. Cataract Refract. Surg.* **1999**, *25*, 316–322. [CrossRef]
4. Fujita, K.; Kitagawa, K.; Ueta, Y.; Nakamura, T.; Miyakoshi, A.; Hayashi, A. Short-term results of canaloplasty surgery for primary open-angle glaucoma in Japanese patients. *Case Rep. Ophthalmol.* **2011**, *2*, 65–68. [CrossRef] [PubMed]
5. Shingleton, B.; Tetz, M.; Korber, N. Circumferential viscodilation and tensioning of Schlemm canal (canaloplasty) with temporal clear corneal phacoemulsification cataract surgery for open-angle glaucoma and visually significant cataract. *J. Cataract Refract. Surg.* **2008**, *34*, 433–440. [CrossRef]
6. Bull, H.; Von Wolff, K.; Körber, N.; Tetz, M. Three-year canaloplasty outcomes for the treatment of open-angle glaucoma: European study results. *Graefe's Arch. Clin. Exp. Ophthalmol.* **2011**, *249*, 1537–1545. [CrossRef]
7. Grieshaber, M.C.; Fraenkl, S.; Schoetzau, A.; Flammer, J.; Orgül, S. Circumferential Viscocanalostomy and Suture Canal Distension (Canaloplasty) for Whites with Open-angle Glaucoma. *J. Glaucoma* **2011**, *20*, 298–302. [CrossRef]
8. Lewis, R.A.; von Wolff, K.; Tetz, M.; Koerber, N.; Kearney, J.R.; Shingleton, B.J.; Samuelson, T.W. Canaloplasty: Three-year results of circumferential viscodilation and tensioning of Schlemm canal using a microcatheter to treat open-angle glaucoma. *J. Cataract Refract. Surg.* **2011**, *37*, 682–690. [CrossRef]
9. Brüggemann, A.; Despouy, J.T.; Wegent, A.; Müller, M. Intraindividual Comparison of Canaloplasty Versus Trabeculectomy With Mitomycin C in a Single-surgeon Series. *J. Glaucoma* **2013**, *22*, 577–583. [CrossRef]
10. Matlach, J.; Dhillon, C.; Hain, J.; Schlunck, G.; Grehn, F.; Klink, T. Trabeculectomy versus canaloplasty (TVC study) in the treatment of patients with open-angle glaucoma: A prospective randomized clinical trial. *Acta Ophthalmol.* **2015**, *93*, 753–761. [CrossRef]
11. Kodomskoi, L.; Kotliar, K.; Schröder, A.C.; Weiss, M.; Hille, K. Suture-Probe Canaloplasty as an Alternative to Canaloplasty Using the iTrack Microcatheter. *J. Glaucoma* **2019**, *28*, 811–817. [CrossRef] [PubMed]
12. Grieshaber, M.C.; Pienaar, A.; Olivier, J.; Stegmann, R. Comparing two tensioning suture sizes for 360° viscocanalostomy (canaloplasty): A randomised controlled trial. *Eye* **2010**, *24*, 1220–1226. [CrossRef] [PubMed]
13. Grieshaber, M.C.; Schoetzau, A.; Grieshaber, H.R.; Stegmann, R. Canaloplasty with Stegmann Canal Expander for primary open-angle glaucoma: Two-year clinical results. *Acta Ophthalmol.* **2017**, *95*, 503–508. [CrossRef] [PubMed]
14. Scharioth, G.B. Risk of circumferential viscodilation in viscocanalostomy. *J. Cataract Refract. Surg.* **2015**, *41*, 1122–1123. [CrossRef]
15. Seuthe, A.-M.; Ivanescu, C.; Leers, S.; Boden, K.; Januschowski, K.; Szurman, P. Modified canaloplasty with suprachoroidal drainage versus conventional canaloplasty—1-year results. *Graefe's Arch. Clin. Exp. Ophthalmol.* **2016**, *254*, 1591–1597. [CrossRef]
16. Gallardo, M.J.; A Supnet, R.; Ahmed, I.I.K. Viscodilation of Schlemm's canal for the reduction of IOP via an ab-interno approach. *Clin. Ophthalmol.* **2018**, *12*, 2149–2155. [CrossRef]
17. Rekas, M.; Konopińska, J.; Byszewska, A.; Mariak, Z. Mini-canaloplasty as a modified technique for the surgical treatment of open-angle glaucoma. *Sci. Rep.* **2020**, *10*, 1–7. [CrossRef]
18. Kicińska, A.K.; Danielewska, M.E.; Byszewska, A.; Lewczuk, K.R.M. Safety and Efficacy of Three Variants of Canaloplasty with Phacoemulsification to Treat Open-Angle Glaucoma: 6-Month Follow Up. In Proceedings of the 13th European Glaucoma Society Congress, Florence, Italy, 19–22 May 2018.
19. Hodapp, E.; Parrish, R.K.; Anderson, D.R. *Clinical Decisions in Glaucoma*; Mosby Incorporated: Maryland Heights, MO, USA, 1993.
20. Battista, S.A.; Lu, Z.; Hofmann, S.; Freddo, T.; Overby, D.; Gong, H. Reduction of the Available Area for Aqueous Humor Outflow and Increase in Meshwork Herniations into Collector Channels Following Acute IOP Elevation in Bovine Eyes. *Investig. Opthalmology Vis. Sci.* **2008**, *49*, 5346–5352. [CrossRef]
21. Lewis, R.A.; von Wolff, K.; Tetz, M.; Korber, N.; Kearney, J.R.; Shingleton, B.; Samuelson, T.W. Canaloplasty: Circumferential viscodilation and tensioning of Schlemm's canal using a flexible microcatheter for the treatment of open-angle glaucoma in adults. *J. Cataract Refract. Surg.* **2007**, *33*, 1217–1226. [CrossRef]
22. Lewis, R.A.; von Wolff, K.; Tetz, M.; Koerber, N.; Kearney, J.R.; Shingleton, B.; Samuelson, T.W. Canaloplasty: Circumferential viscodilation and tensioning of Schlemm canal using a flexible microcatheter for the treatment of open-angle glaucoma in adults: Two-year interim clinical study results. *J. Cataract Refract. Surg.* **2009**, *35*, 814–824. [CrossRef]
23. Peckar, C.O.; Körber, N. Canaloplasty for open angle glaucoma: A three years critical evaluation and comparison with viscocanalostomy. *Spektrum Augenheilkd.* **2008**, *22*, 240–246. [CrossRef]
24. Grieshaber, M.C.; Pienaar, A.; Olivier, J.; Stegmann, R. Canaloplasty for primary open-angle glaucoma: Long-term outcome. *Br. J. Ophthalmol.* **2010**, *94*, 1478–1482. [CrossRef] [PubMed]
25. Grieshaber, M.C.; Pienaar, A.; Olivier, J.; Stegmann, R. Clinical Evaluation of the Aqueous Outflow System in Primary Open-Angle Glaucoma for Canaloplasty. *Investig. Opthalmology Vis. Sci.* **2010**, *51*, 1498–1504. [CrossRef] [PubMed]
26. Körber, N. Ab interno canaloplasty for the treatment of glaucoma: A case series study. *Spektrum Augenheilkd.* **2018**, *32*, 223–227. [CrossRef]
27. Körber, N. Kanaloplastik. *Der Ophthalmol.* **2010**, *107*, 1169–1175. [CrossRef]
28. Armstrong, R.A. When to use the Bonferroni correction. *Ophthalmic Physiol. Opt.* **2014**, *34*, 502–508. [CrossRef]
29. Byszewska, A.; Jünemann, A.; Rękas, M. Canaloplasty versus Nonpenetrating Deep Sclerectomy: 2-Year Results and Quality of Life Assessment. *J. Ophthalmol.* **2018**, *2018*, 1–10. [CrossRef]
30. Koerber, N.J. Canaloplasty in One Eye Compared with Viscocanalostomy in the Contralateral Eye in Patients with Bilateral Open-angle Glaucoma. *J. Glaucoma* **2011**, *21*, 129–134. [CrossRef]

31. Mastropasqua, L.; Agnifili, L.; Salvetat, M.L.; Ciancaglini, M.; Fasanella, V.; Nubile, M.; Mastropasqua, R.; Zeppieri, M.; Brusini, P. In vivo analysis of conjunctiva in canaloplasty for glaucoma. *Br. J. Ophthalmol.* **2012**, *96*, 634–639. [CrossRef]
32. Labbé, A.; Dupas, B.; Hamard, P.; Baudouin, C. In Vivo Confocal Microscopy Study of Blebs after Filtering Surgery. *Ophthalmology* **2005**, *112*, 1979.e1–1979.e9. [CrossRef]
33. Messmer, E.M.; Zapp, D.M.; Mackert, M.J.; Thiel, M.K.A. In vivo confocal microscopy of filtering blebs after trabeculectomy. *Arch. Ophthalmol.* **2006**, *124*, 1095–1103. [CrossRef] [PubMed]
34. Guthoff, R.; Klink, T.; Schlunck, G.G.F. In Vivo Confocal Microscopy of Failing and Functioning Filtering Blebs Results and Clinical Correlations. *J. Glaucoma.* **2006**, *15*, 552–558. [CrossRef] [PubMed]
35. Delarive, T.; Rossier, A.; Rossier, S.; Ravinet, E.; Shaarawy, T.; Mermoud, A. Aqueous dynamic and histological findings after deep sclerectomy with collagen implant in an animal model. *Br. J. Ophthalmol.* **2003**, *87*, 1340–1344. [CrossRef] [PubMed]
36. Klink, T.; Panidou, E.; Kanzow-Terai, B.; Klink, J.; Schlunck, G.; Grehn, F.J. Are There Filtering Blebs After Canaloplasty? *J. Glaucoma* **2011**, *21*, 89–94. [CrossRef]
37. Tian, B.; Kaufman, P.L. A Potential Application of Canaloplasty in Glaucoma Gene Therapy. *Transl. Vis. Sci. Technol.* **2013**, *2*, 2. [CrossRef]
38. Harvey, B.J.; Khaimi, M.A. A review of canaloplasty. *Saudi J. Ophthalmol.* **2011**, *25*, 329–336. [CrossRef]
39. Grieshaber, M.C.; Schoetzau, A.; Flammer, J.; Orgül, S. Postoperative microhyphema as a positive prognostic indicator in canaloplasty. *Acta Ophthalmol.* **2011**, *91*, 151–156. [CrossRef]
40. Damji, K.F. Intraocular pressure following phacoemulsification in patients with and without exfoliation syndrome: A 2 year prospective study. *Br. J. Ophthalmol.* **2006**, *90*, 1014–1018. [CrossRef]
41. Hayashi, K.; Hayashi, H.; Nakao, F.; Hayashi, F. Changes in anterior chamber angle width and depth after intraocular lens implantation in eyes with glaucoma. *Ophthalmology* **2000**, *107*, 698–703. [CrossRef]
42. Suzuki, R.; Tanaka, K.; Sagara, T.; Fujiwara, N. Reduction of Intraocular Pressure after Phacoemulsification and Aspiration with Intraocular Lens Implantation. *Ophthalmologica* **1994**, *208*, 254–258. [CrossRef]
43. Suzuki, R.; Kuroki, S.; Fujiwara, N. Ten-Year Follow-Up of Intraocular Pressure after Phacoemulsification and Aspiration with Intraocular Lens Implantation Performed by the Same Surgeon. *Ophthalmologica* **1997**, *211*, 79–83. [CrossRef] [PubMed]
44. Cekiç, O.B.C. The relationship between capsulorhexis size and anterior chamber depth relation. *Ophthalmic Surg. Lasers.* **1999**, *30*, 185–190. [CrossRef] [PubMed]
45. Tong, J.T.; Miller, K.M. Intraocular pressure change after sutureless phacoemulsification and foldable posterior chamber lens implantation. *J. Cataract Refract. Surg.* **1998**, *24*, 256–262. [CrossRef]
46. Altan, C.; Bayraktar, S.; Altan, T.; Eren, H.; Yilmaz, O.F. Anterior chamber depth, iridocorneal angle width, and intraocular pressure changes after uneventful phacoemulsification in eyes without glaucoma and with open iridocorneal angles. *J. Cataract Refract. Surg.* **2004**, *30*, 832–838. [CrossRef] [PubMed]
47. Rekas, M.; Barchan-Kucia, K.; Konopinska, J.; Mariak, Z.; Żarnowski, T. Analysis and Modeling of Anatomical Changes of the Anterior Segment of the Eye After Cataract Surgery with Consideration of Different Phenotypes of Eye Structure. *Curr. Eye Res.* **2014**, *40*, 1018–1027. [CrossRef]
48. Mansberger, S.L.; Gordon, M.O.; Jampel, H.; Bhorade, A.; Brandt, J.D.; Wilson, B.; Kass, M.A. Reduction in Intraocular Pressure after Cataract Extraction: The Ocular Hypertension Treatment Study. *Ophthalmology* **2012**, *119*, 1826–1831. [CrossRef]
49. Shingleton, B.; Gamell, L.S.; O'Donoghue, M.W.; Baylus, S.L.; King, R. Long-term changes in intraocular pressure after clear corneal phacoemulsification: Normal patients versus glaucoma suspect and glaucoma patients. *J. Cataract Refract. Surg.* **1999**, *25*, 885–890. [CrossRef]
50. Hayashi, K.; Hayashi, H.; Nakao, F.; Hayashi, F. Effect of cataract surgery on intraocular pressure control in glaucoma patients. *J. Cataract Refract. Surg.* **2001**, *27*, 1779–1786. [CrossRef]

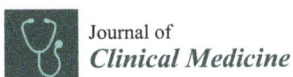

Review

Advances in Canaloplasty—Modified Techniques Yield Strong Pressure Reduction with Low Risk Profile

Peter Szurman [1,2]

[1] Eye Clinic Sulzbach, Knappschaft Hospital Saar, 66280 Sulzbach, Germany; peter.szurman@kksaar.de; Tel.: +49-06897-574-1119
[2] Klaus Heimann Eye Research Institute (KHERI), 66280 Sulzbach, Germany

Abstract: For decades, trabeculectomy (TE) was considered the gold standard for surgical treatment of open-angle glaucoma owing to its powerful intraocular pressure (IOP)-lowering potency. However, owing to the invasive nature and high-risk profile of TE, this standard is changing, and minimally invasive procedures are becoming more preferable. In particular, canaloplasty (CP) has been established as a much gentler alternative in everyday life and is under development as a full-fledged replacement. This technique involves probing Schlemm's canal with a microcatheter and inserting a pouch suture that places the trabecular meshwork under permanent tension. It aims to restore the natural outflow pathways of the aqueous humor and is independent of external wound healing. This physiological approach results in a significantly lower complication rate and allows considerably simplified perioperative management. There is now extensive evidence that canaloplasty achieves sufficient pressure reduction as well as a significant reduction in postoperative glaucoma medications. Unlike MIGS procedures, the indication is not only mild to moderate glaucoma; today, even advanced glaucoma benefits from the very low hypotony rate, which largely avoids a wipeout phenomenon. However, approximately half of patients are not completely medication-free after canaloplasty. As a consequence, a number of canaloplasty modifications have been developed with the goal of further enhancing the IOP-lowering effect while avoiding the risk of serious complications. By combining canaloplasty with the newly developed suprachoroidal drainage procedure, the individual improvements in trabecular facility and uveoscleral outflow facility appear to have an additive effect. Thus, for the first time, an IOP-lowering effect comparable to a successful trabeculectomy can be achieved. Other implant modifications also enhance the potential of canaloplasty or offer additional benefits such as the possibility of telemetric IOP self-measurement by the patient. This article reviews the modifications of canaloplasty, which has the potential to become a new gold standard in glaucoma surgery via stepwise refinement.

Keywords: canaloplasty; trabeculectomy; modifications; telemetric self-measurement; suprachoroidal drainage

1. Introduction

Surgical treatment of glaucoma that cannot be controlled conservatively has undergone rapid transformation in recent years. Trabeculectomy (TE) has long been considered the gold standard globally; however, this surgical filtering technique, which dates back to the 1960s, is increasingly being questioned for several underlying reasons. First, the high risk of filtering bleb scarring can only be reduced with topical antimetabolites. Another disadvantage is the high rate of intra- and postoperative complications, ranging from bulbar hypotony with permanent visual fluctuations [1] and the risk of choroidal hemorrhaging [2], to an increased cataract rate [3] and the relevant lifelong risk of endophthalmitis [4]. These vision-threatening complications are largely due to the creation of an open connection between the anterior chamber and the subconjunctival space (penetrating surgery), which results in nonphysiologic and difficult-to-control bolus-like filtration instead of the desired continuous oozing effect. This is compounded by the time-consuming perioperative management and stressful follow-up care of the filtering bleb [5,6].

For this reason, there has always been a need for procedures with fewer complications and a comparable intraocular pressure (IOP)-lowering effect [7,8]. Although nonpenetrating procedures are, for the most part, significantly less complicating, none of the techniques investigated thus far appear to lower the IOP as effectively as TE. However, the introduction of canaloplasty (CP) and its gradual modifications have changed this picture. In the meantime, modified canaloplasty with additional suprachoroidal drainage (ScD) achieves IOP values similar to those of TE but without its complications.

2. Development and Rationale of Canaloplasty

Non-penetrating procedures are characterized by avoiding a direct connection between the anterior chamber and extraocular subconjunctival spaces in order to avoid the intractable problem of bleb scarring [9]. One of the first non-penetrating procedures was deep sclerectomy (DS), in which a continuous and controlled oozing of aqueous humor from the anterior chamber into an intrascleral pocket was achieved via the trabeculo-descemetic window (TDW) [10]. However, the further outflow remained unclear and was not sufficiently effective.

In parallel, Stegman developed viscocanalostomy (VC), which dilated Schlemm's canal (SC) using a viscoelastic substance [11]. Thus, for the first time, a procedure existed that conceptually aimed to exclusively improve the natural drainage pathways (via SC and the adjacent collector channels).

Described in 2005 by Kearney, CP unites these two techniques: the DS approach allows a continuous ooze to be established using a prepared TDW, and VC is integrated to permanently—rather than temporarily—improve the physiological outflow by using microcatheter technology and a tension thread [12].

Thus, the rationale of CP is to activate and improve natural outflow pathways (trabecular facility) [12]. The IOP-lowering mechanism relies on several effects in the natural outflow tract (Figure 1):

1. The SC is probed using a microcatheter (iTrack 250, Ellex Inc., Eden Prairie, MN, USA) for dilatation of the ostia and lumen of SC, and the adjacent collector channels using a viscoelastic. This effect dilates the canal to almost triple its original size, making it easily visible in the ultrasound biomicroscope (UBM) 50 MHz (Figure 1A).
2. The placement of one or two 10.0 Prolene tensioning sutures results in permanent stretching and tightening of the trabecular meshwork (i.e., surgical "pilocarpine effect") (Figure 1B) [12].
3. Applying tension to the TDW results in the controlled percolation of aqueous humor into the intrascleral cleft formed after resection of the deep flap, which can be enhanced by YAG goniopuncture [13].

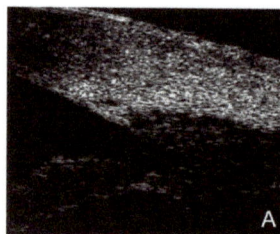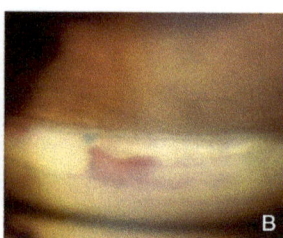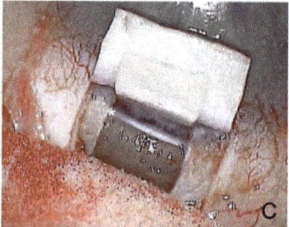

Figure 1. Rationale and mechanisms of action of canaloplasty. (**A**) Viscodilatation of the SC with microcatheter shown in UBM. (**B**) Prolene tension sutures are visible postoperatively on gonioscopy, resulting in permanent stretching of the TMW. (**C**) Controlled percolation of aqueous humor through the TDW.

3. Surgical Technique of Conventional Canaloplasty

The detailed surgical technique has been described before [12]. In brief, the conjunctival opening is created superiorly at the limbus. In contrast to TE, cauterization should be avoided to preserve the episcleral vessels. First, a superficial scleral flap with 1/3 scleral thickness is dissected, with the incision extending to the clear cornea. The SC is unroofed after preparation of a second lamellar flap just above the choroidal plane, simultaneously creating a TDW. The deep scleral lamella is excised, forming an intrascleral lacuna and exposing the two ostia of the SC. After peeling off the juxtacanalicular TMW, the SC is probed and dilated using a 250 µm microcatheter under the constant administration of viscoelastic. The exact position of the catheter tip can be easily tracked via an illuminated laser light fiber located in the catheter, allowing the viscoelastic to be applied with accuracy. This viscodilation is an essential part of the procedure, as it breaks the adhesions within the SC, stretches the TMW, and perforates the intracanalicular septa, thus improving outflow into the collector channels.

After successful circular probing, a non-absorbable suture (Prolene 10.0) is fixed to the distal end of the microcatheter, inserted circularly by withdrawing the catheter into the SC, and knotted under tension. If available, a high-resolution UBM (Figure 1) can be performed at this stage to assess suture tension and dilation of the SC. The superficial flap is sutured to be watertight. Care is taken to avoid microfistulation under the conjunctiva or even the formation of a subconjunctival bleb (Figure 2) [12].

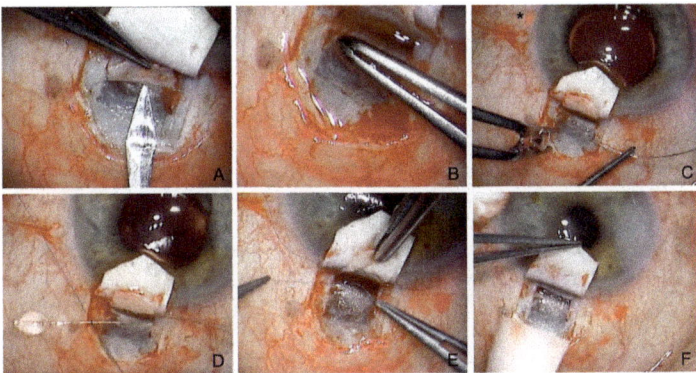

Figure 2. Surgical technique of conventional canaloplasty. (**A**) Unroofing of the SC after the incision of a second deep flap into the TDW. (**B**) Peeling of the juxtacanalicular TMW. (**C**) Probing of the SC with a microcatheter (Asterisk marks illuminated tip). (**D**) Insertion of two Prolene 10.0 sutures. (**E**) Knotting of the tension sutures. (**F**) Controlled percolation of aqueous humor through the TDW into the intrascleral cleft.

4. Spectrum of Severe Glaucomas Treated Using Canaloplasty

The indication for CP now includes all types of open angle glaucoma (OAG), including secondary OAG such as pigment dispersion, pseudoexfoliation, steroid-induced, uveitic, and juvenile glaucoma [14–17]. While earlier publications considered mild to moderate glaucoma as an indication for CP [18], it is increasingly being recognized that especially difficult, advanced, and preoperated glaucoma eyes are good indications for CP. These "difficult" glaucomas are characterized by high-grade pathologies with scarred conjunctiva and very high IOP values, in which all four natural outflow pathways are affected: they have a muddied TMW; a collapsed, fibrotic SC; narrowed collector vessels; and disrupted episcleral veins. At first glance, the high-grade pathology characteristic of severe glaucomas might argue against an intervention aimed at restoring the natural outflow pathway. Nevertheless, these eyes in particular often respond better to CP than to revisional filtering surgery [19,20].

There are several reasons for this: first, the higher the baseline pressure, the higher the IOP-lowering potency of CP [21]. In a study of 1000 canaloplasty patients, the IOP of eyes with a baseline IOP of >30 mmHg was reduced by more than 50% compared with eyes with a baseline IOP of <20 mmHg, which experienced only a 30% reduction [22].

Second, numerous studies have shown that CP can regulate secondary glaucoma as well as primary OAG. In particular, pseudoexfoliation glaucoma shows a very good outcome after CP, even in the long term [17].

Another argument is the very low hypotony rate of CP (<1%). This is particularly important for the often preterminal papillary situation of many difficult glaucomas and may help to prevent the wipeout phenomenon. On the other hand, TE has a very high hypotony rate of more than one-third, of which nearly 20% last longer than 3 months and carry a high risk of long-term damage to the optic nerve fibers [23] (Table 1).

Table 1. Rates of hypotony for different surgical techniques.

Long-Term Hypotony Rate (<5 mmHg for More than 90 Days)	
Canaloplasty	<1% [24]
PreserFlo	<1% [25]
Tubes	2.8% [26]
Trabeculectomy	18.8% [23]

An important new indication is preoperated eyes after failed TE [27–29]. At first glance, this indication seems unpromising because the SC integrity has been breached by TE, making probing difficult. In addition, the SC is known to collapse after filtering surgery and become dysfunctional from lack of use. Nevertheless, good evidence has shown that probing is usually possible even after TE, and the results are promising (Figure 3). In particular, eyes previously subjected to filtering surgery have highly altered conjunctiva, so they especially benefit from a bleb-independent approach.

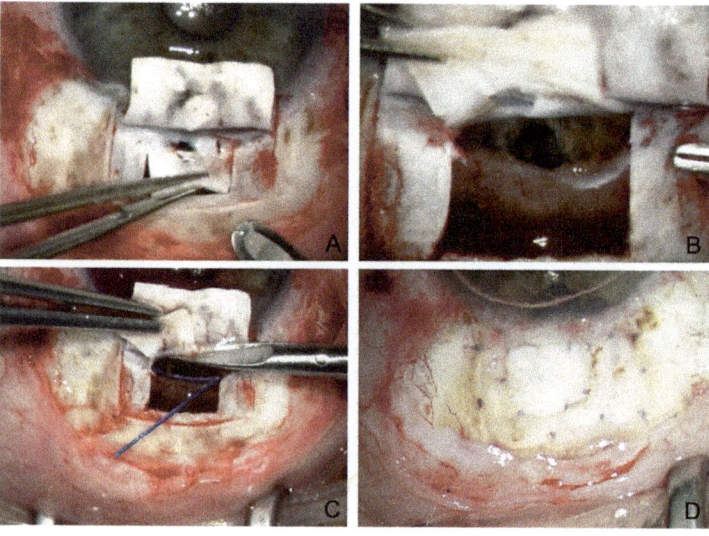

Figure 3. Revision canaloplasty after failed TE. (**A**) Incision and resection of the second deep flap. Note the atrophy in the superficial flap and the defect in the deep flap caused by the previous TE. (**B**) Visualization of the previous TE and iridectomy. (**C**) Probing of the SC on both sides using the suture canaloplasty technique. (**D**) Covering the superficial scleral atrophy with the resected deep scleral flap.

5. Results of Conventional Canaloplasty

Several studies have shown that canaloplasty significantly lowers IOP over the long term with an excellent safety profile [18]. The average IOP reduction is 31–40%, reaching an average final level of 15.0–15.5 mmHg after 3 years [30–32]. There is a linear relationship between suture tension and IOP-lowering efficacy (Figure 4). Eyes with strong suture tension demonstrated in the UBM experienced a 50% greater IOP-lowering effect than eyes with low suture tension [33]. Interestingly, no difference was apparent between phakic and pseudophakic eyes, whereas eyes subjected to a combined phaco-CP (PCP) exhibited significantly lower IOPs with significantly less medication. The combined approach lowers the IOP by an additional 1.9 mmHg compared with using CP alone [34].

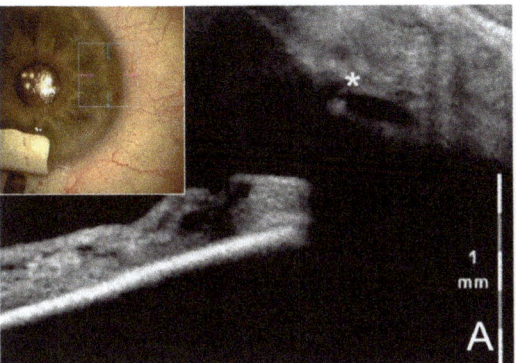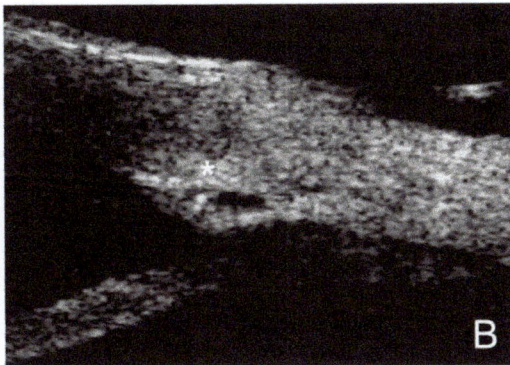

Figure 4. Visible effect of the tension suture stretching the SC. (**A**) Intraoperative visualization of the SC with intraoperative OCT. Asterisk marks the catheter tip within the lumen. (**B**) Postoperative UBM (50 MHz) clearly shows the dilated and stretched SC with knotted suture in the lumen (asterisk).

However, complete success ($\leq$16 mmHg without medication) is achieved in only half the cases. This is because the number of topical glaucoma medications dropped significantly to 1.0–1.5, but only about half of all patients are medication-free after 3 years [14].

Comparative studies with TE confirmed that both methods achieved a sufficient IOP-lowering effect and significant reduction of postoperative glaucoma medications [7,8,23,35]. However, conventional CP (32–39% IOP reduction to 14.5 mmHg) did not reach the IOP level of successful TE (43–55% IOP reduction to 10.8 mmHg). A higher percentage of patients treated with CP rather than TE required postoperative medications (36% vs. 20%), but this did not reach significance [8]. Several meta-analyses confirmed a difference of only 2.3 mmHg between the two procedures at 12 months. However, when an IOP of $\leq$18 mmHg was considered as a criterion for success, no significant difference arose, neither for complete nor qualified success. On the other hand, the rate of visual-acuity-threatening complications was significantly increased in the TE group [20].

In summary, the consensus is that TE leads to a slightly greater reduction of IOP with a higher chance of being medication-free but has a higher risk profile, whereas CP patients required slightly more medication postoperatively but rarely had relevant complications.

These results can be interpreted in two different ways: on the one hand, the studies produced clear evidence that standard CP does not quite achieve the effect of TE in terms of absolute IOP reduction, but on the other hand, it is questionable whether such an extreme IOP reduction of up to 55% is really necessary or useful to these pre-damaged eyes [36]. The often-cited Wurzburg TVC study illustrates this dilemma very well. The authors found a relevantly higher risk profile at 43% IOP reduction after TE, which was accompanied by vision-threatening complications. The risk profile was lower at "only" 32% IOP reduction after CP [23]. In particular, eyes with several months of hypotony showed a high risk for a wipeout effect with permanent visual deterioration. Indeed, in the TE group,

37.5% experienced transient hypotony of <5 mmHg, and 18.8% had hypotony lasting longer than 90 days. Other hypotony-related complications of TE were choroidal detachment (12.5%) and shallow anterior chamber (6.2%). In addition, there were antimetabolite-associated complications such as corneal erosions and avascular filtering blebs [23].

Incidentally, if one excludes these hypotonic eyes in the TVC study, which cannot really be considered a success, the final IOP in the TE group is higher (no longer at 10.8, but at 12.8 mmHg) and does not achieve a better IOP reduction (–9.4 mmHg) than the CP group (–9.3 mmHg) [35]. Since the European Glaucoma Society (EGS) recommends only a 25% IOP reduction in the initial procedure, with an additional 20% reduction in the event of progression, merely aiming to maximize the IOP-lowering potential is too shortsighted [36,37].

This conclusion is also supported by a quality-of-life study that included 327 patients. The study showed higher patient satisfaction after CP compared to TE, which was statistically significant. This was due to better vision quality, fewer second procedures, significantly less stressful follow-up, and less impairment of quality of life [38].

Thus, this study mainly found that CP is not inferior to TE in terms of absolute IOP lowering, but that TE does offer a higher chance of achieving medication-free IOP lowering of <18 mmHg; however, this perk comes at the price of a higher complication rate with longer-term hypotony as well as a more complex follow-up [35].

6. Rationale for Modification of Canaloplasty

Despite the justification given above, it is undisputed that CP would benefit from a somewhat greater and more reliable IOP reduction. If CP could be modified to achieve a mean final IOP of, for example, 13 mmHg instead of 15 mmHg (i.e., within the range of successful TE), CP would likely replace TE as the gold standard owing to its significantly lower risk profile, easier follow-up, and lower impact on patient quality of life [7,23,38].

The goal of numerous scientific efforts, cited below, has been to modify CP in a manner such that it achieves IOP values comparable to those obtained after TE. In fact, numerous approaches have been devised to enhance the IOP-lowering potential of canaloplasty, which are described below.

7. Canaloplasty Combined with Suprachoroidal Drainage

One of the most promising modifications is to combine canaloplasty with an additional suprachoroidal drainage outflow (CP + ScD) to achieve an additive IOP-lowering effect by improving uveoscleral facility [39].

Previous techniques for non-penetrating glaucoma surgery, including conventional CP, have focused only on improving trabecular outflow. However, in addition to conventional trabecular outflow of aqueous humor [40], uveoscleral outflow also plays a significant role and may account for up to 57% of the total aqueous humor outflow under physiologic conditions [41]. It is important to exploit this potential.

Since conventional CP neglects the uveoscleral outflow pathway, the ScD technique was introduced in 2012 [39]. With this Sulzbach modification, the IOP-lowering effect of CP could be significantly enhanced and, for the first time, an IOP reduction comparable to TE could be achieved.

At first glance, the approach is similar to that of conventional CP. The crucial difference is that the deep scleral flap is not dissected lamellarly; instead, it is penetrated down to the choroid. This exposes the ciliary body and completely opens the suprachoroidal space. The deep flap is then dissected toward the limbus until the scleral spur is reached. The SC is safely unroofed and opened through a horizontal incision directly adjacent to the scleral spur (Figure 5). In the following the SC is probed analogously to conventional CP [39].

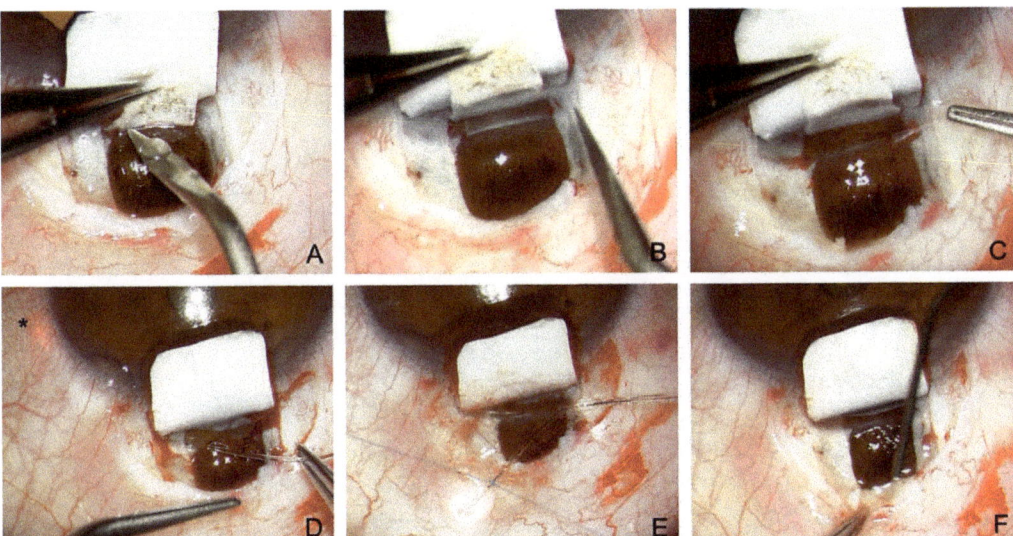

Figure 5. Surgical technique of modified canaloplasty with suprachoroidal drainage. (**A**) Preparation of a second deep flap with incision down to the choroid and incision anterior to the scleral spur. (**B**) Dissection across the scleral spur opens the SC and TDW. (**C**) Peeling of the juxtacanalicular TMW. (**D**) Probing of the SC with a microcatheter. Asterisk marks the laser light of the catheter tip (**E**) Insertion and knotting of two Prolene 10.0 sutures. (**F**) Dilatation of the suprachoroidal space using viscoelastics.

What is the purpose of the additional exposure of the choroidal window? First, the SC is much easier to find because blunt detachment to the scleral spur is simple, and the SC and TDW located directly anterior to the scleral spur can be prepared more reliably (Figure 5A,B). Second, percolation from the SC and TDW occurs not only into the collector vessels (trabecular outflow) but directly into the suprachoroidal space (uveoscleral outflow) via the choroidal window. The choroidal perfusion acts like a powerful water-jet pump and can reabsorb suprachoroidal fluid within minutes. The uveoscleral drainage effect is additive to the trabecular effect of conventional CP.

In a pilot study of 78 eyes, IOP was reduced to a mean of 13.5 mmHg after CP with ScD, with a concomitant reduction of 2.0 medications to 1.0 medication at 12 months. In addition, 52.6% of patients were completely medication-free [39].

These results were confirmed in a comparative, retrospective, two-arm study of 417 eyes over 12 months [24]. The mean IOP reduction after CP with ScD was significantly greater at 35.9% (from 20.9 ± 3.5 mmHg to 13.1 ± 2.5 mmHg) than after conventional canaloplasty at 31.2% (from 20.8 ± 3.6 mmHg to 14.0 ± 2.6 mmHg). The number of medications required was also lower (0.7 ± 1.0). The percentage of patients free of medication after one year was significantly higher in the combined group (56.9%) than in the conventional CP group (45.4%) [24].

Thus, the combination of CP with ScD lowered the IOP significantly more than conventional CP. More importantly, for the first time, the long-term IOP values are close to the IOP-lowering potential of TE, but free of serious complications.

8. Canaloplasty with ScD and Suprachoroidal Collagen Implant

To keep the outflow into the suprachoroidal space open in the long term, the additional implantation of a suprachoroidal collagen implant into the choroidal window was proposed in 2016 [42]. To achieve this, after the usual dissection down to the choroid at the end of surgery, the suprachoroidal space was widened with a viscoelastic, and a 10 × 10 × 2 mm collagen sponge (Ologen, Dahlhausen, Cologne, Germany) was implanted (Figure 6).

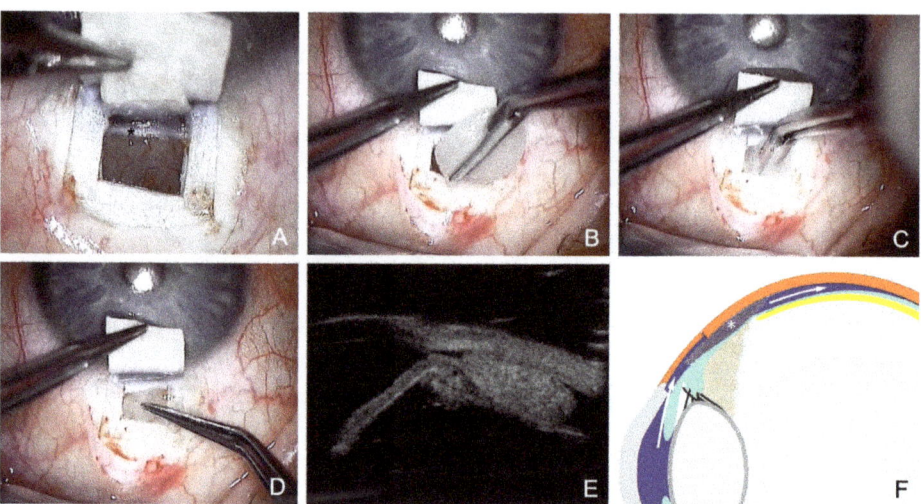

Figure 6. Canaloplasty with ScD and suprachoroidal Ologen sponge. (**A**) Clearly visible choroidal window, the scleral spur (Asterisk) and the TDW anterior to the scleral spur. (**B**) 6 mm Ologen sponge. (**C**) Suprachoroidal implantation of Ologen through the choroidal window. (**D**) Positioning of the Ologen as a placeholder in the suprachoroidal space, keeping the drainage open. (**E**) UBM imaging (50 MHz) of the implanted Ologen; note the suprachoroidal fluid around the implant. (**F**) Schematic showing the mechanism of ScD fluid circulation (arrows) and suprachoroidal Ologen (asterisk). Also marked are the scleral spur (star) and the ciliary body (square).

In a prospective study of 65 eyes over 12 months, the IOP-lowering effect was 35.6% (from 21.0 ± 4.3 mmHg to 13.5 ± 3.0 mmHg); the number of medications decreased from 3.5 to 0.9 [42]. In a recent study of 1034 eyes, this effect also seemed to be stable in the long term; after 2 years, the IOP was even slightly lower (12.9 ± 1.9 mmHg), suggesting a sustained effect [own data, unpublished]. This is remarkable because all large studies on conventional canaloplasty have shown a diminishing effect after 2 or 3 years.

Interestingly, modified CP with ScD and suprachoroidal Ologen also seems to be effective in treating pseudoexfoliation glaucoma. A retrospective study of 111 patients showed a stable IOP reduction of 45.8% to 12.7 ± 2.2 mmHg, even after 4 years. Again, there was no diminishing effect over time after Ologen implantation. This is in marked contrast to conventional CP, which has been judged in several studies to be less suitable for secondary glaucoma. Presumably, especially for secondary glaucoma, a purely trabecular facility improvement (standard CP) is insufficient, and the additional effect of uveoscleral outflow (ScD) is particularly useful [17].

In summary, suprachoroidal implantation of Ologen does not further enhance the IOP-lowering effect of CP with ScD, but the effect of ScD through a space holder in the choroidal window seems to be more sustainable and could maintain the achieved IOP level for at least 4 years.

9. Phacocanaloplasty with ScD

It has been well-acknowledged that combining CP with cataract surgery has an additive IOP-lowering effect. Comparative studies have shown that phacocanaloplasty (PCP) lowers the final pressure by an average of 1.3–1.9 mmHg more than CP alone [30,31]. However, this effect was less pronounced in other studies [32].

This additive effect has also been confirmed in studies employing CP with ScD. In a retrospective comparative study of 328 eyes, CP with ScD alone achieved a 37.0% reduction in IOP at 1 year (from 20.9 ± 3.6 mmHg to 13.2 ± 2.6 mmHg), whereas PCP with ScD produced a significantly greater reduction of 47.4% (from 23.2 ± 5.1 mmHg to 12.2 ± 1.7 mmHg) [43].

This "phaco" effect is independent of axial length and anterior chamber depth, unlike the IOP-lowering effect of cataract surgery in general. Only the preoperative IOP level has been shown to be a strong predictive factor: the higher the preoperative IOP, the greater the postoperative IOP reduction [43].

10. "Filtering" Canaloplasty with Bleb Formation

In CP, the scleral flap should be sutured to be as watertight as possible in order to avoid subconjunctival drainage with formation of a filtering bleb. Instead, drainage via Schlemm's canal alone (and via ScD) is desired. This action makes CP immune to the scarring stimulus of the conjunctiva [44].

However, in clinical practice, a filtering bleb is sometimes formed after canaloplasty. Although it is hardly visible clinically, it can be detected by AC-OCT and UBM [45]. This discrete filtration zone often has no effect on postoperative IOP values but tends to be a negative prognostic factor.

On the other hand, one might assume that by creating an alternative outflow pathway for aqueous humor, an additional decrease in IOP can be achieved. To provide an additional subconjunctival outflow, the superficial scleral flap must be adapted in a dosed manner, similar to TE, to ensure continuous drainage of aqueous humor under the conjunctiva [46].

Technically, this "filtering" CP is not a non-penetrating surgical technique but rather a double-covered TE, which reduces the rate of hypotony but has all the disadvantages of a filtering surgery and so must be managed accordingly [46]. Therefore, to ensure the sustainability of a controlled filtration effect, the use of antimetabolites such as mitomycin C (MMC) as a sponge is reasonable (in analogy to TE). In his study population, Barnebey achieved an average IOP reduction of 42.7% and a reduction in medication from an average of 2.2 drugs to 0 at 12 months. The administered concentrations of MMC (0.025% and 0.03%) did not induce avascular areas, but the rate of postoperative hypotony (15%) was significantly higher than in the control group (1.1%) [46].

MMC can be applied on the superficial sclera, under the scleral flap, or in combination [47,48]. A meta-analysis showed better IOP reduction with MMC (43.56% at 6 months and 42.26% at 36 months) compared with surgery without MMC (39.14% at 6 months and 27.59% at 36 months). Complication rates for wound leakage, hypotony, expulsive hemorrhage, flattening of the anterior chamber, and cataract induction showed no significant differences. The authors conclude that CP with adjunctive use of MMC appears to be a way to improve the efficacy of standard CP [49].

11. Canaloplasty with ScD and Suprachoroidal Eyemate-SC IOP Sensor

In the future, an important modification is the combination of CP with a suprachoroidal IOP sensor for telemetric self-measurement by the patient. Particularly after glaucoma surgery, frequent and reliable measurement of the IOP is crucial to verify successful IOP adjustment in the target range [50,51].

The patented Eyemate-SC (Implandata, Hannover, Germany) is the first available suprachoroidal sensor for telemetric IOP self-measurement. It is placed in the suprachoroidal space during non-penetrating glaucoma surgery, where it remains permanently [52]. The suprachoroidal approach offers several advantages: first, the spatial separation of the IOP measurement from the site of pathology (chamber angle) prevents the causative glaucoma from worsening owing to the diagnostic implantation; second, the procedure can be performed regardless of the lens status and existence of any anterior chamber pathologies; and finally, implantation of the suprachoroidal device can be combined well with glaucoma surgery to monitor the therapeutic success and acts as a placeholder for ScD [50].

Suprachoroidal implantation of the Eyemate-SC IOP sensor (7.5 × 3.5 mm and an outwardly decreasing thickness of 1.3 mm in the center and 0.9 mm on the periphery) can be excellently combined with CP (Figure 7). Both procedures can be consecutively performed using the same access point. This is easiest in CP with ScD, since a choroidal window is prepared anyway, and the sensor can be used as a placeholder in the same way as the Ologen implant (https://youtu.be/F_p9iIGxB9U, accessed on 8 December 2018) [52].

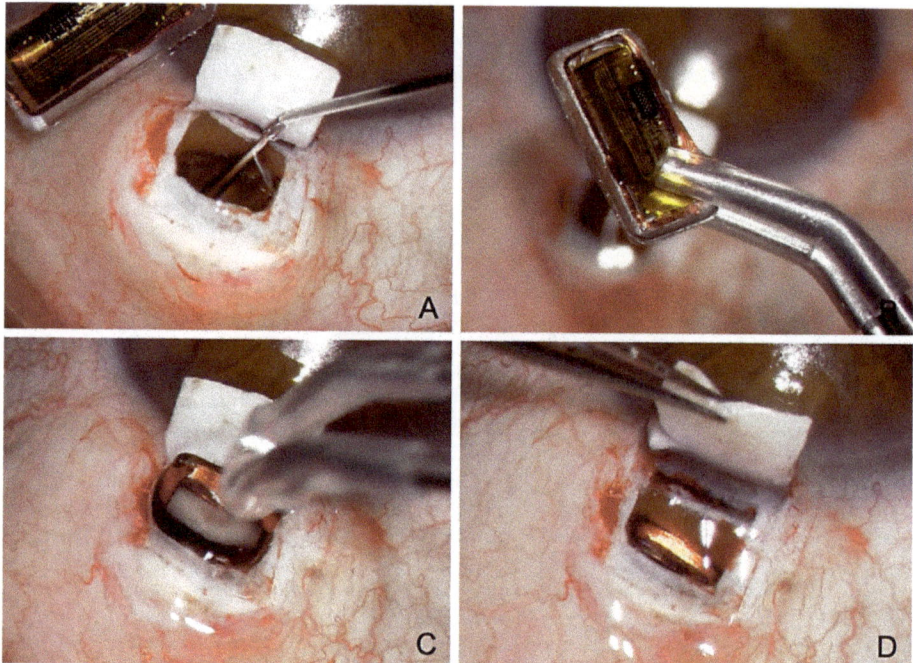

Figure 7. Surgical technique of suprachoroidal implantation of the Eyemate-SC sensor. (**A**) Viscoelastic is injected at the end of the CP with ScD to expand the suprachoroidal space (**B**) The Eyemate-SC sensor is grasped carefully with padded implantation forceps. (**C**) The sensor is implanted into the suprachoroidal space. (**D**) The Eyemate-SC sensor serves as a placeholder for suprachoroidal drainage while allowing continuous IOP monitoring.

Thus, the Eyemate-SC sensor not only serves as a placeholder in the suprachoroidal space but also allows continuous, postoperative IOP-monitoring simultaneously (Figure 8). This is particularly useful for glaucoma surgery patients. Patients undergoing glaucoma surgery usually have advanced visual field defects that require strict control of the mean IOP and diurnal IOP fluctuations. Although the latter have been shown to decrease using this approach, they still persist even after successful glaucoma surgery. Particularly in the postoperative phase (1–3 months), when the IOP fluctuates the most, the validity of Goldmann applanation tonometry (GAT) is limited owing to the altered corneal biomechanics [50,51].

The Eyemate-SC IOP sensor delivers a wireless readout of continuous IOP values. The Mesograph handheld device can store up to 3000 IOP readings. The data can be wirelessly transferred to a secure, web-based platform accessible to the supervising ophthalmologist. Since each measurement is stored with a time stamp, patients can automatically create their individual IOP profile to disclose short- and long-term fluctuations and, if necessary, the therapy can be adapted accordingly [53]. Thus, supervising ophthalmologists can base their therapy decisions on a broad database of many hundreds of measurements instead of only a few measurements per year.

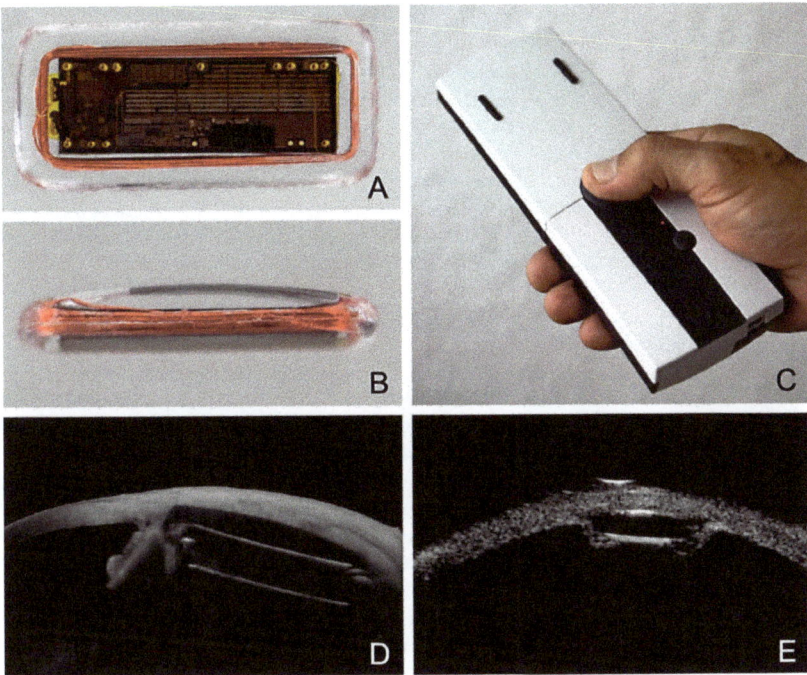

Figure 8. Eyemate-SC sensor looking at the electronics from (**A**) the top and (**B**) the side. (**C**) Mesograph readout device for wireless telemetric IOP measurement. Multimodal imaging 6 months after suprachoroidal implantation of the Eyemate-SC sensor. (**D**) An anterior segment (AC)-OCT visualizes the microelectronics carrier substrate, but not the silicone encapsulation. (**E**) The UBM image (50 MHz) depicts the lens-shaped rounded silicone encapsulation smoothly adapting to the curved scleral shape.

Telemetric self-measurement using an intraocular sensor also has other advantages. The measured values correspond to the true IOP independently of the corneal biomechanics, and the active involvement of the patients as well as the direct treatment response are suitable to improve the poor therapy adherence in glaucoma patients [53,54].

The recently completed European multicenter pivotal study demonstrated excellent safety and reliably reproducible IOP measurements. Except for the early postoperative phase, the GAT and telemetric Eyemate-SC measurements were in excellent agreement, with a mean difference of 0.23 mmHg across all study eyes at 12 months [55].

12. Disadvantages of Modified Canaloplasty

Although one might assume that exposure of the suprachoroidal space could increase the risk of hemorrhage or hypotony, this was not confirmed in the studies. It could be shown that modified canaloplasty (with ScD and Ologen) has a comparably low risk profile as conventional CP. Vision-threatening complications in particular were absent, which seems advantageous compared to TE [24,42,43,55]. Only cutting the perforating vessels can cause intraoperative oozing bleeding temporarily obscuring the view, because cauterization of the choroid should be avoided.

It should be noted, however, that the combination of different outflow pathways makes it difficult to assess the contribution of the individual components. Furthermore, the different outflow pathways influence each other, which becomes most evident in "filtering" CP: When aqueous humor drains outwards, the influence of the other changes (transtrabecular and suprachoroidal) decreases. Filtering CP with MMC also shows, analogously to TE, a significantly increased rate of postoperative hypotony [46].

Costs also differ significantly, as the microcatheter incurs significant additional costs. However, this is counterbalanced by the significantly lower preoperative effort, the lack of costs for MMC, a shorter hospitalization due to the absence of hypotony, and a simpler follow-up without extensive bleb care or bleb revisions (needling, 5-FU injections).

However, the main limitation is the lower scientific evidence (250 vs. 8000 references in PubMed). Most importantly, there are only a few comparative studies and no randomized clinical trials comparing modified CP with TE, so a final weighing of benefits and risks must await.

13. Conclusions

CP is a safe and effective glaucoma surgical procedure that—through various modifications—now achieves an IOP-lowering effect comparable to that associated with successful TE, but without the typical risk profile of TE. The combination of canaloplasty with the newly developed ScD enhances the IOP-lowering effect by adding a new uveoscleral drainage pathway under the choroid. By creating a choroidal window, percolation from the SC and TDW occurs not only into the collector vessels (trabecular outflow) but also directly into the suprachoroidal space (uveoscleral outflow). The choroidal perfusion acts like a powerful water-jet pump and can reabsorb suprachoroidal fluid within a few minutes. Therefore, the combination of CP with ScD lowers the IOP to a significantly greater extent than conventional CP. For the first time, it has been shown that the IOP reduction achieved by CP with ScD is sufficient for the treatment of severe glaucoma, allowing this combined approach to be used a primary procedure instead of TE (Figure 9). This shows that modified CP (+scD+Ologen) is on par with TE in terms of indication spectrum and IOP-lowering potency, clearly differentiating it from the newly emerged MIGS procedures, which show a lower effect on IOP and are reserved for mild to moderate glaucoma. Implant-based modifications implemented using a placeholder in the suprachoroidal space do not further enhance the IOP-lowering effect, but the effect of ScD seems to be more sustainable and could maintain treatment success for at least 4 years. In addition, the novel suprachoroidal IOP sensor allows safe telemetric IOP monitoring after successful canaloplasty.

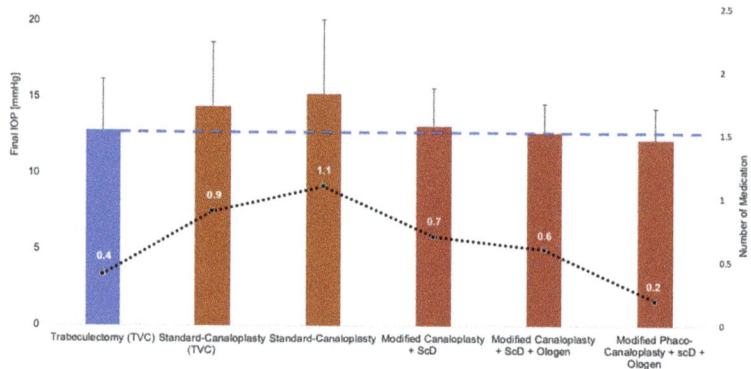

Figure 9. Evolution of canaloplasty modifications to improve the IOP-lowering success and the amount of remaining medication. This continuous refinement, especially the combination with ScD, allows CP to achieve IOP values comparable to TE (dashed line) and a low number of medications (dotted line) for the first time, but without the complications of TE [13,16,22,30,31,41].

Funding: This research received no external funding.

Institutional Review Board Statement: Not applicable.

Informed Consent Statement: Not applicable.

Data Availability Statement: Not applicable.

Conflicts of Interest: Prof. Szurman has an international patent (PCT/EP2015/062976) on the suprachoroidal telemetric intraocular pressure sensor (Eyemate-SC). The author declare no conflict of interest.

References

1. Jampel, H.D.; Musch, D.C.; Gillespie, B.W.; Lichter, P.R.; Wright, M.M.; Guire, K.E.; Collaborative Initial Glaucoma Treatment Study Group. Perioperative complications of trabeculectomy in the collaborative initial glaucoma treatment study (CIGTS). *Am. J. Ophthalmol.* **2005**, *140*, 16–22. [CrossRef] [PubMed]
2. Vaziri, K.; Schwartz, S.G.; Kishor, K.S.; Fortun, J.A.; Moshfeghi, D.M.; Moshfeghi, A.A.; Flynn, H.W., Jr. Incidence of postoperative suprachoroidal hemorrhage after glaucoma filtration surgeries in the United States. *Clin. Ophthalmol.* **2015**, *9*, 579–584.
3. Patel, H.Y.; Danesh-Meyer, H.V. Incidence and management of cataract after glaucoma surgery. *Curr. Opin. Ophthalmol.* **2013**, *24*, 15–20. [CrossRef] [PubMed]
4. Yamamoto, T.; Sawada, A.; Mayama, C.; Araie, M.; Ohkubo, S.; Sugiyama, K.; Kuwayama, Y.; Collaborative Bleb-Related Infection Incidence and Treatment Study Group. The 5-year incidence of bleb-related infection and its risk factors after filtering surgeries with adjunctive mitomycin C: Collaborative bleb-related infection incidence and treatment study 2. *Ophthalmology* **2014**, *121*, 1001–1006. [CrossRef] [PubMed]
5. Rulli, E.; Biagioli, E.; Riva, I.; Gambirasio, G.; De Simone, I.; Floriani, I.; Quaranta, L. Efficacy and safety of trabeculectomy vs nonpenetrating surgical procedures: A systematic review and meta-analysis. *JAMA Ophthalmol.* **2013**, *131*, 1573–1582. [CrossRef]
6. Kim, E.A.; Law, S.K.; Coleman, A.L.; Nouri-Mahdavi, K.; Giaconi, J.A.; Yu, F.; Lee, J.W.; Caprioli, J. Long-Term Bleb-Related Infections After Trabeculectomy: Incidence, Risk Factors, and Influence of Bleb Revision. *Am. J. Ophthalmol.* **2015**, *159*, 1082–1091. [CrossRef]
7. Thederan, L.; Grehn, F.; Klink, T. Comparison of canaloplasty with trabeculectomy. *Klin. Monbl. Augenheilkd.* **2014**, *231*, 256–261.
8. Ayyala, R.S.; Chaudhry, A.L.; Okogbaa, C.B.; Zurakowski, D. Comparison of surgical outcomes between canaloplasty and trabeculectomy at 12 months' follow-up. *Ophthalmology* **2011**, *118*, 2427–2433. [CrossRef]
9. Eldaly, M.A.; Bunce, C.; Elsheikha, O.Z.; Wormald, R. Non-penetrating filtration surgery versus trabeculectomy for open-angle glaucoma. *Cochrane Database Syst. Rev.* **2014**, *15*, CD007059. [CrossRef]
10. Fyodorov, S. Non penetrating deep sclerectomy in open-angle glaucoma. *Eye Microsurg.* **1989**, *2*, 52–55.
11. Stegmann, R.; Pienaar, A.; Miller, D. Viscocanalostomy for open-angle glaucoma in black African patients. *J. Cataract. Refract. Surg.* **1999**, *25*, 316–322. [CrossRef]
12. Cameron, B.; Field, M.; Ball, S.; Kearney, J. Circumferential viscodilation of Schlemm's canal with a flexible microcannula during non-penetrating glaucoma surgery. *Digit. J. Ophthalmol.* **2006**, *12*, 1.
13. Tam, D.Y.; Barnebey, H.S.; Ahmed, I.I. Nd: YAG laser goniopuncture: Indications and procedure. *J. Glaucoma* **2013**, *22*, 620–625. [CrossRef] [PubMed]
14. Brusini, P. Canaloplasty in open-angle glaucoma surgery: A four-year follow-up. *Sci. World J.* **2014**, *2014*, 469609.
15. Brusini, P.; Tosoni, C.; Zeppieri, M. Canaloplasty in corticosteroid-induced glaucoma. Preliminary results. *J. Clin. Med.* **2018**, *7*, 31. [CrossRef] [PubMed]
16. Lommatzsch, C.; Heinz, C.; Heiligenhaus, A.; Koch, J.M. Canaloplasty in patients with uveitic glaucoma: A pilot study. *Graefes. Arch. Clin. Exp. Ophthalmol.* **2016**, *254*, 1325–1330. [CrossRef] [PubMed]
17. Seuthe, A.M.; Szurman, P.; Januschowski, K. Canaloplasty with Suprachoroidal Drainage in Patients with Pseudoexfoliation Glaucoma—Four Years Results. *Curr. Eye Res.* **2021**, *46*, 217–223. [CrossRef]
18. Riva, I.; Brusini, P.; Oddone, F.; Michelessi, M.; Weinreb, R.N.; Quaranta, L. Canaloplasty in the Treatment of Open-Angle Glaucoma: A Review of Patient Selection and Outcomes. *Adv. Ther.* **2019**, *36*, 31–43. [CrossRef] [PubMed]
19. Joshi, A.B.; Parrish, R.K., II; Feuer, W.F. 2002 survey of the American Glaucoma Society: Practice preferences for glaucoma surgery and antifibrotic use. *J. Glaucoma* **2005**, *14*, 172–174. [CrossRef]
20. Lin, Z.J.; Xu, S.; Huang, S.Y.; Zhang, X.B.; Zhong, Y.S. Comparison of canaloplasty and trabeculectomy for open angle glaucoma: A Meta-analysis. *Int. J. Ophthalmol.* **2016**, *9*, 1814–1819.
21. Seuthe, A.M.; Jung, S.; Januschowski, K.; Szurman, P. Predictive factors for the IOP reduction in phacocanaloplasty with suprachoroidal drainage. *Int. Ophthalmol.* **2020**, *40*, 1897–1903. [PubMed]
22. Szurman, P.; Klabe, K. Modifications of canaloplasty: Strong pressure-lowering effect with a low risk profile. *Ophthalmologie* **2022**, *119*, 989–999. [CrossRef] [PubMed]
23. Matlach, J.; Dhillon, C.; Hain, J.; Schlunck, G.; Grehn, F.; Klink, T. Trabeculectomy versus canaloplasty (TVC study) in the treatment of patients with open-angle glaucoma: A prospective randomized clinical trial. *Acta Ophthalmol.* **2015**, *93*, 753–761. [CrossRef] [PubMed]

24. Seuthe, A.M.; Ivanescu, C.; Leers, S.; Boden, K.; Januschowski, K.; Szurman, P. Modified canaloplasty with suprachoroidal drainage versus conventional canaloplasty-1-year results. *Graefes Arch. Clin. Exp. Ophthalmol.* **2016**, *254*, 1591–1597. [PubMed]
25. Erokhina, M.; Seuthe, A.M.; Szurman, P.; Haus, A. One Year Results of PRESERFLOTM MicroShunt Implantation for Refractory Glaucoma. *J. Glaucoma* **2022**, in press.
26. Gedde, S.J.; Schiffman, J.C.; Feuer, W.J.; Herndon, L.W.; Brandt, J.D.; Budenz, D.L.; Tube versus Trabeculectomy Study Group. Treatment outcomes in the Tube Versus Trabeculectomy (TVT) study after five years of follow-up. *Am. J. Ophthalmol.* **2012**, *153*, 789–803.
27. Brusini, P.; Tosoni, C. Canaloplasty after failed trabeculectomy: A possible option. *J. Glaucoma* **2014**, *23*, 33–34. [CrossRef]
28. Korber, N. Canaloplasty after trabeculectomy. *Ophthalmologe* **2015**, *112*, 332–336.
29. Xin, C.; Chen, X.; Shi, Y.; Li, M.; Wang, H.; Wang, N. One-year interim comparison of canaloplasty in primary open-angle glaucoma following failed filtering surgery with primary canaloplasty. *Br. J. Ophthalmol.* **2016**, *100*, 1692–1696. [CrossRef]
30. Bull, H.; von Wolff, K.; Korber, N.; Tetz, M. Three-year canaloplasty outcomes for the treatment of open-angle glaucoma: European study results. *Graefes Arch. Clin. Exp. Ophthalmol.* **2011**, *249*, 1537–1545. [CrossRef]
31. Lewis, R.A.; von Wolff, K.; Tetz, M.; Koerber, N.; Kearney, J.R.; Shingleton, B.J.; Samuelson, T.W. Canaloplasty: Three-year results of circumferential viscodilation and tensioning of Schlemm canal using a microcatheter to treat open-angle glaucoma. *J. Cataract. Refract. Surg.* **2011**, *37*, 682–690. [CrossRef] [PubMed]
32. Khaimi, M.A.; Dvorak, J.D.; Ding, K. An analysis of 3-year outcomes following canaloplasty for the treatment of open-angle glaucoma. *J. Ophthalmol.* **2017**, *2017*, 2904272. [CrossRef] [PubMed]
33. Lewis, R.A.; von Wolff, K.; Tetz, M.; Koerber, N.; Kearney, J.R.; Shingleton, B.J.; Samuelson, T.W. Canaloplasty: Circumferential viscodilation and tensioning of Schlemm canal using a flexible microcatheter for the treatment of open-angle glaucoma in adults: Two-year interim clinical study results. *J. Cataract. Refract. Surg.* **2009**, *35*, 814–824. [CrossRef]
34. Tetz, M.; Koerber, N.; Shingleton, B.J.; von Wolff, K.; Bull, H.; Samuelson, T.W.; Lewis, R.A. Phacoemulsification and intraocular lens implantation before, during, or after canaloplasty in eyes with open-angle glaucoma: 3-year results. *J. Glaucoma* **2015**, *24*, 187–194. [CrossRef] [PubMed]
35. Januschowski, K.; Leers, S.; Haus, A.; Szurman, P.; Seuthe, A.M.; Boden, K.T. Is trabeculectomy really superior to canaloplasty? *Acta Ophthalmol.* **2016**, *94*, e666–e667. [CrossRef]
36. Heijl, A.; Leske, M.C.; Bengtsson, B.; Hyman, L.; Bengtsson, B.; Hussein, M.; Early Manifest Glaucoma Trial Group. Reduction of intraocular pressure and glaucoma progression: Results from the Early Manifest Glaucoma Trial. *Arch. Ophthalmol.* **2002**, *120*, 1268–1279. [CrossRef]
37. Malik, R.; O'Leary, N.; Mikelberg, F.S.; Balazsi, A.G.; LeBlanc, R.P.; Lesk, M.R.; Nicolela, M.T.; Trope, G.E.; Chauhan, B.C.; Canadian Glaucoma Study Group. Neuroretinal Rim Area Change in Glaucoma Patients with Visual Field Progression Endpoints and Intraocular Pressure Reduction. The Canadian Glaucoma Study: 4. *Am. J. Ophthalmol.* **2016**, *163*, 140–147. [CrossRef]
38. Klink, T.; Sauer, J.; Körber, N.J.; Grehn, F.; Much, M.M.; Thederan, L.; Matlach, J.; Salgado, J.P. Quality of life following glaucoma surgery: Canaloplasty versus trabeculectomy. *Clin. Ophthalmol.* **2014**, *9*, 7–16.
39. Szurman, P.; Januschowski, K.; Boden, K.T.; Szurman, G.B. A modified scleral dissection technique with suprachoroidal drainage for canaloplasty. *Graefes Arch. Clin. Exp. Ophthalmol.* **2015**, *254*, 351–354. [CrossRef]
40. Overby, D.R.; Stamer, W.D.; Johnson, J. The changing paradigm of outflow resistance generation: Towards synergistic models of the JCT and inner wall endothelium. *Exp. Eye Res.* **2009**, *88*, 656–670. [CrossRef]
41. Lutjen-Drecoll, E.; Kruse, F.E. Primary open angle glaucoma. Morphological bases for the understanding of the pathogenesis and effects of antiglaucomatic substances. *Ophthalmologe* **2007**, *104*, 167–178.
42. Szurman, P.; Januschowski, K.; Boden, K.T.; Seuthe, A.M. Suprachoroidal drainage with collagen sheet implant—A novel technique for non-penetrating glaucoma surgery. *Graefes Arch. Clin. Exp. Ophthalmol.* **2018**, *256*, 381–385. [PubMed]
43. Seuthe, A.M.; Januschowski, K.; Mariacher, S.; Ebner, M.; Opitz, N.; Szurman, P.; Boden, K. The effect of canaloplasty with suprachoroidal drainage combined with cataract surgery—1-year results. *Acta Ophthalmol.* **2018**, *96*, e74–e78. [PubMed]
44. Grieshaber, M.C.; Pienaar, A.; Olivier, J.; Stegmann, R. Canaloplasty for primary open-angle glaucoma: Long-term outcome. *Br. J. Ophthalmol.* **2010**, *94*, 1478–1482. [CrossRef] [PubMed]
45. Klink, T.; Panidou, E.; Kanzow-Terai, B.; Klink, J.; Schlunck, G.; Grehn, F.J. Are there filtering blebs after canaloplasty? *J. Glaucoma* **2012**, *21*, 89–94. [PubMed]
46. Barnebey, H.S. Canaloplasty with intraoperative low dosage mitomycin C: A retrospective case series. *J. Glaucoma* **2013**, *22*, 201–204. [CrossRef]
47. Liang, Y.; Sun, H.; Shuai, J.; Xu, K.; Ji, F.F.; Sucijanti Yuan, Z.L. Modified viscocanalostomy in the Chinese population with open angle glaucoma: A 10-year follow-up results. *Int. J. Ophthalmol.* **2019**, *12*, 429–435. [PubMed]
48. Elksne, E.; Mercieca, K.; Prokosch-Willing, V. Canaloplasty with mitomycin C after previous combined cataract surgery and Schlemm's canal microstent implantation. *Eur. J. Ophthalmol.* **2022**, *32*, 712–716. [CrossRef]
49. Cheng, J.W.; Cai, J.P.; Li, Y.; Wei, R.L. Intraoperative mitomycin C for nonpenetrating glaucoma surgery: A systematic review and meta-analysis. *J. Glaucoma* **2011**, *20*, 322–326.
50. Szurman, P.; Mansouri, K.; Dick, H.B.; Mermoud, A.; Hoffmann, E.M.; Mackert, M.; Weinreb, R.N.; Rao, H.L.; Seuthe, A.M. Safety and performance of a suprachoroidal sensor for telemetric measurement of intraocular pressure in the EYEMATE-SC trial. *Br. J. Ophthalmol.* **2023**, *107*, 518–524. [CrossRef]

51. Wasielica-Poslednik, J.; Schmeisser, J.; Hoffmann, E.M.; Weyer-Elberich, V.; Bell, K.; Lorenz, K.; Pfeiffer, N. Fluctuation of intraocular pressure in glaucoma patients before and after trabeculectomy with mitomycin C. *PLoS ONE* **2017**, *12*, e0185246. [CrossRef] [PubMed]
52. Szurman, P. Implant for Determining Intraocular Pressure. International Application No. PCT/EP2015/062976, 30 December 2015.
53. Mariacher, S.; Ebner, M.; Januschowski, K.; Hurst, J.; Schnichels, S.; Szurman, P. Investigation of a novel implantable suprachoroidal pressure transducer for telemetric intraocular pressure monitoring. *Exp. Eye Res.* **2016**, *151*, 54–60. [CrossRef] [PubMed]
54. Sleath, B.; Blalock, S.; Covert, D.; Stone, J.L.; Skinner, A.C.; Muir, K.; Robin, A.L. The relationship between glaucoma medication adherence, eye drop technique, and visual field defect severity. *Ophthalmology* **2011**, *118*, 2398–2402. [CrossRef] [PubMed]
55. Szurman, P.; Gillmann, K.; Seuthe, A.M.; Dick, H.B.; Hoffmann, E.M.; Mermoud, A.; Mackert, M.J.; Weinreb, R.N.; Rao, H.L.; Mansouri, K. EYEMATE-SC Trial: Twelve-Month Safety, Performance, and Accuracy of a Suprachoroidal Sensor for Telemetric Measurement of Intraocular Pressure. *Ophthalmology* **2023**, *130*, 304–312. [CrossRef]

Disclaimer/Publisher's Note: The statements, opinions and data contained in all publications are solely those of the individual author(s) and contributor(s) and not of MDPI and/or the editor(s). MDPI and/or the editor(s) disclaim responsibility for any injury to people or property resulting from any ideas, methods, instructions or products referred to in the content.

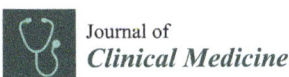

Case Report

Descemet's Membrane Detachment during Phacocanaloplasty: Case Series and In-Depth Literature Review

Marta Orejudo de Rivas [1,*], Juana Martínez Morales [1], Elena Pardina Claver [1], Diana Pérez García [1], Itziar Pérez Navarro [1], Francisco J. Ascaso Puyuelo [1,2,3], Julia Aramburu Clavería [1] and Juan Ibáñez Alperte [1,2]

1. Department of Ophthalmology, Lozano Blesa University Clinic Hospital, 50009 Zaragoza, Spain; jascaso@gmail.com (F.J.A.P.); juanibanezalperte@msn.com (J.I.A.)
2. Aragon Health Research Institute (IIS Aragon), 50018 Zaragoza, Spain
3. Department of Surgery, School of Medicine, University of Zaragoza, 50009 Zaragoza, Spain
* Correspondence: martaoredr@gmail.com

Abstract: This article presents three cases of Descemet's membrane detachment (DMD) occurring during 'ab externo' phacocanaloplasty procedures in three patients with uncontrolled primary open-angle glaucoma (OAG) and discusses the management of this condition by reviewing the available literature. Following a successful 360° cannulation of Schlemm's canal (SC), the microcatheter was withdrawn while an ophthalmic viscosurgical device (OVD) was injected into the canal. During passage through the inferonasal quadrant, a spontaneous separation of the posterior layer of the cornea was observed. Each case was managed differently after diagnosis, with the third case being drained intraoperatively based on experience gained from the previous cases. On the first postoperative day, slit-lamp biomicroscopy (BMC) revealed multiple DMDs in case one and a hyphema in the lower third of a deep anterior chamber. In the other two cases, a single DMD was observed. The second case developed hemorrhagic Descemet membrane detachment (HDMD), while the other two were non-hemorrhagic. In all three cases, anterior segment optical coherence tomography (AS-OCT) revealed the presence of retrocorneal hyperreflective membranes indicative of DMDs. These membranes were located in the periphery of the cornea and did not impact the visual axis. After evaluation, a small incision was made in the inferotemporal DMD of the first case. However, for the two remaining cases, a strategy of watchful waiting was deemed appropriate due to the location and size of the DMDs, as they did not affect the best-corrected visual acuity (BCVA). Over time, the patients demonstrated progressive improvement with a gradual reduction in the size of the DMDs.

Keywords: phacocanaloplasty; Descemet's membrane detachment; open-angle glaucoma; Schlemm's canal

Citation: Orejudo de Rivas, M.; Martínez Morales, J.; Pardina Claver, E.; Pérez García, D.; Pérez Navarro, I.; Ascaso Puyuelo, F.J.; Aramburu Clavería, J.; Ibáñez Alperte, J. Descemet's Membrane Detachment during Phacocanaloplasty: Case Series and In-Depth Literature Review. *J. Clin. Med.* **2023**, *12*, 5461. https://doi.org/10.3390/jcm12175461

Academic Editors: Michele Figus and Karl Mercieca

Received: 26 July 2023
Revised: 17 August 2023
Accepted: 20 August 2023
Published: 23 August 2023

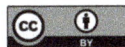

Copyright: © 2023 by the authors. Licensee MDPI, Basel, Switzerland. This article is an open access article distributed under the terms and conditions of the Creative Commons Attribution (CC BY) license (https://creativecommons.org/licenses/by/4.0/).

1. Introduction

Canaloplasty is a well-established surgical technique for nonpenetrating glaucoma surgery that involves circumferential 360° catheterization and viscodilation of Schlemm's canal (SC) to enhance the outflow of aqueous humor through the physiological collector system [1]. This article delves into the subject of iTrack Canaloplasty, also referred to as 'ab externo'. The ab externo canaloplasty technique involves circumferential viscodilation of Schlemm's canal, creating internal tension within the canal through the application of a tension suture. Nevertheless, recent studies have shown that complete 360° viscodilation without the need for sutures also yields favorable outcomes. These findings lend support to the significance of implementing the ab interno variation in this technique, utilizing an angle-based approach that is performed from within the eye [2]. While canaloplasty has shown a higher safety profile compared to conventional techniques, rare intraoperative and postoperative complications have been reported [3]. Konopinska et al. [4] recently reviewed the intraoperative complications of canaloplasty, identifying the most common complication as the inability to pass the microcatheter through SC, with an incidence ranging from 10 to 26%, and Descemet's membrane detachment (DMD) occurring in 1.6 to 9.1%

of patients. Alobeidan et al. [5] reported a 9.5% incidence of DMD in patients undergoing canaloplasty and phacocanaloplasty, noting that most cases of DMD occurred in combination with phacocanaloplasty. In this case report, we present three cases of DMD among a sample of 180 patients who underwent canaloplasty or phacocanaloplasty. These cases highlight the low incidence of this complication (1.67%) and provide additional evidence supporting the higher occurrence of DMD during phacocanaloplasty when compared to standard canaloplasty, particularly in patients with uncontrolled intraocular pressure (IOP) and open-angle glaucoma (OAG). This encompasses secondary glaucomas that present an open angle, such as pseudoexfoliative glaucoma. Additionally, we draw attention to the more frequent manifestation of DMD in the lower quadrants and discuss the management of this condition, given the absence of a consensus.

2. Case Series

2.1. Surgical Method

A standard ab externo SC surgery, known as canaloplasty ab externo, and phacoemulsification were performed under peribulbar anesthesia. Topical vasoconstrictive agents were applied to minimize bleeding. A corneal traction suture (7/0 vicryl) was placed at 12 o'clock to expose the upper area, followed by a limbal peritomy to expose the sclera. Minimal cautery was used for hemostasis, ensuring preservation of the episcleral collector channels. A partial thickness square flap measuring 4 × 4 mm was dissected according to the standard technique, followed by a deeper scleral flap (3 × 3 mm) created at approximately 95% depth, just above the choroidal tissue. At this stage, a standard phacoemulsification and a posterior chamber intraocular lens (AcrySof IQ IOL, Alcon®, Geneva, Switzerland) implantation were performed. The primary corneal incision was sutured using 10/0 nylon. Subsequently, the dissection of the inner scleral flap was continued until the SC was identified, crossing the scleral spur. The sides of the deep flap were dissected forward into the cornea creating a trabeculodescemetic window [6]. An ophthalmic viscosurgical device (OVD) with viscoadaptative properties (Healon GV; Johnson and Johnson, New Brunswick, NJ, USA) was injected through the SC opening on both sides. The canal was probed 360° using a microcatheter (iTrack®; Nova Eye Medical, Adelaide, Australia), with the surgeon tracking the illuminated tip of the catheter, aided by dimmed microscope lights. During the retraction of the catheter, OVD was injected at every 2 clock hours to dilate the canal, as directed by a well-trained assistant surgeon. The injected volume was controlled by a quarter turn of the syringe provided by the company, equivalent to 0.5 µL. While retracting the catheter, at the 6 o'clock position, a DMD was observed, accompanied by significant blood leakage mixed with viscoelastic material in the lower quadrants (inferonasal and inferotemporal quadrants in case 1, inferotemporal quadrant in cases 2 and 3), resembling a possible micro-rupture of the trabecular meshwork. In the third case, intraoperative management involved draining the DMD with a 30-gauge needle and intracameral air injection. Following that, the deeper scleral flap was excised, while the superficial flap was positioned and sutured tightly with 10/0 nylon to ensure closure of the trabeculodescemetic window. The primary objective was to prevent leakage through the filtering bleb instead of facilitating the exit of fluid through the collector channels. The anterior chamber was reformed with a balanced salt solution, and an air bubble was left to occupy the entire anterior chamber (AC). The conjunctiva was closed using a non-absorbable suture (8/0 silk).

All three procedures were performed using the same method and by the same surgeons, with no noticeable variations observed.

All the data regarding intraocular pressure provided below have been measured using Goldmann applanation tonometry, while the best-corrected visual acuity (BCVA) assessments were conducted using the Snellen chart.

2.2. Case 1

A 68-year-old woman, who was being monitored by the glaucoma department due to medically uncontrolled primary OAG, was selected as a candidate for a non-penetrating glaucoma canaloplasty surgery. Prior to the procedure, her BCVA was 1.0 and 0.3 in the right and left eyes (RE and LE), respectively. Ophthalmic refraction showed a slightly hyperopic prescription (+1.50 −0.50 90° in the RE and +0.25 +0.25 180° in the LE). Slit-lamp biomicroscopy (BMC) examination with a Topcon Slit Lamp Imaging System (SL-D701, Topcon Healthcare®, Oakland, NJ, USA) revealed the presence of a corticonuclear cataract in the LE. The IOP measured using Goldmann applanation tonometry while the patient was on maximum topical antiglaucoma medications ranged from 26 to 28 mmHg in the LE. The RE only required a single topical antihypertensive drop, and the IOP was well-controlled. Given the relatively slow progression of the disease and the IOP being below 30 mmHg, canaloplasty was selected as the treatment option [7].

On the first day after the surgery, slit-lamp BMC showed two transparent DMDs in the inferonasal and inferotemporal quadrants, measuring approximately 4 × 4 mm and 4 × 5 mm in diameter, respectively. Additionally, a 3 mm hyphema was observed in the lower region of a well-defined AC, which did not affect the visual axis (Figure 1a). The transparent appearance of the DMDs confirmed the presence of viscoelastic material and aqueous humor within them, and they did not contain hematic material.

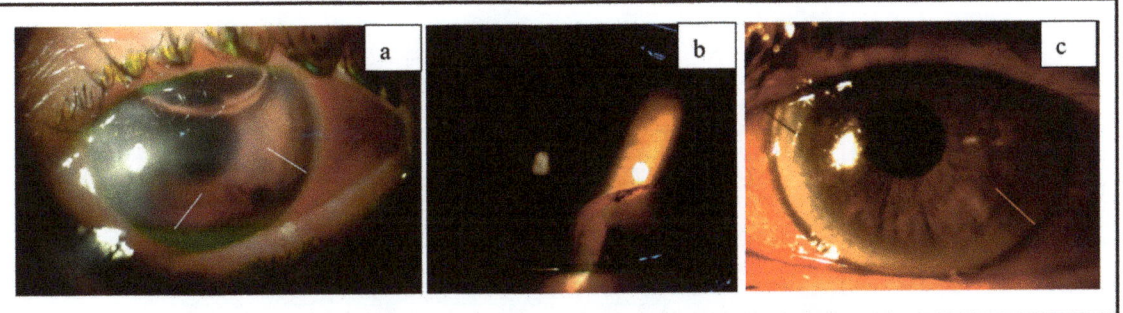

Figure 1. The BMC examination revealed two DMDs in the inferior quadrants, depicted by the white lines, along with a hyphema in the anterior chamber. Additionally, an air bubble was observed in the superior part of the anterior chamber (**a**). The second image (**b**) displays a hemorrhagic Descemet membrane detachment in the inferior temporal quadrant. Finally, the third image (**c**) shows a non-HDMD in the inferior temporal quadrant, indicated by the orange line.

2.3. Case 2

A 55-year-old woman diagnosed with uncontrolled primary OAG was chosen as a candidate for a combined phacocanaloplasty procedure. The patient was receiving treatment with topical prostaglandin analogs, and the Goldmann applanation tonometry measured the IOP at 24 mmHg. In terms of her ophthalmological history, the RE had previously undergone a successful phacoemulsification combined with non-penetrating deep sclerectomy (NPDS) surgery in 2020. Prior to the surgery, the BCVA was 1.0 in the RE and 0.3 in the LE. Slit-lamp BMC examination revealed the presence of a nuclear cataract and mild conjunctival hyperemia.

After a 24-h postoperative assessment, BMC examination showed corneal stromal edema and hemorrhagic Descemet membrane detachment (HDMD) in the lower temporal sector, measuring approximately 4 × 4 mm in diameter. The HDMD did not affect the visual axis, and an air bubble was observed in the upper AC. The IOP measured at this time was 17 mmHg.

2.4. Case 3

A 79-year-old woman was diagnosed with open-angle pseudoexfoliative glaucoma and had a history of trabeculectomy in her RE. Due to progressive glaucoma in her LE with an IOP of 27 mmHg, despite treatment with prostaglandin analogs and topical beta-blockers, it was decided to perform phacocanaloplasty. Slit-lamp BMC examination revealed the presence of a corticonuclear cataract. The BCVA prior to the surgery was 0.6.

On the first day after the surgery, a significant corneal edema was observed, which hindered the clear visualization of the inferior temporal DMD that was noted during the intraoperative period. The IOP measured at this time was 12 mmHg.

In all three cases, a treatment regimen consisting of topical antibiotics and corticosteroids was initiated, along with anti-edematous medication.

Anterior segment optical coherence tomography (AS-OCT) imaging using the Spectralis System from Heidelberg Engineering®, Heidelberg, Germany, displayed the presence of a retrocorneal hyperreflective membrane in all three cases. This membrane formed a pseudo-chamber with sinuous edges and contained a hypointense material corresponding to a DMD (Figure 2a,c). Additionally, in case 2, AS-OCT showed a hyperintense material corresponding to an HDMD (Figure 2b).

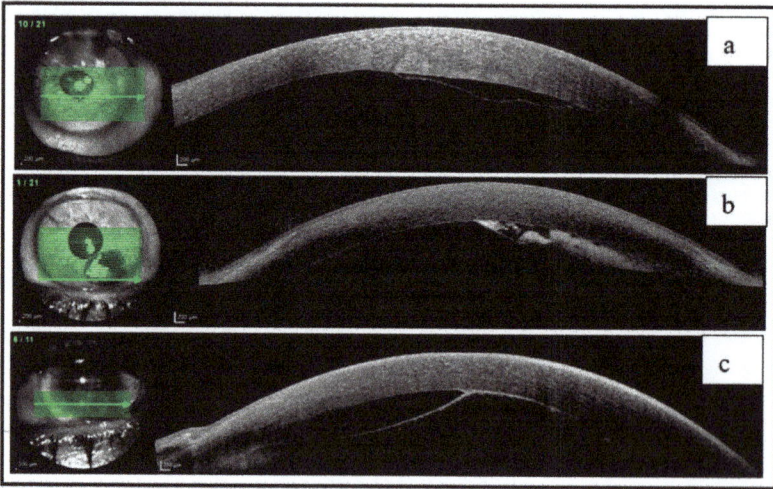

Figure 2. On the first postoperative day, AS-OCT of the LE revealed the presence of distinct DMDs in the inferior quadrants. The green lines represent horizontal cross-sections of the cornea, indicating the precise locations where the OCT scan has been performed.

The peripheral locations of the DMDs observed did not extend to the visual axis. Following the diagnosis, the DMD in the temporal position of case 1, which was larger and closer to the visual axis, was drained using a precise cornea blade. However, for the remaining cases, an initial period of expectant management was deemed suitable since the location and size of the DMDs did not have an impact on BCVA. In case 2, multiple follow-up visits were scheduled to closely monitor the hematic collection.

3. Results

The patients demonstrated positive progress during the 3-month follow-up period, with gradual improvement. In case 1, where the DMD was drained immediately after surgery, a faster resolution was observed. Follow-up examinations with BMC and SA-OCT indicated a gradual reduction in the detachment, eventually leading to its complete reapplication, and the BCVA after 3 months was 0.9 (Figures 3a and 4a). In case 2, the HDMD underwent oxidation, resulting in a residual pre-Descemetic intracorneal orange spot. However, this spot did not have any impact on vision, and the BCVA after 3 months was 1 (Figures 3b and 4b). In case 3, a minor localized disruption of Descemet's membrane was visible, without causing edema or affecting vision, and the BCVA after 3 months was 0.9 (Figures 3c and 4c). Six months post-surgery, the patients achieved a BCVA of 0.9–1, and their IOPs ranged between 12 and 15 mmHg. There was no evidence of structural or functional progression in their glaucoma condition (Table 1).

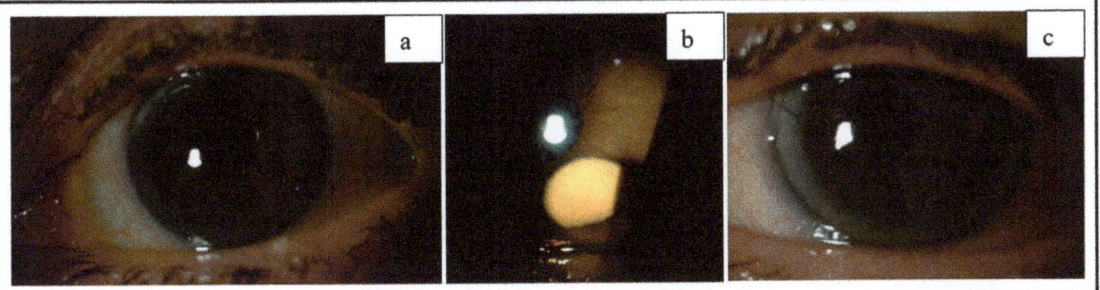

Figure 3. Three months after the surgery, BMC examination shows the progression of the DMDs in the lower corneal segment.

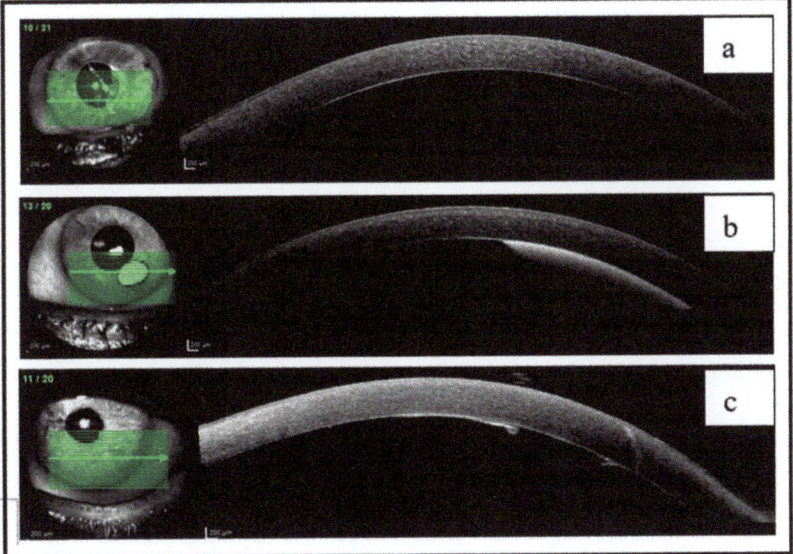

Figure 4. Three months post-surgery, the SA-OCT of the LE reveals different findings: in (**a**), there is a complete reapplication of the Descemet membrane after three months of observation; (**b**) shows a remaining intracorneal stain that does not have an impact on vision; in (**c**), a minor disruption of the DM is observed, but there is no corneal edema present.

Table 1. Baseline clinical features and visual outcome of DMDs.

Subject	Baseline BCVA	Surgery	Type of Dmd	Location of DMD	BCVA after DMD	Intervention	BCVA after 3 Months	Cornea Status
1	0.3	Phacocanaloplasty	Non-HDMD	Infero-nasal and infero-temporal	0.5	Postoperative drainage	0.9	Clear
2	0.4	Phacocanaloplasty	HDMD	Infero-temporal	0.7	Observation	1	Remnants of HDMD
3	0.6	Phacocanaloplasty	Non-HDMD	Infero-temporal	0.6	Intraoperative surgical drainage and air injection	0.9	Disruption of DM with no edema

4. Discussion

This research paper focuses on three cases of DMD that occurred in our center following phacocanaloplasty procedures. It is important to emphasize that this complication was observed exclusively in cases where combined surgery was performed, and it did not arise during standard canaloplasty procedures. It is worth highlighting that our center possesses a wealth of expertise and experience in performing canaloplasty and phacocanaloplasty procedures, having successfully completed a total of 180 interventions of this nature. This extensive experience contributes to our understanding and management of complications such as the DMDs observed in these cases.

Canaloplasty is a minimally invasive surgery for glaucoma that has proven effective in treating mild-to-moderate OAG and has demonstrated an excellent safety record [7]. Numerous studies have compared outcomes and complication rates between various glaucoma treatment techniques. In comparison to trabeculectomy, canaloplasty has shown similar postoperative success rates, lower complication rates, and higher patient satisfaction [3,8–11]. One of the major advantages of canaloplasty is its minimal complications and their limited clinical significance, particularly when compared to the presence of a filtering bleb. The secure closure of the superficial scleral flap eliminates patient discomfort, positive Seidel's test indicating wound leakage, and intraocular infections [7]. Hyphema, characterized by the reflux of blood from the SC towards the AC, is a common occurrence (with reported incidences ranging from 6.1 to 70%) resulting from the difference in intraocular and intravenous pressure [12–14]. This phenomenon is considered an early sign of the procedure's success, as it indicates the patency of natural drainage pathways [12]. DMD is a rare complication following nonpenetrating glaucoma surgery, including canaloplasty. Following standard phacoemulsification, recent reports indicate an occurrence of DMD ranging from 0.044% to 0.52% [15]. The reported incidence of DMD after canaloplasty varies from 1.6 to 9.1% [5,6,12,16–19], which is comparable to the findings of our study. In our center, we have conducted a series of 180 interventions over the past few years. The sample was carefully chosen to ensure comparability, and consisted of a population group that ensured comparability, with an equal distribution of men and women and similar average age. All surgeries were performed by the same surgical team, using a standardized technique and without any reported errors. The learning curve and guidance from the principal surgeon to the assistant surgeon are crucial, as a rapid withdrawal of the microcatheter or excessive pressure during sodium hyaluronate injection in the SC (more than one click or 1/8 turn every 2–3 clock hours) can lead to this complication [5]. Of the 180 surgeries, we observed DMD in three cases (1.67%). As mentioned earlier, the detachments in our study occurred after the withdrawal catheter and viscodilation procedure.

During canaloplasty, the occurrence of DMD is more frequent in one of the inferior quadrants [4], which aligns with our observations. This increased frequency in the inferior region is believed to be attributed to the higher pressure induced in that specific area. There are a few explanations for the different causes of this complication. The most widely supported hypothesis suggests that during the withdrawal of the microcatheter, the viscoelastic material injected may accumulate to a critical mass in the inferior quadrants of the SC, where it cannot exit easily through the ostia of the canal as it does in the upper quadrants. Furthermore, this situation may be exacerbated by a recoil effect in the viscoelastic material following the actuation of the device. The resistance within the canal may exceed the durability of the termination of DM at Schwalbe's line, leading to a prolapse of the viscoelastic material and triggering blood reflux between the corneal stroma and Descemet's membrane (DM) [4,5,20]. This intraluminal overpressure can occur due to obstructions or anatomic factors that make the cornea susceptible to weak adherence [13]. Additionally, bilateral DMD has been documented [21].

In our series of cases, all instances of DMDs occurred in the lower quadrants of the cornea and did not affect the visual axis. This percentage aligns with findings from other published articles [1,4,5].

Furthermore, based on our experience and from the existing literature [5], we have observed that this complication is more commonly seen in cases where combined surgery, specifically phacoemulsification combined with canaloplasty, is performed. This could be attributed to greater intraoperative hypotonia during these combined procedures. Alobeidan et al. [5] reported a 9.5% incidence of DMD in patients undergoing canaloplasty and phacocanaloplasty. Notably, they found that six out of ten cases occurred in combination with phacocanaloplasty and most cases of HDMD were observed in this group (Figure 5). It is worth mentioning that all our cases of DMD were encountered in the context of combined surgery (Figure 6).

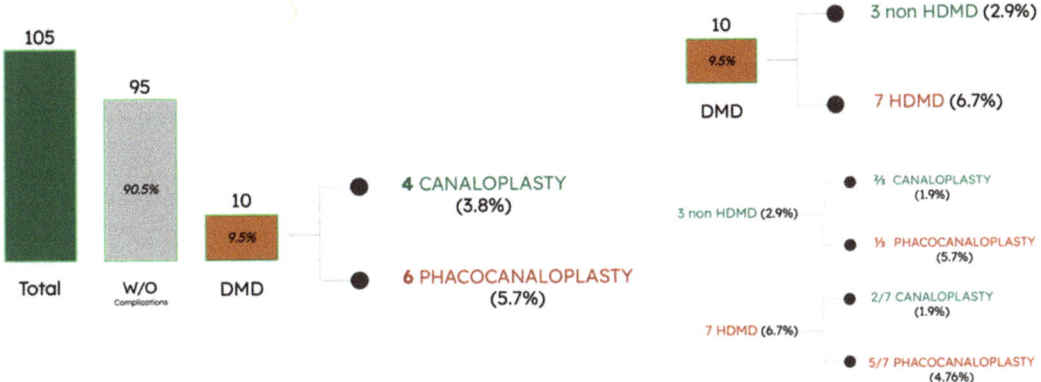

Figure 5. Incidence of DMD described by Alobeidan et al. [5], classified based on the type of surgery performed and the specific type of DMD.

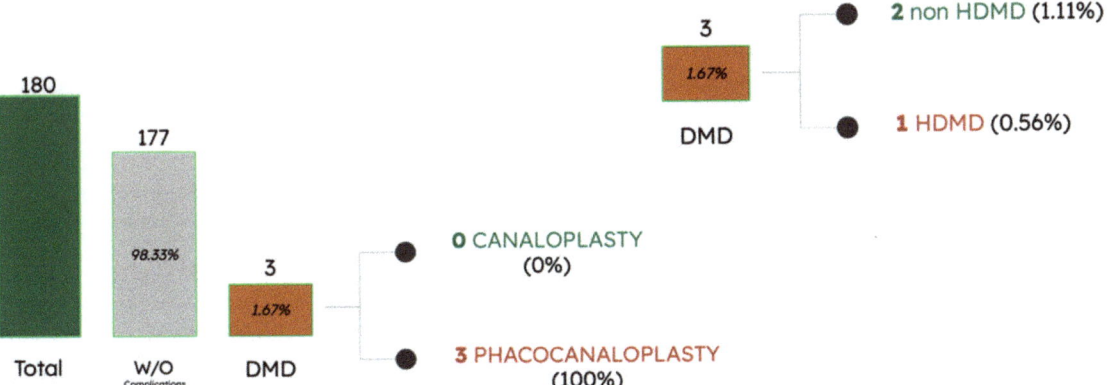

Figure 6. Incidence of DMD in our group, classified based on the type of surgery performed and the specific type of DMD.

These figures aim to illustrate the low frequency of the complication in various series, emphasizing the key significance of the type of surgery performed and the subtype of DMD.

DMDs can be classified into two primary categories: hemorrhagic and non-hemorrhagic. This distinction is crucial in managing this complication. As previously mentioned, DMDs commonly occur in the lower areas of the cornea after canaloplasty. The lower nasal region is particularly rich in collector channels, which connect episcleral veins to the SC [22]. This anatomical arrangement can result in the reflux of blood within the space formed by the DMD.

Another potential factor that can trigger blood reflux from the collector channels and contribute to HDMD is the aforementioned hypotonia during phacoemulsification in the same procedure [5,21]. Additional factors that can contribute to HDMD include the use of anticoagulant medications, anatomical changes in the SC such as changes in diameter and location [23], as well as preexisting stromal adherence to the Descemet membrane [24]. Collectively, these factors influence the development and severity of HDMD.

The management of the DMD depends primarily on its size, location, and content. Kumar et al. [25] proposed the HELP algorithm, which utilizes the height, extent, and relationship to the pupil based on AS-OCT for managing post-phacoemulsification DMD [15]. Non-conservative management is typically required for large detachments, especially those involving the visual axis or containing hemorrhagic DMD, and it is advisable to evaluate the risks/benefits and potentially withdraw anticoagulant medication. Various techniques have been described in the literature, such as neodymium: yttrium–aluminum–garnet (Nd: YAG) laser Descemet membranotomy, which is used to treat pre-Descemet hemorrhage [1,26]. This procedure helps prevent corneal blood staining and preserves corneal endothelium. It should be performed when the cornea appears free from opacities [27]. A recent novel treatment for severe cases of HDMD was described by Hamid et al. [28]. They suggested the use of tissue plasminogen activator (TPA) to quickly resolve the HDMD.

When surgical intervention is required [25], descemetopexy has emerged as the gold standard approach for managing DMD. This surgical technique involves filling the AC with an isoexpansile gas, such as perfluoropropane (C3F8) or sulfur hexafluoride (SF6), using a 26- or 30-gauge needle [29]. It is recommended to perform the paracentesis away from the DMD where the DM is still attached. The procedure begins with continuous drainage of aqueous fluid, followed by the injection of the gas [20]. Initially, descemetopexy was performed with air; however, its rapid absorption led to the adoption of isoexpansile gases [30].

To avoid postoperative pupillary block, the size of the gas bubble should be reduced to two-thirds of the AC. If a complete gas-filled chamber is left, it is advisable to perform an inferior peripheral iridectomy. After the procedure, the patient must maintain a supine position until the gas bubble is reabsorbed and the DM is reattached.

Considering that this procedure might lead to a raised IOP and pupillary block glaucoma in 11.6% of patients [29,30], the use of cycloplegic drops and preoperative laser peripheral iridotomy to prevent this complication could be a prudent approach, especially in glaucomatous patients [15,31].

Conservative therapy for managing the condition involves the use of topical steroids to control inflammation and reduce the fibrosis. Additionally, hyperosmotic agents can be employed to clear corneal edema and improve VA [15].

In our case, due to its broader extension and closer proximity to the central cornea, we chose the less invasive approach for pre-Descemet drainage using a blade incision on the inferotemporal region of the DMD [32,33]. The interface was then rinsed with a balanced saline solution to remove any remaining OVD.

When the type and duration of the OVD used are known, the material gradually disappears, allowing the Descemet's membrane to coapt without further manipulation.

Several authors have recommended expectant management for small detachments with regular edges located in peripheral regions and containing visco-aqueous content, as these cases have been observed to reattach spontaneously [34].

5. Conclusions

In conclusion, Descemet's membrane detachment (DMD) represents a relatively infrequent but significant complication, particularly in the context of glaucoma and cataract surgeries. Despite the advancements in surgical techniques and understanding, the precise etiology of this complication remains elusive. While suspicions exist regarding the potential role of micro-ruptures within Schlemm's canal during viscodilation, further research is required to establish a definitive cause.

To address the challenge of DMD prevention, meticulous attention and caution during viscodilation procedures are paramount. Implementing strategies to minimize the risk of micro-ruptures, such as precise surgical manipulation and controlled pressure application, could potentially contribute to reducing the incidence of DMD.

Furthermore, it is imperative to recognize the considerable advantages that combined surgeries offer in terms of convenience and lowered healthcare expenses. Nevertheless, it is crucial to maintain awareness regarding the potential susceptibility to DMD resulting from postoperative hypotony.

In cases where DMD extends and impacts the visual axis, prompt intervention through external drainage techniques becomes imperative. By ensuring the preservation of best-corrected visual acuity (BCVA) and preventing the progression of visual impairment, these interventions play a critical role in maintaining patients' ocular health and overall quality of life.

For smaller cases of DMD that do not encroach upon the visual axis, an approach of vigilant observation and conservative management is often warranted. Regular monitoring and periodic assessments are essential in order to promptly detect any changes that might necessitate intervention.

Continued research efforts are necessary to deepen our understanding of the mechanisms underlying DMD and to develop more precise preventive measures and effective management strategies. Collaborative endeavors between ophthalmologists and researchers are pivotal in advancing our knowledge and refining clinical practices to further enhance patient outcomes and minimize the impact of Descemet's membrane detachment in ophthalmic surgeries.

Author Contributions: M.O.d.R.: writing—review and editing, investigation, software, conceptualization, project administration; J.M.M.: data curation, resources; E.P.C.: visualization; D.P.G.: formal analysis; I.P.N.: investigation; F.J.A.P.: funding acquisition, writing—review and editing, validation; J.A.C.: visualization; J.I.A.: project administration, supervision, writing—review, and editing, investigation, methodology. All authors have read and agreed to the published version of the manuscript.

Funding: This research received no external funding.

Institutional Review Board Statement: The study did not require ethical approval.

Informed Consent Statement: Informed consent was obtained from all subjects involved in the study. Written informed consent has been obtained from the patients to publish this paper.

Data Availability Statement: Data is unavailable due to privacy.

Acknowledgments: We would like to express our gratitude to the glaucoma department, which guided us throughout this project and inspired us with their work.

Conflicts of Interest: The authors declare no conflict of interest.

References

1. Robert, M.-C.; Harasymowycz, P. Hemorrhagic Descemet Detachment After Combined Canaloplasty and Cataract Surgery. *Cornea* **2013**, *32*, 712–713. [CrossRef] [PubMed]
2. Beres, H.; Scharioth, G.B. Canaloplasty in the spotlight: Surgical alternatives and future perspectives. *Rom. J. Ophthalmol.* **2022**, *66*, 225–232. [CrossRef]
3. Zhang, B.; Kang, J.; Chen, X. A System Review and Meta-Analysis of Canaloplasty Outcomes in Glaucoma Treatment in Comparison with Trabeculectomy. *J. Ophthalmol.* **2017**, *2017*, 2723761. [CrossRef] [PubMed]

4. Konopińska, J.; Mariak, Z.; Rękas, M. Improvement of the safety profile of canaloplasty and phacocanaloplasty: A review of complications and their management. *J. Ophthalmol.* **2020**, *2020*, 8352827. [CrossRef] [PubMed]
5. Alobeidan, S.A.; Almobarak, F.A. Incidence and management of haemorrhagic Descemet membrane detachment in canaloplasty and phacocanaloplasty. *Acta Ophthalmol.* **2015**, *94*, e298–e304. [CrossRef] [PubMed]
6. Grieshaber, M.C. Viscocanalostomy and Canaloplasty: Ab Externo Schlemm's Canal Surgery. *Dev. Ophthalmol.* **2017**, *59*, 113–126. [CrossRef] [PubMed]
7. Byszewska, A.; Konopińska, J.; Kicińska, A.K.; Mariak, Z.; Rękas, M. Canaloplasty in the Treatment of Primary Open-Angle Glaucoma: Patient Selection and Perspectives. *Clin. Ophthalmol.* **2019**, *13*, 2617–2629. [CrossRef]
8. Khaimi, M.A. Canaloplasty: A minimally invasive and maximally effective glaucoma treatment. *J. Ophthalmol.* **2015**, *2015*, 485065. [CrossRef]
9. Vold, S.D.; Williamson, B.K.; Hirsch, L.; Aminlari, A.E.; Cho, A.S.; Nelson, C.; Dickerson, J.E., Jr. Canaloplasty and trabeculotomy with the OMNI system in pseudophakic patients with open-angle glaucoma: The ROMEO study. *Ophthalmol. Glaucoma* **2021**, *4*, 173–181. [CrossRef]
10. Schoenberg, E.D.; Chaudhry, A.L.; Chod, R.; Zurakowski, D.; Ayyala, R.S. Comparison of surgical outcomes between phacocanaloplasty and phacotrabeculectomy at 12 months' follow-up: A longitudinal cohort study. *J. Glaucoma* **2015**, *24*, 543–549. [CrossRef]
11. Brüggemann, A.; Despouy, J.T.; Wegent, A.; Müller, M. Intraindividual comparison of Canaloplasty versus trabeculectomy with mitomycin C in a single-surgeon series. *J. Glaucoma* **2013**, *22*, 577–583. [CrossRef] [PubMed]
12. Lewis, R.A.; von Wolff, K.; Tetz, M.; Korber, N.; Kearney, J.R.; Shingleton, B.; Samuelson, T.W. Canaloplasty: Circumferential viscodilation and tensioning of Schlemm's canal using a flexible microcatheter for the treatment of open-angle glaucoma in adults. *J. Cataract. Refract. Surg.* **2007**, *33*, 1217–1226. [CrossRef] [PubMed]
13. Koch, J.M.; Heiligenhaus, A.; Heinz, C. Canaloplasty and transient anterior chamber haemorrhage: A prognostic factor? *Klin. Monbl. Augenheilkd.* **2011**, *228*, 465–467. [CrossRef] [PubMed]
14. Lopes-Cardoso, I.; Esteves, F.; Amorim, M.; Calvão-Santos, G.; Freitas, M.L.; Salgado-Borges, J. Viscocanalostomía circunferencial con sutura de tensión en el canal de Schlemm (canaloplastia): Un año de experiencia. *Arch. Soc. Esp. Oftalmol.* **2013**, *88*, 207–215. [CrossRef] [PubMed]
15. Singhal, D.; Sahay, P.; Goel, S.; Asif, M.I.; Maharana, P.K.; Sharma, N. Descemet membrane detachment. *Surv. Ophthalmol.* **2020**, *65*, 279–293. [CrossRef] [PubMed]
16. Jaramillo, A.; Foreman, J.; Ayyala, R.S. Descemet membrane detachment after canaloplasty: Incidence and management. *J. Glaucoma* **2014**, *23*, 351–354. [CrossRef] [PubMed]
17. Ayyala, R.S.; Chaudhry, A.L.; Okogbaa, C.B.; Zurakowski, D. Comparison of surgical outcomes between canaloplasty and trabeculectomy at 12 months' follow-up. *Ophthalmology* **2011**, *118*, 2427–2433. [CrossRef] [PubMed]
18. Bull, H.; von Wolff, K.; Körber, N.; Tetz, M. Three-year canaloplasty outcomes for the treatment of open-angle glaucoma: European study results. Graefe s Archive for Clinical and Experimental. *Ophthalmology* **2011**, *249*, 1537–1545. [CrossRef]
19. Brusini, P. Canaloplasty in Open-Angle Glaucoma Surgery: A Four-Year Follow-Up. *Sci. World J.* **2014**, *2014*, 469609. [CrossRef]
20. Djavanmardi, S.; Arciniegas-Perasso, C.A.; Duch, S.; Avila-Marrón, E.; Milla, E. Hemorrhagic Descemet's membrane detachment in nonpenetrating glaucoma surgery: A rare and relevant complication. *J. Glaucoma* **2021**, *30*, 352–356. [CrossRef]
21. Palmiero, P.-M.; Aktas, Z.; Lee, O.; Tello, C.; Sbeity, Z. Bilateral Descemet membrane detachment after canaloplasty. *J. Cataract Refract. Surg.* **2010**, *36*, 508–511. [CrossRef] [PubMed]
22. Bentley, M.D.; Hann, C.R.; Fautsch, M.P. Anatomical variation of human collector channel orifices. *Investig. Ophthalmol. Vis. Sci.* **2016**, *57*, 1153–1159. [CrossRef] [PubMed]
23. Irshad, F.A.; Mayfield, M.S.; Zurakowski, D.; Ayyala, R.S. Variation in schlemm's canal diameter and location by ultrasound biomicroscopy. *Ophthalmology* **2010**, *117*, 916–920. [CrossRef] [PubMed]
24. Rasouli, M.; Mather, R.; Tingey, D. Descemet membrane detachment following viscoelastic injection for posttrabeculectomy hypotony. *J. Cataract Refract. Surg.* **2008**, *43*, 254–255. [CrossRef] [PubMed]
25. Kumar, D.A.; Agarwal, A.; Sivanganam, S.; Chandrasekar, R. Height-, extent-, length-, and pupil-based (HELP) algorithm to manage post-phacoemulsification Descemet membrane detachment. *J. Cataract Refract. Surg.* **2015**, *41*, 1945–1953. [CrossRef] [PubMed]
26. Kim, Y.J.; Kim, M.J.; Tchah, H.; Kim, J.Y. Descemet membranotomy with an Nd:YAG laser can be used to treat pre-Descemet hemorrhage. *Cornea* **2012**, *31*, 206–208. [CrossRef] [PubMed]
27. Weng, Y.; Ren, Y.-P.; Zhang, L.; Huang, X.-D.; Shen-Tu, X.-C. An alternative technique for Descemet's membrane detachment following phacoemulsification: Case report and review of literature. *BMC Ophthalmol.* **2017**, *17*, 109. [CrossRef] [PubMed]
28. Hamid, M.; Thompson, P.; Harasymowycz, P. Novel treatment for hemorrhagic Descemet detachment after canaloplasty. *Cornea* **2015**, *34*, 1611–1612. [CrossRef]
29. Desprendimiento de Membrana de Descemet Postquirúrgico, una Complicación Inusual, Pero Importante. FacoElche. 2019. Available online: Facoelche.com (accessed on 18 April 2023).
30. Jain, R.; Murthy, S.I.; Basu, S.; Ali, M.H.; Sangwan, V.S. Anatomic and visual outcomes of descemetopexy in post-cataract surgery descemet's membrane detachment. *Ophthalmology* **2013**, *120*, 1366–1372. [CrossRef]

31. Fan, N.-W. Outcomes of repeat descemetopexy in post-cataract surgery descemet membrane detachment. *Am. J. Ophthalmol.* **2014**, *157*, 1330–1331. [CrossRef]
32. Chow, V.W.S.; Agarwal, T.; Vajpayee, R.B.; Jhanji, V. Update on diagnosis and management of Descemet's membrane detachment. *Curr. Opin. Ophthalmol.* **2013**, *24*, 356–361. [CrossRef]
33. Freiberg, F.J.; Salgado, J.P.; Grehn, F.; Klink, T. Intracorneal hematoma after canaloplasty and clear cornea phacoemulsification: Surgical management. *Eur. J. Ophthalmol.* **2012**, *22*, 823–825. [CrossRef]
34. Gallego-Pinazo, R.; López-Sánchez, E.; Marín-Montiel, J. Hemorrhagic Descemet's membrane detachment after viscocanalostomy. *Arch. Soc. Esp. Oftalmol.* **2010**, *85*, 110–113. [CrossRef]

Disclaimer/Publisher's Note: The statements, opinions and data contained in all publications are solely those of the individual author(s) and contributor(s) and not of MDPI and/or the editor(s). MDPI and/or the editor(s) disclaim responsibility for any injury to people or property resulting from any ideas, methods, instructions or products referred to in the content.

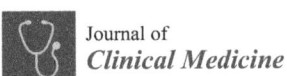

Article

Italian Candidates for the XEN Implant: An Overview from the Glaucoma Treatment Registry (XEN-GTR)

Chiara Posarelli [1,*], Michele Figus [1], Gloria Roberti [2], Sara Giammaria [2], Giorgio Ghirelli [3], Pierpaolo Quercioli [3], Tommaso Micelli Ferrari [4], Vincenzo Pace [4], Leonardo Mastropasqua [5], Luca Agnifili [5], Matteo Sacchi [6], Gianluca Scuderi [7], Andrea Perdicchi [7], Romeo Altafini [8], Maurizio Uva [9], Dino D'Andrea [10], Giuseppe Covello [1], Maria Novella Maglionico [1], Antonio Maria Fea [11], Carmela Carnevale [2] and Francesco Oddone [2]

1. Department of Surgical, Medical, Molecular Pathology and of Critical Area, University of Pisa, 56124 Pisa, Italy
2. IRCCS Fondazione Bietti, 00198 Rome, Italy
3. Ospedale San Pietro, Fatebenefratelli, 00186 Rome, Italy
4. Ospedale Generale Regionale F. Miulli di Acquaviva delle Fonti, 70021 Bari, Italy
5. Ophthalmology Clinic, Department of Medicine and Aging Science, University G. D'Annunzio of Chieti-Pescara, 66100 Chieti, Italy
6. University Eye Clinic, San Giuseppe Hospital, University of Milan, 20162 Milan, Italy
7. Ophthalmology Unit, NESMOS Department, S. Andrea Hospital, Faculty of Medicine and Psychology, University of Rome La Sapienza, 00189 Rome, Italy
8. Ospedale di Dolo, 30031 Venice, Italy
9. Azienda Ospedaliera Universitaria, "Policlinico Vittorio Emanuele", P.O. Gaspare Rodolico, 95123 Catania, Italy
10. Ospedale Dell'Aquila, 67100 L'Aquila, Italy
11. Ophthalmic Eye Hospital, Department of Surgical Sciences, University of Turin, 10122 Turin, Italy
* Correspondence: chiara.posarelli@med.unipi.it; Tel.: +39-050997675

Abstract: Background The Italian XEN Glaucoma Treatment Registry (XEN-GTR) was created to acquire a comprehensive prospective dataset that includes the patient characteristics, intraoperative variables, and postoperative management of glaucoma patients undergoing the XEN gel stent implantation. **Methods** This was a prospective observational, longitudinal clinical study involving 10 centres throughout Italy. The baseline examination included a comprehensive evaluation of demographic parameters (age, sex, ethnicity, and systemic condition), specific ophthalmological parameters, and quality of life questionnaire score collection. **Results** The baseline data of 273 patients were analysed. The median (IQR) age was 72 (65.0 to 78.0) years. Of the 273 patients, 123 (45%) were female and 150 (55%) were male. A total of 86% of the patients had open-angle glaucoma with a mean intraocular pressure of 24 ± 6 (range 12.0–60.0) mmHg. The mean number of medications was 2.7 ± 0.9 at baseline for the patients with a prevalence of prostaglandin analogues combined with a beta-blocker and anhydrase carbonic inhibitor (31.8%). The mean scores of the NEI-VFQ 25 and GSS questionnaires were 78 ± 18 (range 26.5–100) and 85 ± 14 (range 79–93), respectively. Combined XEN/cataract surgeries were scheduled in 73.7% of the patients. The preferred place for the XEN implant was the supero-nasal quadrant (91.6%). **Conclusions** Observing the baseline characteristics of the typical Italian candidates for the XEN gel implant shows that they are patients affected by POAG and cataracts, with moderate to severe glaucoma damage, all of which has an impact on their quality of life.

Keywords: glaucoma; surgical treatment; XEN gel; outcomes; real-life; registry

1. Introduction

Real-world observational studies have become increasingly important in providing evidence of treatment effectiveness in clinical practice. While randomized clinical trials are the gold standard for evaluating the safety and efficacy of new therapeutic strategies, necessarily strict inclusion and exclusion criteria mean that trial populations might limit the generalizability of their results and are often not representative of the target patient population encountered in clinical practice.

Moreover, real-world studies can provide information on the long-term safety and effectiveness of treatments in heterogeneous populations [1], as well as information on utilisation patterns and health and economic outcomes.

It has been well established that glaucoma is associated with a reduction of quality of life (QoL), and that QoL decreases with advancing disease severity [2]. Increased attention to QoL has emerged in recent years and new surgical techniques have been designed to reduce the possible morbidity connected with traditional glaucoma surgery [3,4]. One promising technique involves the use of the XEN gel implant (XEN, Allergan, Dublin, Ireland), which is a biocompatible 6 mm gelatine microtube designed to create a channel from the anterior chamber to the subconjunctival space and to allow aqueous humour outflow, and it has a minimally invasive procedure when inserted through a small corneal incision [5–9].

The purpose of the Italian XEN Glaucoma Treatment Registry (XEN-GTR), an observational, prospective, longitudinal clinical study, is to obtain a comprehensive prospective dataset that includes patients' characteristics, intraoperative variables, and postoperative management patterns for analysis of the effectiveness, safety, quality of life, and cost-effectiveness outcomes of the treatment.

The baseline characteristics of the first 273 Italian patients enrolled are described herein and could represent an overview of the typical Italian candidates for the XEN implant.

2. Materials and Methods

2.1. Study Design and Patient Population

This is a prospective, observational study involving 10 centres throughout Italy. Consecutive patients diagnosed with glaucoma and deemed to be suitable for the XEN implant, according to the normal indications and procedures of the attending ophthalmologist, were considered for inclusion if the following criteria were met: age > 18 years, ability to understand and sign written informed consent, diagnosis of open-angle glaucoma according to the diagnostic criteria of the 5th edition of the Guidelines of the European Glaucoma Society [10], and an indication for treatment with the XEN implant, in the opinion of the ophthalmologist treating the patient, such as glaucoma progression or uncontrolled IOP despite medical treatment. Patients who needed cataract surgery in combination with glaucoma surgery were also included as patients with primary angle closure glaucoma, with indications for the XEN45 implant, only if it was combined with phacoemulsification.

The exclusion criteria included the following: secondary glaucoma (different from pseudoexfoliation and pigmentary glaucoma); the presence of conjunctival scarring or conjunctival pathologies (e.g., pterygium) in the target quadrant; signs of active inflammation (e.g., blepharitis, conjunctivitis, keratitis, or uveitis); active iris neovascularization or the presence of iris neo-vessels within 6 months of the date of surgery; intraocular lenses in the anterior chamber; the presence of intraocular silicone oil; vitreous humor in the anterior chamber; altered episcleral venous drainage (e.g., Sturge–Weber syndrome or nanophthalmos); known or suspected allergy or sensitization to drugs required for the surgical procedure or for some component of the device (e.g., glutaraldehyde or porcine derivatives); and a history of keloid scars. If a patient needed surgery in both eyes, only the data of the first eye were included in the register.

The baseline clinical data were collected before surgery (1 to 4 weeks before surgery, at visit 0) and included the demographic and ophthalmologic variables listed in Table 1. The data collected on the day of surgery (visit 1) were strictly related to the procedure and to the surgeon's habits (Table 1).

Table 1. Reporting form recording the study visits and variables registered at baseline.

Study Visit	Time	Variables Registered	
		Demographic	Ophthalmological
Visit 0	1 to 4 weeks before surgery	• Age • Sex • Ethnicity • Systemic condition	• Type of Glaucoma • Lens state • Previous surgery • BCVA • IOP • Gonioscopy • Medications • VF • RNFL OCT • Indirect ophthalmoscopy • ECC • NEI-VFQ 25 • GSS
Visit 1	Day of surgery		• Type of surgery • Surgeon position • XEN position • OVD • XEN features • Bleb formation • Intra-operative complication • Post-operative treatment

OP, intraocular pressure; BCVA, best-corrected visual acuity; VF, visual field; RNFL OCT, retinal nerve fibre layer thickness optical coherence tomography; ECC, endothelial cell count; NEI-VFQ 25, National Eye Institute Visual Function Questionnaire-25; GSS, Glaucoma Symptoms Scale; OVD, ophthalmic viscosurgical device.

Eligible patients, after signing a written informed consent form, underwent a comprehensive eye examination and medical and ocular history evaluation. The eye examination included a best-corrected visual acuity (BCVA) assessment, a slit lamp evaluation, a gonioscopy, an IOP measurement using Goldmann applanation tonometry (the average of 3 measurements was considered for the analysis), and an indirect dilated ophthalmoscopy with a 90 dioptres lens.

A visual field test (standard white-on-white perimetry), retinal nerve fibre layer thickness optical coherence tomography (OCT), and an endothelial cell count were also performed.

The endothelial cell count was performed by means of non-contact specular microscopy, and the average of 5 measurements was considered for the study purposes.

During the visit, patients were also asked to complete the Italian version of two questionnaires: the NEI-VFQ-25 and the GSS [11,12].

2.2. Statistical Analysis

Continuous data are described as means and standard deviations if normally distributed or as medians and interquartiles if not normally distributed. Categorical and nominal data are described as frequencies.

3. Results

Between January 2018 and October 2020, 273 patients were enrolled.

One hundred and fifty patients were male (55%), while one hundred and twenty-three patients were female (45%). The median (IQR) age was 72.0 (65.0 to 78.0) years, with a frequency of comorbidities such as hypertension (47.6%, 130/273), diabetes (13.6%, 37/273), and autoimmune diseases (5.9%, 16/273). Anticoagulant therapy was being undertaken by 16.5% (45/273) of the patients.

Baseline ophthalmological data are reported in Tables 2 and 3. According to perimetry classification [13], 105/273 (42.7%) patients were classified as having severe glaucoma (mean defect of worse than −12 dB), 66/273 (26.8%) as having moderate glaucoma (mean defect of between -6 to −12 dB), and 58/273 (23.6%) as having early glaucoma (mean defect of better than −6 dB), respectively. The data of 44 patients (16.12%) were not available.

Table 2. Baseline ophthalmological data in the XEN-GTR.

Parameters	Mean Value ± SD	Range
BCVA (decimal)	0.53 ± 0.3	0.1–1
Spherical equivalent (dioptres)	−0.7 ± 2.5	−25.5–4.5
Anterior chamber depth (mm)	3.4 ± 0.8	2–6
Axial length (mm)	24.3 ± 2.4	20–35
Endothelial cell count (cell/mm^2)	2108 ± 461	600–3076
Lens status, no. (%)	127 (46.5%) pseudophakic 145 (53.1%) phakic 1 (0.3%) aphakic	

EN-GTR, XEN Glaucoma Treatment Registry; BCVA, best-corrected visual acuity; SD, standard deviation.

Table 3. Baseline ophthalmological parameters describing the glaucoma condition of the enrolled patients in the XEN-GTR.

Parameters	Mean Value ± SD	Range
IOP (mmHg)	24 ± 6	12–60
Ophthalmoscopic cup/disc ratio	0.7 ± 0.14	0.3–1
CCT (μm)	523 ± 38	424–650
MD (dB)	−12.3 ± 8.6	−33–4
RNFL thickness (μm)	68 ± 19	0.63–120

OP, intraocular pressure; CCT, central corneal thickness; MD, mean deviation; RNFL, retinal nerve fibre layer; SD, standard deviation; XEN-GTR, XEN Glaucoma Treatment Registry.

The patients' previous ocular surgeries and laser procedures are reported in Table 4.

Table 4. Previous ocular surgeries and laser procedures of the patients enrolled in the XEN-GTR (no. (%)).

Previous Ocular Surgeries and Laser Procedures	
None	141 (51.6%)
Cataract surgery	116 (42.5%)
Trabeculectomy	1 (0.4%)
Combined surgery (phacotrabeculectomy)	2 (0.7%)
Selective laser trabeculoplasty/argon laser trabeculoplasty	6 (2.2%)
Retinal detachment	1 (0.4%)
Other	5 (1.8%)
Not answered	1 (0.4%)

EN-GTR, XEN Glaucoma Treatment Registry.

The types of glaucoma of the patients enrolled in the study were primary open-angle glaucoma (87.2%, 238/273), pseudoexfoliative (6.6%, 18/273), primary angle closure glaucoma (2.6%, 7/273), uveitic (2.1%, 6/273), steroid-induced (1.1%, 3/273), and post-traumatic (0.4%, 1/273) glaucoma.

The mean number of medications taken by the patients was 2.7 ± 0.9; however, 42.9% (117/273) of the patients used 3 active compounds, 2.5% (7/273) used 4 active compounds, and 16.1% (44/273) used 5 active compounds (including systemic carbonic anhydrase inhibitors). The patients' drug regimens are represented in Table 5. Thirty-one percent of patients (85/273) were also using systemic carbonic anhydrase inhibitors.

Table 5. Treatment regimens of the patients enrolled in the XEN-GTR (no. (%)).

Compound	N (%)
BBA2	1 (0.3)
CAI	2 (0.7)
BBCAI preserved	3 (1.1)
PGBB preserved	4 (1.4)
A2CAI	4 (1.4)
PG preserved	5 (1.8)
BB	6 (2.2)
A2CAI + BBPG	7 (2.5)
A2CAI + PG	7 (2.5)
PG	15 (5.5)
BBCAI	19 (6.9)
PG + BBA2	23 (8.4)
PGBB	40 (14.6)
PG + BBCAI + A2	44 (16.1)
PG + BBCAI	87 (31.8)
NA	1 (0.3)
No medications	5 (1.8)

B, beta-blocker; PG, prostaglandin analogues; CAI, carbonic anhydrase inhibitors; A2, alfa2 adrenergic agonists; XEN-GTR, XEN Glaucoma Treatment Registry.

The mean score of the NEI-VFQ 25 was 78 ± 18 (range 26.5–100), while the mean score of the GSS was 85 ± 14 (range 79–93), and only 60 patients competed the questionnaires. Linear regression analysis was performed at baseline between the baseline NEI-VFQ 25 score and the MD (Figure 1). The Spearman correlation coefficient was 0.42, with a 95% bootstrap CI: 0.07–0.60 (1000 bootstrap replications). The regression coefficient was 0.80 (p = 0.002). In our series, the patients with a worse MD value presented a lower NEI-VFQ score.

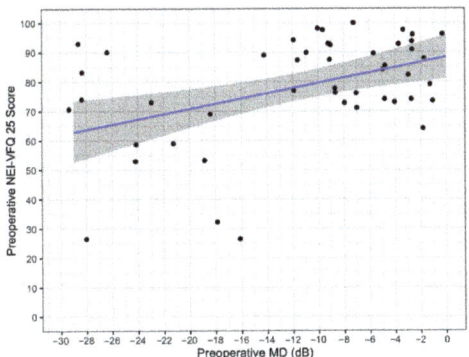

Figure 1. Preoperative NEI VFQ25 vs. preoperative MD.

All the patients (273/273) underwent implantation preceded by a subconjunctival injection of 0.1 mL of mitomycin C (0.2 mg/mL), and 39.9% (109/273) of the implantations were performed in combination with cataract surgeries. The ophthalmic viscosurgical device used was cohesive in 90.11% of the cases (246/273), dispersive in 6.96% of the cases (19/273), and Duovisc® (Alcon Laboratoires, Fort Worth, TX, USA) in 3.14% of patients (8/273). The surgeon's position was mainly superior (178/273), but in 34.79% of the cases, it was temporal.

The implant was in a supero-nasal position in 91.58% of the cases (250/273), nasal in 4.39% of the cases (12/273), superior in 1.47% of the cases (4/273), supero-temporal in 1.47% of the cases (4/273), and temporal in 1.09% of the cases (3/273). The estimated depth was subconjunctival in 89.01% of the cases (243/273). Of the remaining cases, 7.3% (20/273) of the implants were judged as subtenonian and 3.66% (10/273) were judged as undeterminable. The XEN subconjunctival course immediately after implantation was linear in 86.45% (236/273) of the patients, curved in 1.47% (4/273), and undeterminable in 12.09% (33/273).

The implant was visible in the anterior chamber in 90.10% of the patients' eyes (246/273). In 4.03% (11/273) of the patients, the XEN was visible in the anterior chamber only gonioscopically, and in 5.86% (16/273) of the patients, it was not visible at all.

Bleb formation was noted in 87.67% (239/273) of the patients; a flat bleb was observed in 12.45% (34/273) of the patients.

Intraoperative complications were seen in 39.93% of the cases (109/273), consisting of microscopic hyphema (73/273), mild hyphema (Grade I; 34/273), and conjunctival tears (2/273).

One week after surgery, 4/273 patients were treated with an active compound (3 patients with BB and 1 with PG) and 3/273 with two active compounds (BB and CAI).

4. Discussion

When a new surgical intervention becomes available, questions regarding its effectiveness and safety in comparison with established techniques and questions regarding the ideal patient candidate are required to be answered to determine its best placement in the therapeutic algorithm of a specific disease.

Disease progression, worsening QoL, and poor adherence should guide glaucoma specialists toward changing from a maximal tolerated medical treatment to selective laser trabeculoplasty, an MIGS, or a traditional surgery [10].

The XEN-GTR represents a national prospective glaucoma surgery registry in Italy, and it has been designed to prospectively collect multicentre, real-world data about the indications and use, alone or in combination with cataract surgery, of the XEN gel implant across a time-frame of 36 months. The XEN gel implant is a device designed for a minimally invasive surgical treatment of glaucoma and has been available in Italy since the year 2016. It represents the first ab-interno device designed for the subconjunctival filtration of the aqueous humour by acting as a shunt between the anterior chamber and the subconjunctival space, thus bypassing the outflow resistance of the trabecular meshwork and beyond [5–9].

From the data, is clear that the time of surgical indication may be adjusted based on the stage of the disease, the glaucoma therapy-related ocular surface disease, and the quality of life of the patient, and this has already been demonstrated in previous publications [14–17].

Among the potential advantages of the XEN gel implant over other established techniques such as trabeculectomy, there is a significantly reduced surgical time and a lack of conjunctival incisions, with potential advantages in terms of reduced inflammation and scarring [8,18–23].

The basal profile of the candidate patient for this kind of surgery within the Italian XEN-GTR is characterized by an average IOP of 24.0 mmHg with a wide variation spanning from 12 to 60 mmHg and by an average visual field defect, as expressed by the MD of -12 dB, and again with a wide variation spanning from -4 dB to -33 dB. Interestingly, the XEN gel implant in Italy has been proposed not only in patients with early to moderate glaucoma, but also in patients with severe glaucoma who are traditionally candidates for trabeculectomy.

Most of the enrolled population was represented by POAG (90%), and a smaller proportion of patients with secondary glaucoma was also enrolled and included pseudoexfoliative, uveitic, steroid-induced, and post-traumatic glaucoma. Considering that those categories of patients do not represent the primary indications of the XEN gel implant, it will be of great interest to explore the effectiveness and safety results in such challenging cases over the 36 months of planned follow-up for the study.

The preservation of QoL at a sustainable cost is the ultimate goal of any glaucoma treatment [10], and within the XEN-GTR, QoL measures such as the NEI VFQ-25 and GSS were recorded at baseline and will be monitored over time. It is noteworthy that collecting QoL data in our clinical practice represents an important limit because it takes time and our patients did not fully comprehend the significance of that information. Our preliminary data showed how patients with worse MD values presented lower NEI-VFQ scores. Therefore, it is fundamental to raise awareness about this topic and to stress the importance of collecting such data using questionnaires.

It is interesting to highlight that the XEN was implanted as a unique intervention in 164 (60.1%) patients, of which 10 were phakic, and in which 109 (39.9%) received the implant in combination with cataract surgery, thus indicating either that the XEN as a solo procedure in phakic eyes is not a procedure of choice for most surgeons in Italy or that the coexistence of glaucoma and cataracts is highly prevalent.

Despite the surgical technique for the XEN gel implant being standardized, some variations were undertaken within the XEN-GTR cohort, mainly regarding the implant location, in which a minority of cases (8.42%, 23/273) was different from the recommended supero-nasal quadrant and the type of ophthalmic viscosurgical device used, which was, in a majority of the cases, cohesive (90.11%).

When the XEN device is implanted, even by an expert surgeon, its depth with respect to the conjunctival and tenonian planes is known to be hardly predictable, even though a consistent surgical technique is demanded. Within the XEN-GTR cohort, in 89.01% of the cases, the depth of the implant was judged as subconjunctival, while in the remaining cases, it was judged as subtenonian. In 10 cases, it was judged as not determinable.

When the implant is released, its course may be found to be linear or curved under the tissues again, even if a consistent surgical technique is used. The linearity of the implant is likely to be related to the presence of subconjunctival tissue at the tip of the implant, which prevents its distension over the underlying tissue planes. Within the XEN-GTR, while immediately after implantation, the device was found to be clearly curved under the tissues in only 1.47% of the cases, in 12.09%, the course was undeterminable, most likely because of the deep subtenonian position of the implant itself.

Again, despite a consistent implanting technique of a given surgeon, some implants may result in being clearly and directly visible in the anterior chamber, while other implants will be visible only gonioscopically or not visible at all.

It is not known thus far whether the observed variations in the surgical technique or in the device placement within the eye tissues are able to influence the efficacy and safety outcomes over time, and this will be part of the associative analysis that will be performed after medium and long-term follow-up data become available

Maximum medical therapy is considered by most authors as the combination of three hypotensive agents or three drops per day, usually a prostaglandin analogue in association with a non-prostaglandin fixed combination [10]. In addition, an increased number of hypotensive topical medications with their preservatives has been shown to be associated with a reduced success rate of conventional filtering surgery [24].

The baseline results of the XEN-GTR indicate that, in Italy, 62% of the glaucoma surgical population is treated with three or more hypotensive agents, and thirty-one percent of patients (85/273) were also using systemic carbonic anhydrase inhibitors, suggesting a tendency to overtreat before undergoing surgery, with potential consequences on the outcome, which will be the objective of future investigations.

Indeed, compared to previous prospective studies, our study's patients were enrolled without restrictions in terms of the type of glaucoma, baseline IOP value, visual field defect, or central corneal thickness [20,25–30], reflecting a real-world clinical scenario. This will allow for the evaluation of the XEN in a broader spectrum of patients with glaucoma, such as that seen in daily practice.

Moreover, the design of the XEN-GTR as a surgical registry is aimed at making all data available for the scientific community with an interest in performing post-hoc analysis for clinical, economic, or health purposes.

5. Conclusions

In conclusion, based on the preliminary registered evidence, the typical Italian candidate for the XEN gel implant is a patient with POAG, on maximum medical therapy, and with moderate to severe visual field damage with no difference regarding the lens status. Comparing the Italian candidate with the recommended patients for the XEN gel implant, we can observe some relevant differences: most of the Italian patients scheduled for the implant were on a maximum medical therapy, which is different from a maximum tolerated medical therapy, and, ultimately, only 5% of the patients had a previous glaucoma surgery but not a MIGS.

One year follow-up results regarding the efficacy and the safety of the implant will be published shortly, and they will integrate this preliminary evidence.

Author Contributions: Conceptualization, M.F. and F.O.; methodology, M.F, F.O. and C.P.; software, S.G. and G.R.; validation, M.F., G.R., F.O., A.M.F., L.A., M.S. and S.G.; formal analysis, S.G. and C.P.; investigation, G.C., M.N.M., G.G., P.Q., T.M.F., V.P., L.M., L.A., G.S., A.P., R.A., M.U., D.D. and C.C.; data curation, S.G., C.P., F.O. and M.F.; writing—original draft preparation, C.P.; writing—review and editing, F.O., M.F., L.A. and M.S.; supervision, F.O., M.F and A.M.F. All authors have read and agreed to the published version of the manuscript.

Funding: Unrestricted grant by Abbvie.

Institutional Review Board Statement: The study was conducted in accordance with the Declaration of Helsinki and obtained Local Ethical Committee approval from the Comitato Etico Area Vasta Nord Ovest on 15 March 2018, protocol number 17107 (EC register number for 11040_FIGUS). In accordance with the Declaration of Helsinki, all patients gave written informed consent after having been fully informed about the details of the study's purposes.

Informed Consent Statement: Informed consent was obtained from all subjects involved in the study.

Data Availability Statement: The data presented in this study are available on request from the corresponding author after the authorization of the scientific committee of the Italian XEN Glaucoma Treatment Registry. The data are not publicly available because they are property of members of the Italian XEN Glaucoma Treatment Registry (XEN-GTR) and the study is still ongoing.

Conflicts of Interest: The authors declare no conflict of interest.

References

1. Fea, A.M.; Bron, A.M.; Economou, M.A.; Laffi, G.; Martini, E.; Figus, M.; Oddone, F. European Study of the Efficacy of a Cross-Linked Gel Stent for the Treatment of Glaucoma. *J. Cataract. Refract. Surg.* **2020**, *46*, 441–450. [CrossRef]
2. Floriani, I.; Quaranta, L.; Rulli, E.; Katsanos, A.; Varano, L.; Frezzotti, P.; Rossi, G.C.M.; Carmassi, L.; Rolle, T.; Ratiglia, R.; et al. Health-Related Quality of Life in Patients with Primary Open-Angle Glaucoma. An Italian Multicentre Observational Study. *Acta Ophthalmol.* **2016**, *94*, e278–e286. [CrossRef]
3. Kirwan, J.F.; Lockwood, A.J.; Shah, P.; Macleod, A.; Broadway, D.C.; King, A.J.; McNaught, A.I.; Agrawal, P. Trabeculectomy in the 21st Century. *Ophthalmology* **2013**, *120*, 2532–2539. [CrossRef] [PubMed]
4. Jiang, L.; Eaves, S.; Dhillon, N.; Ranjit, P. Postoperative Outcomes following Trabeculectomy and Nonpenetrating Surgical Procedures: A 5-Year Longitudinal Study. *Clin. Ophthalmol.* **2018**, *12*, 995–1002. [CrossRef] [PubMed]
5. Grover, D.S.; Flynn, W.J.; Bashford, K.P.; Lewis, R.A.; Duh, Y.-J.; Nangia, R.S.; Niksch, B. Performance and Safety of a New Ab Interno Gelatin Stent in Refractory Glaucoma at 12 Months. *Am. J. Ophthalmol.* **2017**, *183*, 25–36. [CrossRef] [PubMed]
6. Lewis, R.A. Ab Interno Approach to the Subconjunctival Space Using a Collagen Glaucoma Stent. *J. Cataract. Refract. Surg.* **2014**, *40*, 1301–1306. [CrossRef]
7. Sheybani, A.; Dick, H.B.; Ahmed, I.I.K. Early Clinical Results of a Novel Ab Interno Gel Stent for the Surgical Treatment of Open-Angle Glaucoma. *J. Glaucoma* **2016**, *25*, e691–e696. [CrossRef]
8. Chaudhary, A.; Salinas, L.; Guidotti, J.; Mermoud, A.; Mansouri, K. XEN Gel Implant: A New Surgical Approach in Glaucoma. *Expert Rev. Med. Devices* **2018**, *15*, 47–59. [CrossRef]
9. Sheybani, A.; Reitsamer, H.; Ahmed, I.I.K. Fluid Dynamics of a Novel Micro-Fistula Implant for the Surgical Treatment of Glaucoma. *Investig. Opthalmol. Vis. Sci.* **2015**, *56*, 4789. [CrossRef]

10. European Glaucoma Society. Terminology and Guidelines for Glaucoma, 5th Edition. *Br. J. Ophthalmol.* **2021**, *105* (Suppl. S1), 1–169. [CrossRef]
11. Lee, B.L. The Glaucoma Symptom Scale. *Arch. Ophthalmol.* **1998**, *116*, 861. [CrossRef] [PubMed]
12. Rossi, G.C.M.; Pasinetti, G.M.; Scudeller, L.; Milano, G.; Mazzone, A.; Raimondi, M.; Bordin, M.; Lanteri, S.; Bianchi, P.E. The Italian Version of the Glaucoma Symptom Scale Questionnaire. *J. Glaucoma* **2013**, *22*, 44–51. [CrossRef] [PubMed]
13. Mills, R.P.; Budenz, D.L.; Lee, P.P.; Noecker, R.J.; Walt, J.G.; Siegartel, L.R.; Evans, S.J.; Doyle, J.J. Categorizing the Stage of Glaucoma from Pre-Diagnosis to End-Stage Disease. *Am. J. Ophthalmol.* **2006**, *141*, 24–30. [CrossRef] [PubMed]
14. Nijm, L.M.; de Benito-Llopis, L.; Rossi, G.C.; Vajaranant, T.S.; Coroneo, M.T. Understanding the Dual Dilemma of Dry Eye and Glaucoma: An International Review. *Asia-Pac. J. Ophthalmol.* **2020**, *9*, 481–490. [CrossRef]
15. Holló, G.; Katsanos, A.; Boboridis, K.G.; Irkec, M.; Konstas, A.G.P. Preservative-Free Prostaglandin Analogs and Prostaglandin/Timolol Fixed Combinations in the Treatment of Glaucoma: Efficacy, Safety and Potential Advantages. *Drugs* **2018**, *78*, 39–64. [CrossRef] [PubMed]
16. Pflugfelder, S.C.; Baudouin, C. Challenges in the Clinical Measurement of Ocular Surface Disease in Glaucoma Patients. *Clin. Ophthalmol.* **2011**, *5*, 1575–1583. [CrossRef] [PubMed]
17. Baudouin, C.; Aragona, P.; Messmer, E.M.; Tomlinson, A.; Calonge, M.; Boboridis, K.G.; Akova, Y.A.; Geerling, G.; Labetoulle, M.; Rolando, M. Role of Hyperosmolarity in the Pathogenesis and Management of Dry Eye Disease: Proceedings of the OCEAN Group Meeting. *Ocul. Surf.* **2013**, *11*, 246–258. [CrossRef]
18. Schlenker, M.B.; Gulamhusein, H.; Conrad-Hengerer, I.; Somers, A.; Lenzhofer, M.; Stalmans, I.; Reitsamer, H.; Hengerer, F.H.; Ahmed, I.I.K. Efficacy, Safety, and Risk Factors for Failure of Standalone Ab Interno Gelatin Microstent Implantation versus Standalone Trabeculectomy. *Ophthalmology* **2017**, *124*, 1579–1588. [CrossRef]
19. Galal, A.; Bilgic, A.; Eltanamly, R.; Osman, A. XEN Glaucoma Implant with Mitomycin C 1-Year Follow-Up: Result and Complications. *J. Ophthalmol.* **2017**, *2017*, 5457246. [CrossRef]
20. Mansouri, K.; Guidotti, J.; Rao, H.L.; Ouabas, A.; D'Alessandro, E.; Roy, S.; Mermoud, A. Prospective Evaluation of Standalone XEN Gel Implant and Combined Phacoemulsification-XEN Gel Implant Surgery. *J. Glaucoma* **2018**, *27*, 140–147. [CrossRef]
21. Hohberger, B.; Welge-Lüßen, U.-C.; Lämmer, R. MIGS: Therapeutic Success of Combined Xen Gel Stent Implantation with Cataract Surgery. *Graefe's Arch. Clin. Exp. Ophthalmol.* **2018**, *256*, 621–625. [CrossRef] [PubMed]
22. Reitsamer, H.; Sng, C.; Vera, V.; Lenzhofer, M.; Barton, K.; Stalmans, I. Two-Year Results of a Multicenter Study of the Ab Interno Gelatin Implant in Medically Uncontrolled Primary Open-Angle Glaucoma. *Graefe's Arch. Clin. Exp. Ophthalmol.* **2019**, *257*, 983–996. [CrossRef] [PubMed]
23. Schlenker, M.B.; Durr, G.M.; Michaelov, E.; Ahmed, I.I.K. Intermediate Outcomes of a Novel Standalone Ab Externo SIBS Microshunt with Mitomycin C. *Am. J. Ophthalmol.* **2020**, *215*, 141–153. [CrossRef] [PubMed]
24. Boimer, C.; Birt, C.M. Preservative Exposure and Surgical Outcomes in Glaucoma Patients. *J. Glaucoma* **2013**, *22*, 730–735. [CrossRef] [PubMed]
25. Coleman, A.L.; Richter, G. Minimally Invasive Glaucoma Surgery: Current Status and Future Prospects. *Clin. Ophthalmol.* **2016**, *2016*, 189–206. [CrossRef]
26. Ansari, E. An Update on Implants for Minimally Invasive Glaucoma Surgery (MIGS). *Ophthalmol. Ther.* **2017**, *6*, 233–241. [CrossRef]
27. Gillmann, K.; Bravetti, G.E.; Mermoud, A.; Rao, H.L.; Mansouri, K. XEN Gel Stent in Pseudoexfoliative Glaucoma. *J. Glaucoma* **2019**, *28*, 676–684. [CrossRef]
28. Smith, M.; Charles, R.; Abdel-Hay, A.; Shah, B.; Byles, D.; Lim, L.-A.; Rossiter, J.; Kuo, C.-H.; Chapman, P.; Robertson, S. 1-Year Outcomes of the Xen45 Glaucoma Implant. *Eye* **2019**, *33*, 761–766. [CrossRef]
29. Ibáñez-Muñoz, A.; Soto-Biforcos, V.S.; Rodríguez-Vicente, L.; Ortega-Renedo, I.; Chacón-González, M.; Rúa-Galisteo, O.; Arrieta-Los Santos, A.; Lizuain-Abadía, M.E.; del Río Mayor, J.L. XEN Implant in Primary and Secondary Open-Angle Glaucoma: A 12-Month Retrospective Study. *Eur. J. Ophthalmol.* **2020**, *30*, 1034–1041. [CrossRef] [PubMed]
30. Karimi, A.; Lindfield, D.; Turnbull, A.; Dimitriou, C.; Bhatia, B.; Radwan, M.; Gouws, P.; Hanifudin, A.; Amerasinghe, N.; Jacob, A. A Multi-Centre Interventional Case Series of 259 Ab-Interno Xen Gel Implants for Glaucoma, with and without Combined Cataract Surgery. *Eye* **2019**, *33*, 469–477. [CrossRef]

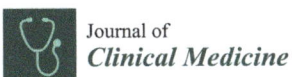

Article

Safety and Efficacy of Ab Interno XEN 45 Gel Stent in Patients with Glaucoma and High Myopia

Matteo Sacchi [1,*,†], Antonio M. Fea [2,†], Gianluca Monsellato [1], Elena Tagliabue [3], Edoardo Villani [1,4], Stefano Ranno [5] and Paolo Nucci [6]

1. University Eye Clinic, San Giuseppe Hospital, IRCCS Multimedica, University of Milan, 20123 Milan, Italy
2. Department of Ophthalmology, University of Turin, 10124 Turin, Italy
3. MultiMedica IRCCS, 20099 Milan, Italy
4. Department of Clinical Sciences and Community Health, University of Milan, 20122 Milan, Italy
5. Ophthalmology Department, Circolo and Fondazione Macchi Hospital, ASST Sette Laghi, 21100 Varese, Italy
6. Department of Biomedical, Surgical and Dental Sciences, University of Milan, 20122 Milan, Italy
* Correspondence: matteosacchi.hsg@gmail.com; Tel.: +39-0285994975; Fax: +39-0229415945
† These authors contributed equally to this work.

Abstract: This study reports on the safety and efficacy of Xen 45 in patients with glaucoma and high myopia. It was a retrospective study including patients with high myopia (>6D) who underwent Xen implant with 2 years of follow-up. The primary outcome was to report the incidence of hypotony (IOP ≤ 5 mmHg) and hypotony-related complications. Patients with high myopia treated with mitomycin-C-augmented trabeculectomy were included as a control group. We included 14 consecutive patients who underwent Xen implant (seven eyes) and trabeculectomy (seven eyes). The mean myopia was −14.71 ± 5.36 and −15.07 ± 6.11 in the trabeculectomy and Xen groups, respectively ($p > 0.05$). The success rate and the mean IOP at 1 and 2 years from the intervention were statistically comparable between the two groups. The group undergoing trabeculectomy showed a higher incidence of hypotony (six eyes (85.71%) vs. two eyes (28.57%)) and hypotony maculopathy (three eyes (42.86%) vs. zero eyes (0%)) and required more postoperative procedures. Patients with high myopia were at higher risk of hypotony-related complications after trabeculectomy. The Xen implant can achieve an IOP control comparable to trabeculectomy with a significantly better safety profile and can be considered as an option for the management of patients with high myopia and glaucoma.

Keywords: glaucoma; glaucoma surgery; stent gel implant; Xen; trabeculectomy; hypotony; hypotony maculopathy

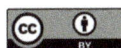

1. Introduction

The only proven treatment for the management of glaucoma is to decrease intraocular pressure (IOP). In the glaucoma treatment algorithm, the surgical approach is considered after the failure of medication and laser. Indications for surgery are uncontrolled IOP, progressing disease despite apparent IOP control, and intolerance to active agents. Although several surgical options are available, and mini-invasive glaucoma surgeries are rising in popularity, trabeculectomy is still the most performed glaucoma surgical technique [1–3].

Although trabeculectomy can effectively lower IOP, significant complications can occur postoperatively, including hypotony [4].

The term hypotony refers to an IOP value of 5 mmHg or less [5].

In clinical practice, hypotony occurring within 3 months after surgery is defined as "early," whereas hypotony still persistent 3 months after surgery is defined as "chronic" [6–8].

Hypotony is one of the most common complications [9], potentially leading to clinically significant and sigh-threatening conditions such as choroidal effusion, optic nerve edema, and maculopathy [5]. Since the 1990s, myopia has been associated with the development of hypotony maculopathy after filtering surgery [10–12], and a large retrospective study confirmed that myopia was significantly associated with hypotony maculopathy [5].

In order to improve the predictability and the safety profile of glaucoma surgery, several minimally invasive glaucoma surgical (MIGS) techniques have been studied and developed in the last years and are nowadays available [13,14].

The Xen 45 gelatin stent (Allergan, Dublin, Ireland) is a 6 mm device implant with a 45 µm internal lumen designed to create a conjunctival filtering bleb [15].

The advantages of this less invasive, bleb-forming technique are a more controlled aqueous humor outflow; less tissue manipulation; quick recovery; and a lower incidence of complication, including hypotony, compared to trabeculectomy [16,17].

In this retrospective study, we report the efficacy and safety of Xen 45 in consecutive patients with uncontrolled glaucoma and concomitant high myopia (>6D). We included in the analysis consecutive patients with glaucoma and high myopia who underwent trabeculectomy as a control group.

2. Methods

We conducted a retrospective medical chart review using the hospital's electronic database (e4cure, Exprivia, Molfetta, BA, Italy). The search period was between 1 January 2016, and 1 January 2020, and patients referred to the glaucoma service were screened.

Consecutive patients with myopia >6 D, 18 years or older, with available data at the established post-operative time points and with a follow-up of at least two years who underwent filtration surgery (Xen implant or trabeculectomy) between 1 January 2016, and 1 January 2020, were included in the study. All the surgeries had to be performed by the same glaucoma-trained surgeon (MS), and both standalone and combined surgery with phacoemulsification were considered eligible for the analysis. Patients who underwent laser trabeculoplasty at least six months before the surgery were also considered eligible.

Patients underwent surgery according to the clinical judgment when meeting one of the following criteria: (a) unmet target intraocular pressure (IOP) despite maximum tolerated medical therapy (including oral acetazolamide) and laser; (b) a significant perimetric progression confirmed on three consecutive reliable visual fields (VF) (Humphrey field analyzer II 750-Carl Zeiss Meditec Inc.; Dublin, CA-30-2 test, full-threshold); (c) intolerance to medical therapy.

Exclusion criteria were previous surgery, except for cataract surgery, if performed at least 6 months before the Xen implant; anterior chamber intraocular lens; neovascular, uveitic, angle-closure, and syndromic glaucoma.

We used the threshold of >6D for the definition of high myopia [18], and the threshold of ≤5 mmHg for the definition of hypotony [5].

For our analysis, the following demographic and clinical data were collected: age, gender, diabetes status, refraction, axial length, best-corrected visual acuity (BCVA), lens status, type of glaucoma, baseline IOP, corneal thickness, number of glaucoma medications, VF mean deviation.

The primary outcome of the analysis was to report the incidence of hypotony and hypotony-related complications, including maculopathy in patients with glaucoma and high myopia after Xen 45 ab interno implant and after trabeculectomy. Secondary outcomes were to report other major and minor complications, assess the IOP lowering efficacy, and compare the safety profile and the efficacy of Xen 45 with trabeculectomy.

The success of the procedures was defined as an IOP between 5 and 15 mmHg at any follow-up visit. As stated by the World Glaucoma Association consensus group, the success was complete if without medicines and qualified if with drugs [19].

Patients undergoing other IOP lowering procedures were considered failures.

The study was carried out at the Ophthalmic Clinic, San Giuseppe Hospital, IRCCS Multimedica, University of Milan. This study was approved by the Institutional Review Board (San Giuseppe Hospital, Milan—IRCCS Multimedica) and adhered to the tenets of the Declaration of Helsinki. We informed the patients about processing personal data, and we obtained consent from all the patients before their data were part of this analysis.

2.1. Surgical Technique

2.1.1. Trabeculectomy

The trabeculectomy technique has been previously described [20].

Briefly, trabeculectomy was performed under a peribulbar block. After a traction suture was passed through the cornea, a fornix-based conjunctival flap was dissected, and a partial-thickness scleral flap was fashioned. A total of 0.3 mg/mL mitomycin (MMC) was applied with sponges left for 2.5 min under the Tenon-conjunctival layer.

After MMC was carefully washed-out with a balanced salt ophthalmic solution, a punch was used to perform sclerotomy, and peripheral iridectomy was performed in each patient. The scleral flap was sutured with two-four 10-0 nylon sutures, and the conjunctiva and Tenon's layer were closed with polyglactin sutures. A 10-0 nylon suture was used to close the Tenon-conjunctival layers to the cornea.

2.1.2. Xen Implant

Xen surgeries were performed under topical anesthesia. After 0.1 mL of mitomycin-C (MMC), 0.2 mg/mL was injected within the upper bulbar conjunctiva, the main and the side port corneal incisions were made, and the anterior chamber was filled with viscoelastic (Healon GV®PRO, Johnson & Johnson Surgical Vision, Inc. 1700 E. St. Andrew Place Santa Ana, CA 92705 USA 1-877-266-4543); the Xen was placed in the superior nasal quadrant. The surgeon's goal was to obtain the Xen gel implant to be positioned following the "3:2:1 rule": 3 mm under the conjunctiva, 2 mm intrascleral, and 1 mm left in the anterior chamber. At the end of the surgery, the proper placement of the Xen in the anterior chamber was verified using a goniolens and viscoelastic washed-out.

Patients were instructed to withdraw topical and systemic ocular hypotensive medications on the day of surgery. Postoperative therapy for both groups consisted of a topical steroid/antibiotic combination for the first two weeks, then switched to a topical steroid, tapered in 4–6 months. Cyclopentolate was prescribed after trabeculectomy twice a day for the first two weeks and then according to the physician's judgment.

2.2. Statistical Analysis

Data were summarized as mean ± standard deviation, if continuous, or frequencies and percentages, if categorical. Differences between trabeculectomy and Xen were evaluated for each variable by the non-parametric Wilcox test, if continuous, or Fisher's exact test, if categorical. As efficacy outcomes, IOP values were collected at the following time points after surgery: 1 day, 1 week, 1 month, 3 months, 6 months, 12 months, and 24 months. Values were then compared between groups by the non-parametric Wilcoxon test and longitudinally by mixed models. Kaplan–Meier curves were drawn to graphically represent differences between groups in the probability of success, defined as IOP values between 5 and 15 mmHg, and the log-Rank test was used to evaluate the differences between the curves.

3. Results

In total, 18 eyes of 18 patients were identified: 9 eyes received a Xen, and 9 underwent trabeculectomy. We excluded two patients per group for insufficient follow-up, one patient in the trabeculectomy group for previous glaucoma surgery, and one patient in the Xen group for diagnosis of uveitic glaucoma.

A total of 14 eyes, 7 in the Xen and 7 in the trabeculectomy group, were examined. The follow-up was 2 years. The mean age and mean deviation in the Xen group were lower compared to the trabeculectomy group (52.96 ± 10.15 vs. 63.99 ± 13.06, and −10.88 ± 5.59 vs. −16.17 ± 5.68 in the Xen and trabeculectomy groups, respectively); however, these differences were not statistically significant. All patients met the diagnostic criteria of primary open-angle glaucoma. Other baseline characteristics were comparable (Table 1).

Table 1. Preoperative data.

	Trabeculectomy (n = 7)	XEN Gel Stent (n = 7)	p Value *
Age (years)	63.9 ± 13.06	52.96 ± 10.15	0.1252
Sex (M/F), n (%)	1/6 (14.29/85.71%)	3/4 (42.86/57.14%)	0.5594 ^
Diabetes status (yes), n	1/7	1/7	- - -
Refraction (Sphere, D)	−14.71 ± 5.36	−15.07 ± 6.11	0.4776
Axial length (mm)	30.28 ± 2.38	30.85 ± 3.00	0.2225
BCVA (logMAR)	0.19 ± 0.13	0.43 ± 0.36	0.5261
Pseudophakic, n	5/7	4/7	0.5770
Type of glaucoma, n POAG	7/7	7/7	- - -
Intraocular pressure (mmHg)	22.00 ± 1.52	22.14 ± 4.88	0.3592
Pachymetry (μm)	519.71 ± 38.57	535.71 ± 26.03	0.5649
Glaucoma medications (N)	3.57 ± 0.53	3.14 ± 0.38	0.1246
Mean deviation (dB)	−16.17 ± 5.68	−10.88 ± 5.59	0.1252

Data are presented as mean ± standard deviation or frequencies and percentages. * Non-parametric Wilcoxon test; ^ Fisher's exact test.

One patient per group received simultaneous glaucoma and cataract surgery. Eyes treated with trabeculectomy had a lower IOP throughout the follow-up than those treated with Xen. The difference was statistically significant from 1 week to 6 months after surgery in favor of trabeculectomy, while it was comparable after 1 and 2 years from intervention (10.00 ± 2.83 vs. 12.00 ± 1.90, p 0.22, and 12.83 ± 4.62 vs. 14.83 ±3.97, p 0.8717, trabeculectomy vs. Xen at 1 and 2 years, respectively; Table 2).

Table 2. Postoperative IOP values.

IOP (mmHg)	Trabeculectomy (n = 7)	XEN Gel Stent (n = 7)	p Value
1 day after surgery	5.43 ± 2.30	7.00 ± 1.41	0.1185
1 week after surgery	5.43 ± 2.44	8.43 ± 2.44	0.0440 *
1 month after surgery	5.43 ± 2.51	10.71 ± 1.25	0.0042 *
3 months after surgery	8.00 ± 2.58	13.00 ± 3.61	0.0324 *
6 months after surgery	8.50 ± 2.26 ^	14.50 ± 2.35	0.0059 *
1 year after surgery	10.00 ± 2.83 ^	12.00 ± 1.90	0.2240
2 year after surgery	12.83 ± 4.62	14.83 ±3.97	0.8717
p-value	<0.0001 #	<0.0001 #	

IOP = intraocular pressure. * Significant p-value (non-parametric Wilcoxon test). # Compared to baseline. ^ Fisher's exact test.

Xen and trabeculectomy showed an equal probability of success at 2 years of follow-up (41.31% ± 1.96 vs. 42.23% ± 1.96, p 0.3925, log-Rank test; Figure 1).

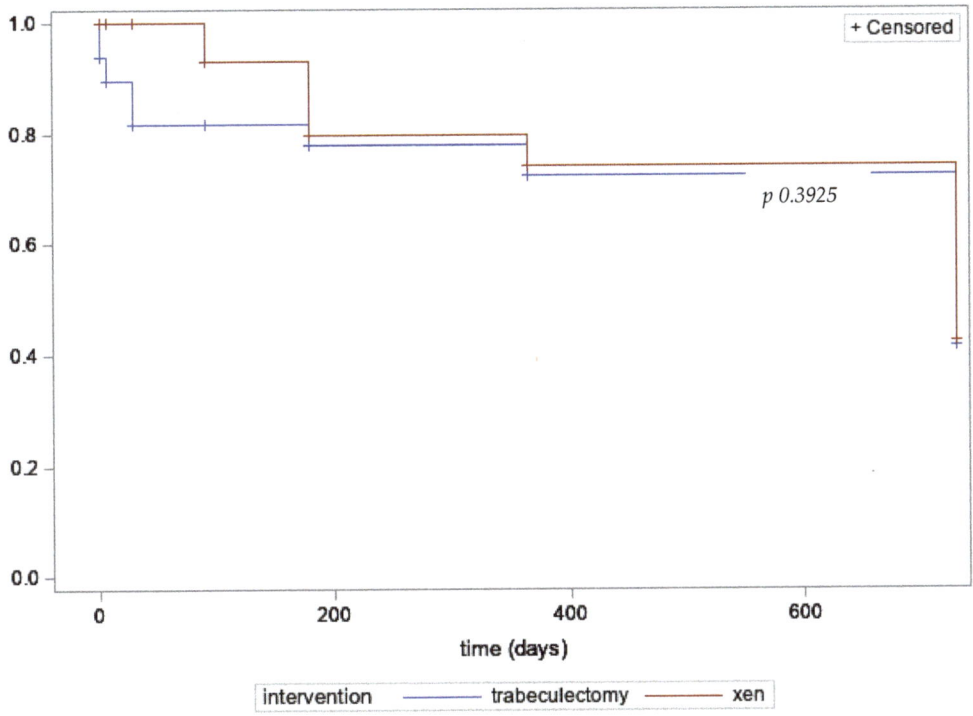

Figure 1. Kaplan–Meier curves for success of estimated probability (%).

At the last follow-up, and starting from 1 year after surgery, one patient per group was using a prostaglandin analogue, and one patient per group was under a fixed combination of timolol and dorzolamide. The number of hypotony and hypotony-related complications was significantly higher in the trabeculectomy group. Hypotony maculopathy was recorded in 42.86% of eyes after trabeculectomy, whereas none of the eyes in the Xen group experienced this complication (Table 3). All the cases of hypotony maculopathy occurred in the first month after surgery.

Table 3. Postoperative complications.

	Trabeculectomy (n = 7)	XEN Gel Stent (n = 7)	Total (n = 14)
Hypotony	6 (85.71%)	2 (28.57%)	8 (57.14%)
Hypotony maculopathy	3 (42.86%)	0	3 (21.43%)
Choroidal detachment	4 (57.14%)	1 (14.29%)	5 (35.71%)
Flat anterior chamber	2 (28.57%)	0	2 (14.29%)
Hyphema	0	1 (14.29%)	1 (7.14%)
Bleb leakage	1 (14.29%)	0	1 (7.14%)
Endophthalmitis	0	0	0

Patients in the trabeculectomy group required more post-operative procedures (Table 4).

Table 4. Postoperative management.

	Trabeculectomy (n = 7)	XEN Gel Stent (n = 7)	Total (n = 14)
Bleb needling	2 (28.57%)	2 (28.57%)	4 (28.57%)
Intrableb autologous blood injection	3 (42.86%)	0	3 (21.43%)
Laser suture lysis	1 (14.29%)	0	1 (7.14%)
AC viscoelastic injection	2 (28.57%)	0	2 (14.29%)
Surgical bleb revision	1 (14.29%)	1 (14.29%)	2 (14.29%)

AC = anterior chamber.

Patients requiring bleb needlings and surgical bleb revision were similar in the two groups, but more myopic patients undergoing trabeculectomy required intrableb autologous blood injection and AC refilling with viscoelastic compared to patients who underwent Xen implant (42.86% vs. 0% and 28.57% vs. 0% in trabeculectomy and Xen groups, respectively; Table 4).

4. Discussion

To the best of our knowledge, this is the first study reporting a dataset of the safety and efficacy of ab interno Xen 45 and trabeculectomy in a subset of patients with high myopia. Recently, we published a retrospective, multicenter study on Xen implant in patients with high myopia [21]. In the current study, we introduced as a control group consecutive patients with uncontrolled glaucoma and high myopia (>6D) who underwent trabeculectomy.

The primary outcome of our analysis was to report the incidence of hypotony and hypotony-related complications.

Overall, throughout 2 years of follow-up, Xen 45 implant showed a lower incidence of complications compared to trabeculectomy. None of the patients with glaucoma and high myopia treated with ab interno Xen 45 implant experienced hypotony maculopathy, in contrast to what we observed in the trabeculectomy group.

The incidence of hypotony after trabeculectomy varies greatly in the literature, and it has been reported in up to 42% of patients. In a retrospective, 5-year study involving 123 patients, late hypotony occurred in 42.2% of eyes, hypotony maculopathy in 8.9%, and 14.9% of eyes had a significant loss of vision (four lines of visual acuity) [22]. A large retrospective study involving nine centers in the UK and 395 patients followed up for at least 2 years reported the presence of late hypotony (>6 months) in 7.2% of cases. Patients who experienced hypotony had a significantly higher risk of losing vision than the whole group (10% vs. 6%) [4]. The TVT study, a large RCT comparing the safety and efficacy of tubes with trabeculectomy, showed similar results, reporting persistent hypotony (>3 months) in 12.3% of patients who underwent trabeculectomy [6]. Different exposure times, concentrations, and areas of application of MMC and the use of different sutures (adjustable, releasable) can at least partially explain the wide range of hypotony reported in the literature [4].

Myopia has been recognized as a risk factor for hypotony after glaucoma surgery since the 1990s [10–12], and more recently, large retrospective studies [5] and reports [23,24] confirmed the link between the onset of hypotony [5] and hypotony maculopathy [23,24] after trabeculectomy in patients with glaucoma and myopia.

As described by Gass, hypotony maculopathy is caused by the sclera bending inward, associated with retinal and choroidal folds over the posterior pole [25]. Both levels of IOP and biomechanical properties of the sclera are considered crucial in the development of hypotony maculopathy. Myopic eyes have a thinner sclera, particularly at the posterior pole, due to the loss of extracellular matrix and the reduction in collagen fibril diameter [26]. These biomechanical changes lead to an overall reduced scleral stiffness in myopic eyes [27]. Due to the lower thickness and rigidity, the myopic eyeball is more likely to collapse, making myopic patients at higher risk of hypotony maculopathy in cases of hypotony after filtering surgery [28]. Published studies reported a rate of hypotony maculopathy up to 20% after trabeculectomy [29,30]. In our work, we found a rate of 42.86% of hypotony maculopathy after trabeculectomy in a high-risk population of highly myopic eyes. The populations and the methods of these studies were different compared to our work as they did not include patients with high myopia, and they did not use optical coherence tomography (OCT) for the detection of hypotony maculopathy. As there are no studies having as the first outcome the rate of hypotony and hypotony-related complications in patients with high myopia who underwent trabeculectomy, it is hard to compare our finding with published data. We used OCT as a routine postoperative examination in any patients who underwent glaucoma surgery. It is likely that the use of OCT has increased our diagnostic power as we were able to detect even subtle signs of hypotony maculopathy. Taking these considerations together, we can speculate that the reported rate of hypotony maculopathy up to 20% in non-highly myopic eyes can be compared with our rate of 42% of hypotony maculopathy detected by a high-resolution imaging technique in a population at high risk of hypotony-related complications.

The Xen 45 implant is a less invasive glaucoma surgical technique, leading to a filtering bleb by an ab interno approach. This device was designed to prevent hypotony, as the length/lumen ratio theoretically controls the aqueous outflow, according to the Hagen–Poiseuille equation [31]. Xen 45 and trabeculectomy have been compared in 12- and 24-month retrospective studies. Overall, the Xen 45 showed a safer postoperative profile compared to trabeculectomy. The incidence of hypotony ranged from 0% to 2.4% after Xen 45 and from 6.7% to 10.5% after trabeculectomy. In the retrospective study by Wagner and coauthors involving 82 cases of XEN implant and 89 cases of trabeculectomy, hypotony was reported in 6.7% of patients in the trabeculectomy and 2.4% of patients in the Xen group [32]. In a 24-month retrospective study, patients in the Xen 45 group experienced a significantly lower incidence of wound leak (0% vs. 15.8%), bleb leak (0% vs. 6%), and hypotony (1.8% vs. 10.5%) compared to trabeculectomy [17], and a retrospective study comparing trabeculectomy with Xen implant, both in combination with phacoemulsification, reported a higher incidence of hypotony after trabeculectomy (7.7% vs. 0%) [33]. In two retrospective Xen vs. trabeculectomy studies, the incidence of hypotony was not reported; however, the anterior chamber flattening, a condition commonly related to hypotony, was greatly more frequent in the trabeculectomy compared to the Xen group (19.6% vs. 1.5% and 14.7% vs. 0%, trabeculectomy vs. Xen, respectively) [34,35]. In one study, no late hypotony and hypotony maculopathy occurred after the first month of follow-up [36], and one study reported a similar incidence of choroidal folds and hypotony maculopathy in the two groups (hypotony maculopathy 1.1% Xen, trabe 0.6%) [16]. In a large, comparative retrospective study between standalone Xen 45 and standalone trabeculectomy [16], the authors reported a significantly lower percentage of patients with a vision loss of >2 lines in the Xen group.

The second outcome of our analysis was to report the efficacy of the two techniques.

Xen implant and trabeculectomy achieved a significant IOP reduction at 2 years of follow-up with a comparable survival curve. Although the IOP lowering efficacy was superior in the trabeculectomy group, we did not find a statistically significant difference at 1 and 2 years between the two techniques. The lower mean IOP we observed during the first 6 months in the trabeculectomy group is likely correlated with the higher proportion of hypotony that occurred in the trabeculectomy group. The mean IOP in the Xen 45 group was 12.43 and 15.0 at 1- and 2-year follow-ups. We found 28% and 7% of cases needing a needling procedure and a surgical revision, respectively. In large retrospective multicenter [37,38] and single-center [39,40] European studies, the mean IOP ranged from 14.6 to 15.5 and from 14.2 to 14.8 throughout the first and the second year of follow-up. The proportion of patients who underwent needling procedures ranged from 36% to 62% [37–40]. As none of these studies reported sub-analysis about patients with myopia or high myopia, it is hard to compare our results with existing literature.

We recently published a multicenter, retrospective study reporting the effectiveness and safety of Xen 45 in eyes with open-angle glaucoma (OAG) and high myopia [21]. Overall, the study by Fea et al. and the current study reported a significant reduction of

IOP compared to baseline and a good safety profile in patients with glaucoma and high myopia who received a Xen implant. The IOP achieved at 1 year of follow-up and the rate of hypotony was similar in the two studies (12.6 mmHg vs. 12.0 mmHg, and 28.6% vs. 28.5%, Fea et al. and the current study, respectively).

Compared to the current study, the study by Fea and colleagues is multicentric and has a larger sample size but lacked a control group.

The baseline characteristics were similar between the studies in terms of mean deviation and number of antiglaucoma drugs (11.8 dB vs. 10.88 dB, and 3.0 vs. 3.14, Fea et al. [21] and the current study, respectively), but patients in the Fea et al. study were older and had a higher baseline IOP, as well as a lower mean refraction (62.1 years vs. 52.9 years, 24.5 mmHg vs. 22.1 mmHg, −13.2 D vs. −15.07, Fea et al. [21] and the current study, respectively).

We are aware of the limitations of our study. First, the design of our work carries the limitations of any retrospective analysis.

The risk of selection bias due to the lack of randomization is counterbalanced by the lack of significant differences in the baseline characteristics of the two groups. As in any retrospective work, the rate of complications, specifically choroidal detachment and hypotony maculopathy, could be underestimated. However, this bias involves both groups equally. In addition, the threshold of attention in patients with high myopia is exceptionally high. Patients underwent a dilated funduscopic examination at any postoperative visit and an optical coherence tomography retina exam in the case of low visual acuity recovery and complaint of visual changes. Among the limitations, we are aware that the small sample size reduces the power of the study. However, our preliminary work aimed to explore the safety and efficacy of the Xen 45 implant in patients with glaucoma and high myopia, a relatively uncommon condition. As expected, the refractive characteristics we used as inclusion criteria of our analysis narrowed the sample size.

We also want to point out to be cautious in generalizing the results of this study and that the interpretation of our findings should be restricted to patients with similar baseline characteristics and in a similar setting.

Among the strengths, we defined strict inclusion and exclusion criteria using the hospital's electronic database, and a single surgeon treated all the patients, thus minimizing the bias related to the surgical technique. We extended the follow-up to 2 years and included patients with the same refractive characteristics (high myopia) treated by trabeculectomy as a control group.

In conclusion, we report for the first time the safety and efficacy of Xen 45 implant in comparison with trabeculectomy in patients with concomitant glaucoma and high myopia. Myopic eyes are at higher risk of hypotony maculopathy after glaucoma surgery due to the sclera's weakened biomechanical properties, including scleral thinning and reduced scleral stiffness. Xen implant showed a favorable safety profile, with a lower incidence of postoperative hypotony maculopathy compared to patients with similar characteristics treated with trabeculectomy. The safety results of our study after the Xen 45 implant agree with the available literature. Although the retrospective nature of our work and the limited sample size, we suggest considering Xen 45 implant in patients with high myopia requiring glaucoma surgery.

We hope this explorative work can draw attention to the management of patients with concomitant glaucoma and high myopia and will encourage further, larger works investigating this topic.

Author Contributions: Conceptualization, M.S., G.M. and A.M.F.; methodology, M.S. and A.M.F.; software, G.M., E.T. and E.V; validation, M.S., E.T., E.V. and P.N.; formal analysis, E.T.; investigation, M.S., G.M. and S.R.; resources, M.S.; data curation, M.S., G.M. and S.R.; writing—original draft preparation, M.S.; writing—review and editing, M.S., A.M.F., E.V. and P.N.; visualization, M.S.; supervision, P.N. All authors have read and agreed to the published version of the manuscript.

Funding: This research received no external funding.

Institutional Review Board Statement: The study was conducted in accordance with the Declaration of Helsinki and obtained Local Ethical Committee approval from the Comitato Etico IRCCS-Multimedica, Milan on 12 April 2022, protocol number 534.2022.

Informed Consent Statement: Informed consent was obtained from all subjects involved in the study. Written informed consent was obtained from the patients to publish this paper.

Data Availability Statement: The data presented in this study are available on request from the corresponding author. The data are not publicly available due to privacy restrictions.

Conflicts of Interest: The authors declare no conflict of interest.

References

1. European Glaucoma Society Terminology and Guidelines for Glaucoma, 5th Edition. *Br. J. Ophthalmol.* **2021**, *105*, 1–169. [CrossRef] [PubMed]
2. Vinod, K.; Gedde, S.J.; Feuer, W.J.; Panarelli, J.F.; Chang, T.C.; Chen, P.P.; Parrish, R.K. Practice Preferences for Glaucoma Surgery. *J. Glaucoma* **2017**, *26*, 687–693. [CrossRef] [PubMed]
3. Iwasaki, K.; Arimura, S.; Takamura, Y.; Inatani, M. Clinical practice preferences for glaucoma surgery in Japan: A survey of Japan Glaucoma Society specialists. *Jpn. J. Ophthalmol.* **2020**, *64*, 385–391. [CrossRef] [PubMed]
4. Kirwan, J.F.; Lockwood, A.J.; Shah, P.; Macleod, A.; Broadway, D.C.; King, A.J.; McNaught, A.I.; Agrawal, P. Trabeculectomy in the 21st Century. *Ophthalmology* **2013**, *120*, 2532–2539. [CrossRef] [PubMed]
5. Fannin, L.A.; Schiffman, J.C.; Budenz, D.L. Risk factors for hypotony maculopathy. *Ophthalmology* **2003**, *110*, 1185–1191. [CrossRef]
6. Gedde, S.J.; Schiffman, J.C.; Feuer, W.J.; Herndon, L.W.; Brandt, J.D.; Budenz, D.L.; Tube versus Trabeculectomy Study Group. Treatment Outcomes in the Tube Versus Trabeculectomy (TVT) Study After Five Years of Follow-up. *Am. J. Ophthalmol.* **2012**, *153*, 789–803.e2. [CrossRef]
7. Budenz, D.L.; Barton, K.; Gedde, S.J.; Feuer, W.J.; Schiffman, J.; Costa, V.P.; Godfrey, D.G.; Buys, Y.M. Five-Year Treatment Outcomes in the Ahmed Baerveldt Comparison Study. *Ophthalmology* **2014**, *122*, 308–316. [CrossRef]
8. Gedde, S.J.; Feuer, W.J.; Lim, K.S.; Barton, K.; Goyal, S.; Ahmed, I.I.; Brandt, J.D. Treatment Outcomes in the Primary Tube Versus Trabeculectomy Study after 3 Years of Follow-up. *Ophthalmology* **2019**, *127*, 333–345. [CrossRef]
9. Tan, H.; Kang, X.; Lu, S.; Liu, L.; Xin, K. Comparison of Ahmed Glaucoma Valve Implantation and Trabeculectomy for Glaucoma: A Systematic Review and Meta-Analysis. *PLoS ONE* **2015**, *10*, e0118142. [CrossRef]
10. Suñer, I.J.; Greenfield, D.S.; Miller, M.P.; Nicolela, M.T.; Palmberg, P.F. Hypotony maculopathy after filtering surgery with mitomycin-C. Incidence and treatment. *Ophthalmology* **1997**, *104*, 207–214. [CrossRef]
11. Jampel, H.D.; Pasquale, L.R.; Dibernardo, C. Hypotony Maculopathy Following Trabeculectomy with Mitomycin C. *Arch. Ophthalmol.* **1992**, *110*, 1049–1050. [CrossRef] [PubMed]
12. Stamper, R.L.; McMenemy, M.G.; Lieberman, M.F. Hypotonous Maculopathy After Trabeculectomy with Subconjunctival 5-Fluorouracil. *Am. J. Ophthalmol.* **1992**, *114*, 544–553. [CrossRef] [PubMed]
13. Saheb, H.; Ahmed, I.I.K. Micro-invasive glaucoma surgery. *Curr. Opin. Ophthalmol.* **2012**, *23*, 96–104. [CrossRef] [PubMed]
14. LaVia, C.; Dallorto, L.; Maule, M.M.; Ceccarelli, M.; Fea, A.M. Minimally-invasive glaucoma surgeries (MIGS) for open angle glaucoma: A systematic review and meta-analysis. *PLoS ONE* **2017**, *12*, e0183142. [CrossRef] [PubMed]
15. Sacchi, M.; Agnifili, L.; Brescia, L.; Oddone, F.; Villani, E.; Nucci, P.; Mastropasqua, L. Structural imaging of conjunctival filtering blebs in XEN gel implantation and trabeculectomy: A confocal and anterior segment optical coherence tomography study. *Graefe's Arch. Clin. Exp. Ophthalmol.* **2020**, *258*, 1763–1770. [CrossRef] [PubMed]
16. Schlenker, M.B.; Gulamhusein, H.; Conrad-Hengerer, I.; Somers, A.; Lenzhofer, M.; Stalmans, I.; Reitsamer, H.; Hengerer, F.H.; Ahmed, I.I.K. Standalone Ab Interno Gelatin Stent versus Trabeculectomy. *Ophthalmol. Glaucoma* **2018**, *1*, 189–196. [CrossRef]
17. Wanichwecharungruang, B.; Ratprasatporn, N. 24-month outcomes of XEN45 gel implant versus trabeculectomy in primary glaucoma. *PLoS ONE* **2021**, *16*, e0256362. [CrossRef]
18. Flitcroft, D.I.; He, M.; Jonas, J.B.; Jong, M.; Naidoo, K.; Ohno-Matsui, K.; Rahi, J.; Resnikoff, S.; Vitale, S.; Yannuzzi, L. IMI—Defining and Classifying Myopia: A Proposed Set of Standards for Clinical and Epidemiologic Studies. *Investig. Ophthalmol. Vis. Sci.* **2019**, *60*, M20–M30. [CrossRef]
19. Shaarawy, T.; Sherwood, M.B.; Grehn, F. *Guidelines on Design and Reporting of Glaucoma Surgical Trials*; Kugler Publications: Amsterdam, The Netherlands, 2009; pp. 1–83.
20. Sacchi, M.; Monsellato, G.; Villani, E.; Lizzio, R.A.U.; Cremonesi, E.; Luccarelli, S.; Nucci, P. Intraocular pressure control after combined phacotrabeculectomy versus trabeculectomy alone. *Eur. J. Ophthalmol.* **2021**, *32*, 327–335. [CrossRef]
21. Fea, A.; Sacchi, M.; Franco, F.; Laffi, G.L.; Oddone, F.; Costa, G.; Serino, F.; Giansanti, F. Effectiveness and Safety of XEN45 in Eyes with High Myopia and Open-angle Glaucoma. *J. Glaucoma* **2023**, *32*, 178–185. [CrossRef]
22. Bindlish, R.; Condon, G.P.; Schlosser, J.D.; D'Antonio, J.; Lauer, K.B.; Lehrer, R. Efficacy and safety of mitomycin-C in primary trabeculectomy: Five-year follow-up. *Ophthalmology* **2002**, *109*, 1336–1341. [CrossRef] [PubMed]
23. Silva, R.A.; Doshi, A.; Law, S.K.; Singh, K. Postfiltration Hypotony Maculopathy in Young Chinese Myopic Women with Glaucomatous Appearing Optic Neuropathy. *Eur. J. Gastroenterol. Hepatol.* **2010**, *19*, 105–110. [CrossRef] [PubMed]

24. Kao, S.-T.; Lee, S.-H.; Chen, Y.-C. Late-onset Hypotony Maculopathy After Trabeculectomy in a Highly Myopic Patient with Juvenile Open-angle Glaucoma. *J. Glaucoma* **2017**, *26*, e137–e141. [CrossRef]
25. Gass, J. Hypotony maculopathy. *Contemp Ophthalmol.* **1972**, *34*, 343–366.
26. Curtin, B.J.; Iwamoto, T.; Renaldo, D.P. Normal and Staphylomatous Sclera of High Myopia. *Arch. Ophthalmol.* **1979**, *97*, 912–915. [CrossRef]
27. McBrien, N.A.; Cornell, L.M.; Gentle, A. Structural and ultra-structural changes to the sclera in a mammalian model of high myopia. *Investig. Ophthalmol. Vis. Sci.* **2001**, *42*, 2179–2187.
28. Costa, V.P.; Arcieri, E.S. Hypotony maculopathy. *Acta Ophthalmol. Scand.* **2007**, *85*, 586–597. [CrossRef]
29. Shields, M.B.; Scroggs, M.W.; Sloop, C.M.; Simmons, R.B. Clinical and Histopathologic Observations Concerning Hypotony After Trabeculectomy with Adjunctive Mitomycin C. *Am. J. Ophthalmol.* **1993**, *116*, 673–683. [CrossRef]
30. Tsai, J.-C.; Chang, H.-W.; Kao, C.-N.; Lai, I.-C.; Teng, M.-C. Trabeculectomy with Mitomycin C versus Trabeculectomy Alone for Juvenile Primary Open-Angle Glaucoma. *Ophthalmologica* **2003**, *217*, 24–30. [CrossRef]
31. Sheybani, A.; Reitsamer, H.; Ahmed, I.I.K. Fluid Dynamics of a Novel Micro-Fistula Implant for the Surgical Treatment of Glaucoma. *Investig. Ophthalmol. Vis. Sci.* **2015**, *56*, 4789–4795. [CrossRef]
32. Wagner, F.M.; Schuster, A.K.-G.; Emmerich, J.; Chronopoulos, P.; Hoffmann, E.M. Efficacy and safety of XEN®—Implantation vs. trabeculectomy: Data of a "real-world" setting. *PLoS ONE* **2020**, *15*, e0231614. [CrossRef] [PubMed]
33. Kee, A.R.M.; Yip, C.H.M.V.; Chua, C.H.B.; Ang, C.H.M.B.; Hu, Y.M.J.; Guo, X.M.; Yip, W.L.M.L. Comparison of Efficacy and Safety of XEN45 Implant Versus Trabeculectomy in Asian Eyes. *J. Glaucoma* **2021**, *30*, 1056–1064. [CrossRef] [PubMed]
34. Parra, M.T.M.; López, J.A.S.; Grau, N.S.L.; Ceausescu, A.M.; Santonja, J.J.P. XEN implant device versus trabeculectomy, either alone or in combination with phacoemulsification, in open-angle glaucoma patients. *Graefe's Arch. Clin. Exp. Ophthalmol.* **2019**, *257*, 1741–1750. [CrossRef] [PubMed]
35. Cappelli, F.; Cutolo, C.A.; Olivari, S.; Testa, V.; Sindaco, D.; Pizzorno, C.; Ciccione, S.; Traaverso, C.E.; Iester, M. Trabeculectomy versus Xen gel implant for the treatment of open-angle glaucoma: A 3-year retrospective analysis. *BMJ Open Ophthalmol.* **2022**, *7*, e000830. [CrossRef] [PubMed]
36. Theilig, T.; Rehak, M.; Busch, C.; Bormann, C.; Schargus, M.; Unterlauft, J.D. Comparing the efficacy of trabeculectomy and XEN gel microstent implantation for the treatment of primary open-angle glaucoma: A retrospective monocentric comparative cohort study. *Sci. Rep.* **2020**, *10*, 19337. [CrossRef] [PubMed]
37. Fea, A.M.; Bron, A.M.; Economou, M.A.M.; Laffi, G.; Martini, E.; Figus, M.M.; Oddone, F.M. European study of the efficacy of a cross-linked gel stent for the treatment of glaucoma. *J. Cataract. Refract. Surg.* **2020**, *46*, 441–450. [CrossRef]
38. Reitsamer, H.; Vera, V.; Ruben, S.; Au, L.; Vila-Arteaga, J.; Teus, M.; Lenzhofer, M.; Shirlaw, A.; Bai, Z.; Balaram, M.; et al. Three-year effectiveness and safety of the XEN gel stent as a solo procedure or in combination with phacoemulsification in open-angle glaucoma: A multicentre study. *Acta Ophthalmol.* **2021**, *100*, e233–e245. [CrossRef]
39. Gabbay, I.E.; Goldberg, M.; Allen, F.; Lin, Z.; Morley, C.; Pearsall, T.; Muraleedharan, V.; Ruben, S. Efficacy and safety data for the Ab interno XEN45 gel stent implant at 3 Years: A retrospective analysis. *Eur. J. Ophthalmol.* **2021**, *32*, 1016–1022. [CrossRef]
40. Rauchegger, T.; Angermann, R.; Willeit, P.; Schmid, E.; Teuchner, B. Two-year outcomes of minimally invasive XEN Gel Stent implantation in primary open-angle and pseudoexfoliation glaucoma. *Acta Ophthalmol.* **2020**, *99*, 369–375. [CrossRef]

Disclaimer/Publisher's Note: The statements, opinions and data contained in all publications are solely those of the individual author(s) and contributor(s) and not of MDPI and/or the editor(s). MDPI and/or the editor(s) disclaim responsibility for any injury to people or property resulting from any ideas, methods, instructions or products referred to in the content.

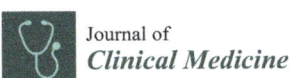

Article

XEN®-63 Compared to XEN®-45 Gel Stents to Reduce Intraocular Pressure in Glaucoma

Charlotte Evers [1,*], Daniel Böhringer [1], Sara Kallee [1], Philip Keye [1], Heiko Philippin [1,2], Timothy Piotrowski [1], Thomas Reinhard [1] and Jan Lübke [1]

[1] Eye Center, Medical Center—University of Freiburg, Faculty of Medicine, University of Freiburg, 79106 Freiburg, Germany

[2] International Centre for Eye Health, Faculty of Infectious & Tropical Diseases, London School of Hygiene & Tropical Medicine, London WC1E 7HT, UK

* Correspondence: charlotte.evers@uniklinik-freiburg.de

Abstract: The XEN® gel stent reduces intraocular pressure (IOP) in glaucoma. XEN®-45 is widely used; the newer XEN®-63 has a larger lumen targeting potentially lower IOP outcomes. We retrospectively compared the first 15 XEN®-63 cases to 15 matched XEN®-45 controls. With a preoperative IOP of 18.1 ± 3.9 mmHg (mean ± SD) and a final IOP of 9.1 ± 2.0 mmHg, XEN®-63 implantation resulted in an IOP reduction of 44.6 ± 16.5%. Similarly, with a preoperative IOP of 18.3 ± 4.5 mmHg and a final IOP of 10.3 ± 2.1 mmHg, XEN®-45 implantation resulted in an IOP reduction of 40.1 ± 17.2%. The median follow-up period was 204 days (range 78–338 days) for the XEN®-63 group and 386 days (range 99–1688 days) for the XEN®-45 group. In total, 5/15 eyes of each group underwent open conjunctival bleb revision within the period of observation. Three eyes of the XEN®-63 group had secondary glaucoma surgery. One eye in the XEN®-63 group and three eyes in the XEN®-45 group required a restart of antiglaucomatous medication. In conclusion, both stents effectively lower IOP and medication. XEN®-63 achieved a slightly lower IOP over a short follow-up. Complication and revision rates were similar.

Keywords: XEN®-63 gel stent; glaucoma; bleb revision

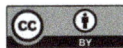

1. Introduction

A XEN® gel stent is a hollow cylindrical implant made of cross-linked collagen derived from porcine gelatin. Implanted ab interno through the sclera, the stent drains fluid from the anterior chamber to the subconjunctival space [1]. The XEN®-45 gel stent has been used successfully to treat primary open-angle glaucoma [2–7], as well as other forms of glaucoma [2–7], by reducing intraocular pressure (IOP) and the number of antiglaucomatous medications required. Compared to classic glaucoma filtration surgery, XEN® implantation is less invasive and may have a better safety profile [8]. However, most studies show a high rate of needling [2,7,9–11] or bleb revision [4,12,13] after XEN®-45 implantation. In the long run, trabeculectomy can achieve lower IOP values [14]. XEN®-45 has a lumen of 45 μm and XEN®-63 a lumen of 63 μm. Both are 6 mm long and are implanted with a 27G injector. XEN®-45 has an outer diameter of 150 μm while XEN®-63 has an outer diameter of 170 μm. Real-world data for XEN®-45 implantation after 1–3 years show postoperative mean IOP levels of 14–16 mmHg [2–4,7,9–11,13,15]. Due to its lower outflow resistance compared to XEN®-45 (2–3 mmHg for XEN®-63 versus 6–8 mmHg for XEN®-45), XEN®-63 was designed to achieve a lower IOP level. So far, there are few studies on the current version of XEN®-63. Previously, studies reported on an earlier, non-marketed version with an inner diameter of 63 μm but an outer diameter of 240 μm, implanted with a 25G injector [16–18]. Fea et al. were the first to report on the newly marketed XEN®-63 [19,20]. Hussien et al. recently compared the novel 63 μm microstent to the conventional 45 μm microstent [21]. We herein present our data of XEN®-63 compared to XEN®-45 for different types of glaucoma in a tertiary center in Germany.

2. Materials and Methods

We conducted a retrospective analysis of the first 15 consecutive XEN®-63 implantations at our tertiary Eye Center at the University of Freiburg, Germany, compared to a matched group of XEN®-45 implantations. This study was performed in accordance with the principles of the Declaration of Helsinki. Approval was granted by the Ethics Committee of the University of Freiburg (No 21-1202_02).

Study patients: XEN®-63 gel stent (Allergan, an AbbVie company, Irvine, CA, USA) was implanted in 15 eyes of 13 patients with medically uncontrolled glaucoma. The control group consisted of 15 eyes of 15 patients who had received a XEN®-45 gel stent (Allergan, an AbbVie company, Irvine, CA, USA) implantation. Both groups were matched for age and type of glaucoma. Eyes with XEN®-45 implantation were selected from a quality control database using propensity matching based on age and type of glaucoma.

We obtained intraocular pressure using Goldmann applanation tonometry (GAT).

The surgical technique was as follows: Either XEN®-45 or XEN®-63 gel stent was implanted ab interno via a clear corneal incision without conjunctival dissection. Prior to the implantation, a very small amount of balanced salt solution was injected subconjunctivally in the target quadrant. At the end of the procedure, 4 mg of dexamethasone was administered intracamerally, and 0.1 mL of 0.2% mitomycin C was injected subconjunctivally. We did neither inject subconjunctival viscoelastic for bleb preparation nor leave any viscoelastic in the anterior chamber to prevent early hypotony. To reduce trauma to the conjunctiva, we did not perform conjunctival dissection in any of the primary procedures. Primary needling was performed if the subconjunctival portion of the XEN® stent demonstrated restricted mobility. Postoperative treatment consisted of glucocorticoid eye drops (usually 1 mg/mL dexamethasone) 5 times daily, which were gradually reduced depending on the degree of postoperative conjunctival injection and intraocular inflammation (usually fortnightly reduction). There were no postoperative subconjunctival 5-fluorouracil injections given in any of the primary procedure cases. IOP-lowering drugs were stopped on the day of surgery.

Postoperative needling was performed in the case of a subconjunctivally encapsulated XEN® stent, which at the discretion of the surgeon, could likely be released by needling alone. Criteria for bleb revision were signs of a dysfunctional bleb due to fibrotic tissue inhibiting the outflow through the subconjunctival part of the XEN® stent or (impending) perforation of the XEN® stent through the conjunctiva. A restart of topical antiglaucomatous treatment was resumed if the postoperative IOP exceeded the target level for that individual patient and the patient declined additional surgical interventions.

For open conjunctival bleb revision, we started with a conjunctival peritomy at the limbus followed by careful dissection of fibrotic tissue around the XEN®. After verification of good flow through the XEN® stent, it was placed underneath Tenon's fascia. Finally, the conjunctiva was closed using 7-0 vicryl sutures, and 0.1 mL of dexamethasone 4 mg/mL was injected subconjunctivally.

After postoperative needling and after bleb revision, patients received postoperative subconjunctival 5-fluorouracil injections (1 mL of 1% 5-fluorouracil) for three consecutive days following surgery and again glucocorticoid eye drops (usually 1 mg/mL dexamethasone) 5 times daily tapered fortnightly by one drop.

Analysis: The success of XEN®-63 versus XEN®-45 implantation was determined using descriptive statistics, including mean values, standard deviation, range, and median if differing substantially from the mean. Furthermore, we included Kaplan–Meier survival estimations. Criteria for failure in the Kaplan–Meier analysis were revision surgery with conjunctival dissection or secondary glaucoma intervention. To compare results between XEN®-63 and XEN®-45, an unpaired two-tailed t-test was performed.

We also analyzed IOP success rates according to the following criteria: Success was defined as a final IOP of ≤15 mmHg (≤12 mmHg) but ≥6 mmHg and an IOP reduction of ≥20% without (complete success) or with ocular hypotensive medications (qualified success) and without secondary glaucoma surgery. Failure was defined as an IOP level above the upper limit or below the lower limit or an IOP reduction < 20%. Complete failure was defined as a necessity for further glaucoma surgical intervention. Needling and bleb revision in this analysis were not recorded as evidence for failure.

3. Results

3.1. Patient Age and Type of Glaucoma

At the time of XEN®-implantation, patients in the XEN®-63 group were between 55 and 86 years old (mean age ± standard deviation: 75.3 ± 9.4 years), and patients in the XEN®-45 group were between 54 and 86 years old (mean age ± standard deviation: 74.8 ± 8.6 years).

The XEN®-63 group comprised five male patients (38.5%), two of whom received XEN®-63 implantation in both eyes and eight female patients (61.5%) who underwent XEN®-63 implantation in one eye. The XEN®-45 group comprised six male (40.0%) and nine female (60.0%) patients. Only one eye of each patient in this group was included in the study.

In both groups, 9/15 (60%) eyes had normal-tension glaucoma, 2/15 (13.3%) had primary open-angle glaucoma, 3/15 (20%) had pseudoexfoliation glaucoma, and 1/15 (6.6%) had uveitic glaucoma.

3.2. Preoperative IOP, Medications, and Previous Glaucoma Treatment

The mean preoperative IOP was 18.1 ± 3.9 mmHg (range 8–34 mmHg) in the XEN®-63 group and 18.3 ± 4.5 mmHg (range 10–35 mmHg) in the XEN®-45 group (no statistically significant difference, $t = -0.12$; $df = 28$; $p = 0.9$). The range of mean preoperative IOP per eye was 11–25 mmHg in the XEN®-63 group and 13–29.2 mmHg in the XEN®-45 group.

Preoperatively, all eyes in both groups were on topical hypotensive agents. Eyes in the XEN®-63 group were on an average of 3.3 substances, and eyes in the XEN®-45 group were on an average of 2.5 substances. In 2/15 cases (13.3%) in the XEN®-63 group and 1/15 cases (0.1%) in the XEN®-45 group, patients received additional oral acetazolamide in varying dosages.

In the XEN®-63 group, 6/15 eyes (40%) had previous glaucoma surgery, some with multiple interventions, including 4 Trabectome® surgeries, 2 MINIject® implantations, 2 cyclophotocoagulations, and 3x selective laser trabeculoplasties. The mean number of glaucoma procedures per eye in this group was 0.9. In case of previous cyclophotocoagulation, this was performed in the inferior quadrants and did not alter the condition of the superior conjunctiva where the bleb forms after XEN® implantation. There were no cases of previous conjunctival incisional surgery.

In the XEN®-45 group, 4/15 eyes (27%) had previous glaucoma surgery. Two eyes had only selective laser trabeculoplasty. Another two eyes had selective laser trabeculoplasty and Trabectome® surgery prior to XEN®-45 implantation.

In case of previous Trabectome® surgery, gonioscopy showed the absence of the trabecular meshwork in the nasal iridocorneal angle, sometimes replaced by some scar tissue.

In both groups, 10 eyes were pseudophakic, and 5 eyes were phakic.

3.3. Postoperative Outcomes

The mean IOP within 4 days (mean 2.3 days) after XEN®-63 implantation was 7.7 ± 3.0 mmHg. IOP values within 4 days after XEN®-63 implantation ranged between 1–46 mmHg (range of mean IOP per eye 4.2–12.5 mmHg). XEN®-63 implantation resulted in a mean IOP reduction of 10.4 ± 3.8 mmHg (range 3.3–14.8 mmHg), or 56.5% (range 22.0–77.9%).

The mean IOP within 4 days (mean 2.6 days) after XEN®-45 implantation was 8.5 ± 3.1 mmHg. IOP values within 4 days after XEN®-45 implantation ranged between 1–39 mmHg (range of mean IOP per eye 3.3–13.1 mmHg). XEN®-45 implantation resulted in a mean IOP reduction of 9.7 ± 6.0 mmHg (range 0.9–22.6 mmHg), or 50.4% (range 6.4–86.6%).

Furthermore, immediate postoperative IOP-lowering medication could be discontinued in all eyes in both groups.

In 10/15 eyes (66.7%) in the XEN®-63 group, the postoperative IOP was <6 mmHg at least once, and in 4 eyes (26.7%), this lasted for over 1 week. In the XEN®-45 group, 8/15 eyes (53.3%) had a postoperative IOP < 6 mmHg, but in only 1 eye (0.07%) did this last for over 1 week.

There were no cases of choroidal effusion in the XEN®-63-group. In the XEN®-45 group, two cases showed transitional choroidal effusion immediately postoperatively associated with an IOP < 6 mmHg. In each group, among the patients with an IOP < 6 mmHg, there was one case of transient choroidal folds in the macular area.

Postoperative anterior chamber hemorrhage was observed in 8/15 eyes (53.3%) in the XEN®-63 group and 10/15 eyes (66.7%) in the XEN®-45 group. In most eyes, anterior chamber hemorrhage resolved within 2–3 weeks. In the XEN®-45 group, one of the eyes with anterior chamber hemorrhage had a transient IOP spike of 39 mmHg, and in another eye, resolution of the hyphema took five weeks. In both groups, three eyes with postoperative anterior chamber hemorrhage later underwent bleb revision. In the XEN®-63 group, one of these eyes also had secondary glaucoma surgery.

One patient in the XEN®-63 group had a suprachoroidal hemorrhage, which occurred on the first postoperative day. As a result, the IOP increased from 3 mmHg initially to a maximum of 46 mmHg, and antiglaucomatous treatment was restarted. Twelve days after surgery, choroidal drainage was performed in this patient. In addition, 40 days after surgery, the patient received secondary glaucoma intervention in the form of cyclophotocoagulation. Preoperative visual acuity was 20/32 or logMAR 0.22, and visual acuity at the last follow-up was 20/160 or logMAR 0.92 (133 days postoperatively). At the time of XEN®-63 implantation, this patient was 86 years old, and the eye undergoing XEN® implantation had a diagnosis of pseudoexfoliation glaucoma for 18 years with a maximum IOP of 50 mmHg. The mean IOP on the day before surgery in this eye was 25.0 mmHg. Immediately postoperative, the IOP was 24 mmHg, but it dropped to 3 mmHg on the first postoperative day. The eye was pseudophakic and had previous myopia of −7 diopters. Before XEN® implantation, the eye underwent selective laser trabeculoplasty, Trabectome® surgery, as well as mild cyclophotocoagulation (inferior quadrants). The patient did not have other general diseases than a diagnosis of depression. In particular, the patient did not have arterial hypertension and was not on anticoagulants, antiplatelet drugs, or other cardiovascular drugs. The risk factors for suprachoroidal hemorrhage in this patient were the postoperative drop in IOP, resulting in a very low IOP, high myopia, long-term uncontrolled ocular hypertension glaucoma, previous intraocular surgeries, and the advanced age of the patient.

Suprachoroidal hemorrhage did not occur in any of the matched XEN®-45 eyes.

3.4. Follow-Up Period

The mean postoperative follow-up period was 199.1 ± 85.5 days (range 78–338 days; median 204 days) for the XEN®-63 group and 734.7 ± 619.8 days (range 99–1688 days; median 386 days) for the XEN®-45 group.

3.5. Post-XEN® Interventions (Figure 1)

In the XEN®-63 group, 5/15 eyes (33.3%) underwent open conjunctival bleb revision an average of 45 days after surgery (range 28–74 days; median 39 days) due to impaired drainage from occlusion of the stent lumen with Tenon's fascia or subconjunctival scarring.

One of these patients had previous unsuccessful needling 6 days before bleb revision (50 days after XEN implantation). There was no primary needling in the XEN®-63 group.

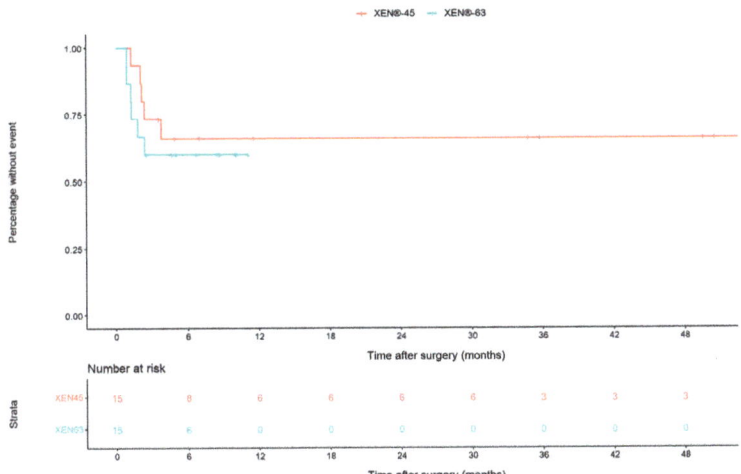

Figure 1. Kaplan–Meier curve for time to bleb revision or secondary glaucoma intervention over time. Steps indicate events, and ticks indicate eyes lost to follow-up. The follow-up period in this graphic is limited to 48 months. There was one additional open conjunctival bleb revision around 4.5 years after surgery in the XEN®-45 group. All other interventions occurred within 4 months of XEN® implantation.

In the XEN®-45 group, the same percentage of eyes (33.3%) underwent open conjunctival bleb revision an average of 330 days after surgery (range 39–1624 days; median 70 days). Only one of these bleb revisions took place more than four months after XEN®-45 implantation (namely 1624 days or about 4.5 years) and was due to impending perforation of the conjunctiva by the XEN® stent. In the XEN®-45 group, primary needling was performed in two eyes at the time of implantation. One of these eyes later underwent bleb revision 73 days postoperatively. Additionally, one eye in the XEN®-45 group had successful postoperative needling performed 63 days after implantation.

Apart from the aforementioned patient with suprachoroidal hemorrhage, who subsequently underwent cyclophotocoagulation, two other patients in the XEN®-63 group underwent PreserFlo® surgery as secondary glaucoma intervention 32 days and 196 days after XEN® implantation, respectively. Four days before PreserFlo® implantation, one of these patients underwent XEN® revision for an encapsulated bleb. After this bleb revision, IOP increased to 45 mmHg due to XEN® obstruction by iris incarceration. The XEN®-63 implant was then replaced with a PreserFlo®. None of the XEN®-45 patients required secondary glaucoma intervention within the follow-up period.

3.6. Restart of Topical Treatment

No other patient in the XEN®-63 group besides the aforementioned one with suprachoroidal hemorrhage had antiglaucomatous treatment restarted within the follow-up period (three topical drugs plus oral acetazolamide).

In the XEN®-45 group, there was one patient who had to restart topical antiglaucomatous treatment (two agents) 302 days after XEN® implantation or 263 days after bleb revision. Two other patients in the XEN®-45 group restarted topical antiglaucomatous treatment without previous bleb-revision 386 days (one agent) and 638 days (initially one agent, but later extended to four agents) post-surgery, respectively.

The mean number of topical antiglaucomatous agents at the end of follow-up was 0.2 ± 0.8 in the XEN®-63 group and 0.5 ± 1.1 in the XEN®-45 group. Compared to the baseline, the mean number of topical antiglaucomatous agents was reduced by 3.1 ± 0.9 agents (94.0%) in the XEN®-63 group and by 2.1 ± 1.8 agents (81.6%) in the XEN®-45 group.

3.7. IOP at Final Follow-Up

For IOP analysis at the final follow-up, we excluded all eyes with secondary glaucoma surgery. Eyes that underwent bleb revision but no secondary glaucoma surgery were included.

In the XEN®-63 group, the mean IOP at the final follow-up was 9.1 mmHg (range 6–12 mmHg). The mean IOP reduction was 7.9 mmHg (range 2.8–13.2 mmHg), or 44.6% (range 18.9–68.8) in the XEN®-63 group.

In the XEN®-45 group, the mean IOP at the final follow-up was 10.5 mmHg (range 7–15 mmHg). The mean IOP reduction was 7.8 mmHg (range 2.0–16.7 mmHg), or 39.8% (range 15.4–67.9%).

The following tables provide a summary of the main results for IOP values (Table 1), topical antiglaucomatous medication (Table 2), postoperative interventions (Table 3), and success rates (Table 4).

Table 1. IOP values.

	XEN®-63 (15 Eyes of 13 Patients)		XEN®-45 (15 Eyes of 15 Patients)	
	Mean	Range	Mean	Range
At baseline: IOP	18.1 mmHg	8–34 mmHg	18.3 mmHg	10–35 mmHg
Within 1–4 days after XEN® implantation: IOP	7.7 mmHg range of mean IOP per eye: 4.2–12.5 mmHg	1–46 mmHg	8.5 mmHg range of mean IOP per eye: 3.3–13.1 mmHg	1–39 mmHg
IOP reduction	10.4 mmHg 56.5%	3.3–14.8 mmHg 22.0–77.9%	9.7 mmHg 50.4%	0.9–22.6 mmHg 6.43–86.6%
Follow-up period	199.1 ± 85.5 days (median 204 days)	78–338 days	734.7 ± 619.8 days (median 386 days)	99–1688 days
At final follow-up: (excluding patients with secondary glaucoma surgery) IOP IOP reduction	9.1 mmHg 7.9 mmHg 44.6%	6–12 mmHg 2.8–13.2 mmHg 18.9–68.8%	10.5 mmHg 7.8 mmHg 39.8%	7–15 mmHg 2–16.7 mmHg 15.4–67.9%

Table 2. Topical antiglaucomatous medication.

	XEN®-63 (15 Eyes of 13 Patients)	XEN®-45 (15 Eyes of 15 Patients)
At baseline:		
• mean number of topical antiglaucomatous agents	3.3 agents	2.5 agents
• eyes on topical treatment	15/15 eyes (100%)	15/15 eyes (100%)
At final follow-up:		
• mean number of topical antiglaucomatous agents	0.2 agents	0.5 agents
• eyes on topical treatment	1/15 eyes (6.7%)	3/15 eyes (20.0%)
• reduction of topical treatment	−3.1 ± 0.9 (−93.9%)	−2.1 ± 1.8 (−81.6%)

Table 3. Postoperative interventions.

	XEN®-63 (15 Eyes of 13 Patients)		XEN®-45 (15 Eyes of 15 Patients)	
• Postoperative needling	1/15 eyes	6.7%	1/15 eyes	6.7%
• Bleb revision	5/15 eyes	33.3%	5/15 eyes	33.3%
• Bleb revision within 6 months	5/15 eyes	33.3%	4/15 eyes	26.7%
• Interval between XEN® implantation and bleb revision	45 days (mean) 39 days (median)	range 28–74 days	330 days (mean) 70 days (median)	range 39–1624 days
• Secondary glaucoma surgery	3/15 patients	20.0%	--	--
• Interval between XEN® implantation and secondary glaucoma surgery	89.3 days	range 32–196 days	--	--

Table 4. Success rates at final follow-up.

	XEN®-63 (15 Eyes of 13 Patients)		XEN®-45 (15 Eyes of 15 Patients)	
Complete success (without ocular hypotensive medications, without secondary glaucoma surgery)	11/15 eyes	73.3%	10/15 eyes	66.7%
• Final IOP ≤ 15 mmHg ≥ 6 mmHg	12/15 eyes	80.0%	12/15 eyes	80.0%
• Final IOP ≤ 12 mmHg ≥ 6 mmHg	12/15 eyes	80.0%	10/15 eyes	66.7%
• IOP reduction ≥ 20%	11/15 eyes	73.3%	10/15 eyes	66.7%
Qualified success (with ocular hypotensive medications, without secondary glaucoma surgery)	--	--	2/15 eyes	13.3%
• Final IOP ≤ 15 mmHg	--	--	3/15 eyes	20.0%
• Final IOP ≤ 12 mmHg	--	--	2/15 eyes	13.3%
• IOP reduction ≥ 20%	--	--	2/15 eyes	13.3%
Failure (IOP reduction < 20%)	1/15 eyes	6.7%	3/15 eyes	20.0%
Complete Failure (Secondary glaucoma surgery)	3/15 eyes	20.0%	--	--

In the XEN®-63 group, 11/15 eyes (73.3%) showed complete success with a final IOP of not only ≤15 mmHg but also ≤12 mmHg and ≥6 mmHg as well as an IOP reduction of ≥20% without ocular hypotensive medications. One eye in the XEN®-63 group (6.7%) was censored as a failure despite having a final IOP of 12 mmHg because the IOP reduction from baseline was <20%. Three other eyes in the XEN®-63 group (20.0%) were censored as complete failure due to secondary glaucoma surgery.

In the XEN®-45 group, 10/15 eyes (66.7%) showed complete success with a final IOP of ≤15 mmHg and ≥6 mmHg, as well as an IOP reduction of ≥20% without ocular hypotensive medications. Only one of these eyes had a final IOP > 12 mmHg but an IOP reduction of >20%. Two eyes in the XEN®-45 group (13.3%) achieved qualified success with a final IOP ≤ 12 mmHg and ≥6 mmHg, as well as an IOP reduction of ≥20% with ocular hypotensive medications. Three other eyes in the XEN®-45 group (20.0%) were censored as a failure because the IOP reduction from baseline was <20%. The final IOP in these eyes was 15 mmHg, 13 mmHg, and 11 mmHg, respectively.

There was no statistically significant difference in baseline and final IOP or IOP reduction between the two groups (Table 5). This may be due to the small sample size.

Table 5. Results of unpaired *t*-test comparing IOP outcomes between XEN®-63 and XEN®-45.

	t	df	*p*
• IOP at baseline	−0.12	28	0.90
• IOP within a few days after XEN® implantation	−0.74	28	0.47
• IOP reduction within a few days after XEN® implantation (total)	0.35	28	0.72
• IOP reduction within a few days after XEN® implantation (percentage)	0.87	28	0.39
• IOP at final follow-up	−1.64	25	0.11
• IOP reduction at final follow-up (total)	0.06	25	0.95
• IOP reduction at final follow-up (percentage)	0.7	25	0.49

4. Discussion

4.1. Effectivity

Our study shows effective IOP reduction after XEN®-63 implantation with mitomycin C. Compared to XEN®-45, the percentage IOP reduction at the end of follow-up was more pronounced (44.6% versus 39.8%), and the absolute IOP at the last visit was slightly lower (mean IOP of 9.1 mmHg versus 10.5 mmHg). These results are clinically relevant and favor XEN®-63, but due to the small sample size, they are not statistically significant. Furthermore, both XEN®-63 and XEN®-45 in our study showed high effectiveness in reducing medical treatment, with all but one patient off treatment at the end of follow-up in the XEN®-63 group and three patients having restarted topical treatment at the end of follow-up in the XEN®-45 group.

However, the follow-up period was short and differed between the two groups, with a median of 204 days (range 78–338 days) in the XEN®-63 group and a median of 386 days (range 99–1688 days) in the XEN®-45 group, which may influence the comparability of the two groups.

When interpreting our study results, it should also be considered that a high percentage of patients had normal-tension glaucoma. This distribution may limit how well the findings generalize to primary open-angle glaucoma populations. However, the fact that in a majority of cases, we observed substantial IOP reduction of ≥20% in a cohort dominated by normal-tension glaucoma suggests efficacy could potentially be even greater in cohorts comprising only primary open-angle glaucoma patients.

Fea et al. [19], in a retrospective study of XEN®-63 implantation with mitomycin C (n = 23) for primary open-angle glaucoma, found similar results after 3 months, with a slightly higher mean IOP (12.2 ± 3.4 mmHg) and slightly lower IOP reduction (40.8 ± 23.5%) at the end of follow-up (baseline IOP 27.0 ± 7.8 mmHg). They also found an effective reduction in the number of hypotensive medications. After 18 months [20], they reported a mean IOP of 14.1 ± 3.4 mmHg without hypotensive medication.

In their recently published retrospective cohort study, Hussien et al. [21] compared outcomes between XEN®-63 and XEN®-45 (*n* = 42 eyes of 41 patients per group) at 12 months post-surgery. They found a significantly higher complete success rate with XEN®-63 compared to XEN®-45 (59.5% vs. 28.6%, *p* = 0.009), although the qualified success rate was not significantly different between groups (66.7% vs. 45.2%, *p* = 0.08). The XEN®-63 group demonstrated a lower mean IOP (12.7 ± 4.8 vs. 15.5 ± 5.1 mmHg, *p* = 0.001) and required fewer medication classes (0.6 ± 1.1 vs. 1.7 ± 1.6 agents, *p* = 0.0005) compared to the XEN®-45 group. While the final IOP was lower in both of our study groups, our follow-up period was shorter compared to the study by Hussien et al. Additionally, unlike our study, they utilized both closed and open conjunctival approaches with ab interno XEN® stent placement. Their cohort also included eyes with combined cataract surgery and previous subconjunctival surgery, which differed from our study population.

4.2. Safety

We observed more cases of hypotony < 6 mmHg lasting over one week after XEN®-63 implantation (4/15, 26.7%) compared to XEN®-45 implantation (1/15, 6.7%). Associated with hypotony, in the XEN®-45 group, 2/15 eyes (13.3%) showed transient choroidal effusion. In the XEN®-63 group, there was one case of suprachoroidal hemorrhage, a rare sight-threatening complication after XEN® implantation, for which there are only a few case reports in the literature following or during XEN®-45 implantation [22–24].

Similarly, Hussien et al. [21] reported more distinct adverse events in the XEN®-63 group compared to XEN®-45 (34 vs. 19 events), though most were early and transient.

Fea et al. [19,20] reported a rate of 17.4% for both transient hypotony and choroidal detachment after XEN®-63 implantation.

4.3. Needling/Revision/Secondary Surgery

In both of our study groups, one-third of the eyes underwent open conjunctival bleb revision. In 9/10 eyes, this bleb revision was due to impaired drainage and occurred 2–4 months after XEN® implantation. Therefore, impaired outflow in our study frequently occurred after implantation of both XEN® types and quite early after XEN® implantation (within 4 months). Only in one eye of the XEN®-45 group did it occur several years after implantation and was due to impending conjunctival perforation. Therefore, the short and differing follow-up periods between the two XEN® groups may not be as relevant in this regard.

However, the shorter follow-up period for the XEN®-63 may artificially favor its outcome by providing insufficient time for failures or complications to manifest. The high rate of bleb revision required in both XEN® groups may limit the success of this technique and should be considered when comparing XEN® implantation to alternative glaucoma interventions.

A high revision rate has been reported for XEN®-45 in the literature [2,4,7,9–13]. To reduce postoperative needling and revision rates, open conjunctival or semi-open techniques have been proposed for XEN® implantation [25–27]. For XEN® implantation, we prefer an ab interno, closed conjunctiva approach, which it is designed for. In cases where an ab externo approach with open conjunctival dissection is favorable, we opt to use the PreserFlo® micro shunt instead.

Secondary glaucoma intervention in this study was more frequent in the XEN®-63 group. However, this was due to rare complications that can also occur after XEN®-45 implantation. Given the small sample size, this difference cannot be considered evidence of a significant difference between the two XEN® types.

In the study by Fea et al. [20], 17.4% underwent needling after a mean of 42.9 ± 11.2 days (one due to elevated IOP). Furthermore, 17.4% of their study required additional surgery: two trabeculectomies (8.7%), one XEN® replacement with XEN®-45 (4.3%), one high-intensity focused ultrasound cyclodestruction (HIFU), and one more patient needed needling or additional surgery at the final follow-up.

There are several studies reporting promising results for needling or bleb revision after XEN®-45 implantation [28–32], some favoring bleb revision over needling [31,32], as we do in the case of bleb fibrosis. Studies on an older, non-marketed version of XEN®-63 after 1–5 years of follow-up reported an IOP reduction of 18–40% and a needling rate of 0–53% [16–18,33].

In the Hussien et al. study [21], the needling rate was 11.9% in each group done as an in-clinic intervention at the slit-lamp. The number of postoperative interventions (28 vs. 21, including needlings) and rate of reoperation (9 (21.4%) versus 6 (14.3%)) were higher in the XEN®-63 group compared to XEN®-45. Reoperations, considered failures in their study, included in-operating room revision surgeries.

4.4. Limitations

Our study is limited by its retrospective nature and relatively small sample size. The follow-up period was short and differed between the two groups. Our study may serve as an orientation for designing a prospective study comparing XEN®-63 versus XEN®-45.

5. Conclusions

XEN®-63 implantation with mitomycin C may lead to even lower IOP levels compared to XEN®-45 implantation over a short follow-up period. Larger studies with longer follow-ups are needed to confirm if this difference persists over time. The rates of complications and required revisions appear to be largely comparable. Further research is needed to evaluate the safety, efficacy, and role of XEN®-63 relative to XEN®-45 and other glaucoma procedures.

Author Contributions: Conceptualization, C.E. and J.L.; Data curation, C.E. and S.K.; Formal analysis, C.E., D.B., S.K., P.K., H.P., T.P., T.R. and J.L.; Investigation, C.E., P.K., H.P. and J.L.; Methodology, C.E., D.B., H.P. and J.L.; Software, D.B.; Supervision, T.R. and J.L.; Validation, C.E., D.B. and J.L.; Visualization, C.E. and D.B.; Writing—original draft, C.E.; Writing—review & editing, D.B., S.K., P.K., H.P., T.P., T.R. and J.L. All authors have read and agreed to the published version of the manuscript.

Funding: This research received no external funding. We acknowledge support by the Open Access Publication Fund of the University of Freiburg.

Institutional Review Board Statement: The study was conducted according to the guidelines of the Declaration of Helsinki and approved by the Ethics Committee of the University of Freiburg (No. 21-1202_02).

Informed Consent Statement: Patient consent was waived because it was not required by law for this study.

Data Availability Statement: The data presented in this study are available on request from the corresponding author. The data are not publicly available due to ethical restrictions.

Conflicts of Interest: C.E. has received a travel grant, and J.L. has received an honorary from Allergan/Abbvie. All other authors declare no conflict of interest.

References

1. Lewis, R.A. Ab Interno Approach to the Subconjunctival Space Using a Collagen Glaucoma Stent. *J. Cataract. Refract. Surg.* **2014**, *40*, 1301–1306. [CrossRef]
2. Hengerer, F.H.; Auffarth, G.U.; Yildirim, T.M.; Conrad-Hengerer, I. Ab Interno Gel Implant in Patients with Primary Open Angle Glaucoma and Pseudoexfoliation Glaucoma. *BMC Ophthalmol.* **2018**, *18*, 339. [CrossRef] [PubMed]
3. Mansouri, K.; Gillmann, K.; Rao, H.L.; Guidotti, J.; Mermoud, A. Prospective Evaluation of XEN Gel Implant in Eyes with Pseudoexfoliative Glaucoma. *J. Glaucoma* **2018**, *27*, 869–873. [CrossRef]
4. Widder, R.A.; Dietlein, T.S.; Dinslage, S.; Kühnrich, P.; Rennings, C.; Rössler, G. The XEN45 Gel Stent as a Minimally Invasive Procedure in Glaucoma Surgery: Success Rates, Risk Profile, and Rates of Re-Surgery after 261 Surgeries. *Graefes Arch. Clin. Exp. Ophthalmol.* **2018**, *256*, 765–771. [CrossRef] [PubMed]
5. Sng, C.C.; Wang, J.; Hau, S.; Htoon, H.M.; Barton, K. XEN-45 Collagen Implant for the Treatment of Uveitic Glaucoma. *Clin. Exp. Ophthalmol.* **2018**, *46*, 339–345. [CrossRef]
6. Qureshi, A.; Jones, N.P.; Au, L. Urgent Management of Secondary Glaucoma in Uveitis Using the Xen-45 Gel Stent. *J. Glaucoma* **2019**, *28*, 1061–1066. [CrossRef]
7. Schargus, M.; Theilig, T.; Rehak, M.; Busch, C.; Bormann, C.; Unterlauft, J.D. Outcome of a Single XEN Microstent Implant for Glaucoma Patients with Different Types of Glaucoma. *BMC Ophthalmol.* **2020**, *20*, 490. [CrossRef]
8. Marcos Parra, M.T.; Salinas López, J.A.; López Grau, N.S.; Ceausescu, A.M.; Pérez Santonja, J.J. XEN Implant Device versus Trabeculectomy, Either Alone or in Combination with Phacoemulsification, in Open-Angle Glaucoma Patients. *Graefes Arch. Clin. Exp. Ophthalmol.* **2019**, *257*, 1741–1750. [CrossRef]
9. Galal, A.; Bilgic, A.; Eltanamly, R.; Osman, A. XEN Glaucoma Implant with Mitomycin C 1-Year Follow-Up: Result and Complications. *J. Ophthalmol.* **2017**, *2017*, 5457246. [CrossRef] [PubMed]
10. Reitsamer, H.; Sng, C.; Vera, V.; Lenzhofer, M.; Barton, K.; Stalmans, I. Apex Study Group Two-Year Results of a Multicenter Study of the Ab Interno Gelatin Implant in Medically Uncontrolled Primary Open-Angle Glaucoma. *Graefes Arch. Clin. Exp. Ophthalmol.* **2019**, *257*, 983–996. [CrossRef]

11. Reitsamer, H.; Vera, V.; Ruben, S.; Au, L.; Vila-Arteaga, J.; Teus, M.; Lenzhofer, M.; Shirlaw, A.; Bai, Z.; Balaram, M.; et al. Three-Year Effectiveness and Safety of the XEN Gel Stent as a Solo Procedure or in Combination with Phacoemulsification in Open-Angle Glaucoma: A Multicentre Study. *Acta Ophthalmol.* **2022**, *100*, e233–e245. [CrossRef]
12. Schlenker, M.B.; Gulamhusein, H.; Conrad-Hengerer, I.; Somers, A.; Lenzhofer, M.; Stalmans, I.; Reitsamer, H.; Hengerer, F.H.; Ahmed, I.I.K. Efficacy, Safety, and Risk Factors for Failure of Standalone Ab Interno Gelatin Microstent Implantation versus Standalone Trabeculectomy. *Ophthalmology* **2017**, *124*, 1579–1588. [CrossRef]
13. Tan, S.Z.; Walkden, A.; Au, L. One-Year Result of XEN45 Implant for Glaucoma: Efficacy, Safety, and Postoperative Management. *Eye* **2018**, *32*, 324–332. [CrossRef]
14. Marcos-Parra, M.T.; Mendoza-Moreira, A.L.; Moreno-Castro, L.; Mateos-Marcos, C.; Salinas-López, J.A.; Figuerola-García, M.B.; González-Alonso, Á.; Pérez-Santonja, J.J. 3-Year Outcomes of XEN Implant Compared with Trabeculectomy, with or without Phacoemulsification for Open Angle Glaucoma. *J. Glaucoma* **2022**, *31*, 826–833. [CrossRef] [PubMed]
15. Poelman, H.J.; Pals, J.; Rostamzad, P.; Bramer, W.M.; Wolfs, R.C.W.; Ramdas, W.D. Efficacy of the XEN-Implant in Glaucoma and a Meta-Analysis of the Literature. *J. Clin. Med.* **2021**, *10*, 1118. [CrossRef] [PubMed]
16. Sheybani, A.; Lenzhofer, M.; Hohensinn, M.; Reitsamer, H.; Ahmed, I.I.K. Phacoemulsification Combined with a New Ab Interno Gel Stent to Treat Open-Angle Glaucoma: Pilot Study. *J. Cataract. Refract. Surg.* **2015**, *41*, 1905–1909. [CrossRef] [PubMed]
17. Lenzhofer, M.; Kersten-Gomez, I.; Sheybani, A.; Gulamhusein, H.; Strohmaier, C.; Hohensinn, M.; Burkhard Dick, H.; Hitzl, W.; Eisenkopf, L.; Sedarous, F.; et al. Four-Year Results of a Minimally Invasive Transscleral Glaucoma Gel Stent Implantation in a Prospective Multi-Centre Study. *Clin. Exp. Ophthalmol.* **2019**, *47*, 581–587. [CrossRef] [PubMed]
18. Lavin-Dapena, C.; Cordero-Ros, R.; D'Anna, O.; Mogollón, I. XEN 63 Gel Stent Device in Glaucoma Surgery: A 5-Years Follow-up Prospective Study. *Eur. J. Ophthalmol.* **2021**, *31*, 1829–1835. [CrossRef]
19. Fea, A.M.; Menchini, M.; Rossi, A.; Posarelli, C.; Malinverni, L.; Figus, M. Early Experience with the New XEN63 Implant in Primary Open-Angle Glaucoma Patients: Clinical Outcomes. *J. Clin. Med.* **2021**, *10*, 1628. [CrossRef]
20. Fea, A.M.; Menchini, M.; Rossi, A.; Posarelli, C.; Malinverni, L.; Figus, M. Outcomes of XEN 63 Device at 18-Month Follow-Up in Glaucoma Patients: A Two-Center Retrospective Study. *J. Clin. Med.* **2022**, *11*, 3801. [CrossRef]
21. Hussien, I.M.; De Francesco, T.; Ahmed, I.I.K. Intermediate Outcomes of the Novel 63 μm Gelatin Microstent versus the Conventional 45 μm Gelatin Microstent. *Ophthalmol. Glaucoma* **2023**, *in press*. [CrossRef]
22. Prokosch-Willing, V.; Vossmerbaeumer, U.; Hoffmann, E.; Pfeiffer, N. Suprachoroidal Bleeding After XEN Gel Implantation. *J. Glaucoma* **2017**, *26*, e261–e263. [CrossRef]
23. Liu, J.C.; Green, W.; Sheybani, A.; Lind, J.T. Intraoperative Suprachoroidal Hemorrhage during Xen Gel Stent Implantation. *Am. J. Ophthalmol. Case Rep.* **2020**, *17*, 100600. [CrossRef] [PubMed]
24. Wang, K.; Wang, J.C.; Sarrafpour, S. Suprachoroidal Hemorrhage after XEN Gel Implant Requiring Surgical Drainage. *J. Curr. Glaucoma Pract.* **2022**, *16*, 132–135. [CrossRef] [PubMed]
25. Dangda, S.; Radell, J.E.; Mavrommatis, M.A.; Lee, R.; Do, A.; Sidoti, P.A.; Panarelli, J.F. Open Conjunctival Approach for Sub-Tenon's Xen Gel Stent Placement and Bleb Morphology by Anterior Segment Optical Coherence Tomography. *J. Glaucoma* **2021**, *30*, 988–995. [CrossRef] [PubMed]
26. Do, A.; McGlumphy, E.; Shukla, A.; Dangda, S.; Schuman, J.S.; Boland, M.V.; Yohannan, J.; Panarelli, J.F.; Craven, E.R. Comparison of Clinical Outcomes with Open Versus Closed Conjunctiva Implantation of the XEN45 Gel Stent. *Ophthalmol. Glaucoma* **2021**, *4*, 343–349. [CrossRef]
27. Kong, Y.X.G.; Chung, I.Y.; Ang, G.S. Outcomes of XEN45 Gel Stent Using Posterior Small Incision Sub-Tenon Ab Interno Insertion (Semi-Open) Technique. *Eye* **2022**, *36*, 1456–1460. [CrossRef]
28. Linton, E.; Au, L. Technique of Xen Implant Revision Surgery and the Surgical Outcomes: A Retrospective Interventional Case Series. *Ophthalmol. Ther.* **2020**, *9*, 149–157. [CrossRef]
29. Midha, N.; Gillmann, K.; Chaudhary, A.; Mermoud, A.; Mansouri, K. Efficacy of Needling Revision After XEN Gel Stent Implantation: A Prospective Study. *J. Glaucoma* **2020**, *29*, 11–14. [CrossRef] [PubMed]
30. José, P.; Teixeira, F.J.; Barão, R.C.; Sens, P.; Abegão Pinto, L. Needling after XEN Gel Implant: What's the Efficacy? A 1-Year Analysis. *Eur. J. Ophthalmol.* **2021**, *31*, 3087–3092. [CrossRef]
31. Ventura-Abreu, N.; Dotti-Boada, M.; Muniesa-Royo, M.J.; Izquierdo-Serra, J.; González-Ventosa, A.; Millá, E.; Pazos, M. XEN45 Real-Life Evaluation: Survival Analysis with Bleb Needling and Major Revision Outcomes. *Eur. J. Ophthalmol.* **2022**, *32*, 984–992. [CrossRef] [PubMed]
32. Steiner, S.; Resch, H.; Kiss, B.; Buda, D.; Vass, C. Needling and Open Filtering Bleb Revision after XEN-45 Implantation-a Retrospective Outcome Comparison. *Graefes Arch. Clin. Exp. Ophthalmol.* **2021**, *259*, 2761–2770. [CrossRef] [PubMed]
33. Fernández-García, A.; Zhou, Y.; García-Alonso, M.; Andrango, H.D.; Poyales, F.; Garzón, N. Comparing Medium-Term Clinical Outcomes Following XEN® 45 and XEN® 63 Device Implantation. *J. Ophthalmol.* **2020**, *2020*, 4796548. [CrossRef] [PubMed]

Disclaimer/Publisher's Note: The statements, opinions and data contained in all publications are solely those of the individual author(s) and contributor(s) and not of MDPI and/or the editor(s). MDPI and/or the editor(s) disclaim responsibility for any injury to people or property resulting from any ideas, methods, instructions or products referred to in the content.

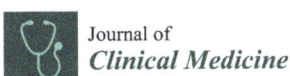

Case Report

XEN Gel Stent for Conjunctiva with Minimal Mobility Caused by Scleral Encircling: A Case Report

Yuri Kim [1], Myungjin Kim [1], Dai Woo Kim [2] and Seungsoo Rho [1,*]

[1] Department of Ophthalmology, Bundang CHA Medical Center, CHA University, Seongnam 13496, Republic of Korea; kimyuri0550@gmail.com (Y.K.); brandmjeyes@gmail.com (M.K.)
[2] Department of Ophthalmology, School of Medicine, Kyungpook National University, Daegu 41944, Republic of Korea; proector97@gmail.com
* Correspondence: harryrho@gmail.com; Tel.: +82-31-780-5330

Abstract: This case report describes the successful use of a XEN gel stent for controlling intraocular pressure (IOP) in a patient who had previously undergone scleral encircling for rhegmatogenous retinal detachment. The patient had very limited mobile conjunctiva due to scarring caused by the earlier surgery, which limited their options for glaucoma surgery. The XEN gel stent, a minimally invasive glaucoma surgery (MIGS) procedure that does not require opening the conjunctiva, was implanted in the subconjunctival space using an ab interno approach. Postoperative blebs were imaged using anterior segment optical coherence tomography, and IOP was monitored over six months. This study found that the XEN gel stent effectively controlled the IOP, and there were no complications during or after surgery. This case report may expand the indication for the XEN gel stent, which could be considered a viable option for patients who have undergone scleral buckling and have limited mobile conjunctiva.

Keywords: MIGS; XEN gel stent; scleral buckling; blebs

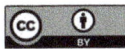

1. Introduction

Minimally invasive glaucoma surgery (MIGS) represents a collection of conjunctival-sparing, ab interno procedures to control intraocular pressure (IOP) in primary open-angle glaucoma or pseudoexfoliation glaucoma eyes [1]. In particular, the bleb-forming glaucoma procedure necessitates the use of conjunctiva; therefore, the more mobile the conjunctiva, the better the outcome. Rhegmatogenous retinal detachment is the most common retinological emergency threatening vision, with an incidence of 1 in 10,000 persons per year, which can cause blindness in the affected eye without proper treatment [2,3]. However, there is no valid justification for refraining from conducting retinal detachment surgery solely based on the presence of mobile conjunctiva, which may potentially be involved in glaucoma surgery at a later point in time. In particular, scleral buckling causes scarring due to damage to the conjunctiva and creates more fibrotic conjunctiva with less mobile area, which reduces the selection width of glaucoma surgical options.

We would like to report a case that successfully formed blebs using a XEN gel stent through the least mobile conjunctiva remaining in the eyes owing to previous scleral buckling. To the best of our knowledge, this is the first report that describes that a XEN gel stent implantation using an ab interno approach can control the IOP in an eye with previous scleral buckling history. This report also offers the morphologic evaluation of the bleb for six months using anterior segment optical coherence tomography (AS-OCT) and might help endeavors to expand the indication for the XEN gel stent in eyes with minimally mobile conjunctiva.

2. Case Presentation

A 49-year-old female was referred to glaucoma service for IOP control. She first visited our hospital for further surgical management of the right eye fourteen years ago. Due to rhegmatogenous retinal detachment, the eye underwent scleral encircling with a 360-degree conjunctiva peritomy using a 4 mm thick sponge, cryopexy (performed between 10:30 and 1:30 o'clock), and pars plana vitrectomy. After one month, the silicone sponge was removed due to uncontrolled IOP. IOP normalized after the sponge was removed. After five years, the patient had undergone cataract surgery in the same eye. The IOP was around 20 mmHg despite maximally tolerated medical treatment, which included preservative-free dorzolamide and timolol, preservative-free 0.15% brimonidine tartrate, and preservative-free latanoprost eye drops. At the time of presentation to glaucoma service, which was thirteen years after the encircling, her best-corrected visual acuity in the right eye remained 20/20, but the IOP was 25 mmHg. The axial length was 26.53 mm, which implies a highly myopic eye. One year after, the visual field index fell from 79% to 71% in the last year (Figure 1). Apart from the uncontrolled IOP and progressing visual field deterioration, surgical intervention was considered, since her eye became allergic and she complained of eyelid change to brimonidine and bimatoprost eye drops, respectively. As possible surgical options, an Ahmed glaucoma valve, trabeculectomy, or a XEN gel stent were prepared. The surgeon had a scrutinized preoperative interview with the patient on the best, most possible option, which would be decided according to the result of the conjunctival mobility check using an injection of air, lidocaine, etc.

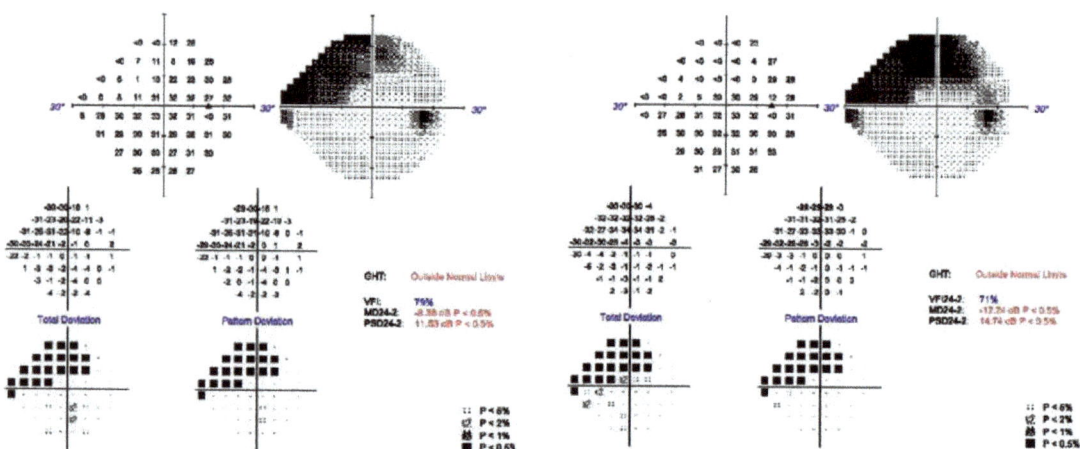

Figure 1. Visual field change before XEN gel stent implantation. Note that the visual field index decreased from 79% (left) to 71% (right) in the last year before the decision for surgery.

Surgical procedures were performed by a skilled surgeon (S.R.) as described elsewhere [4]. Briefly, after topical anesthesia, air and ocular viscoelastics were injected into subconjunctival space to dissect the conjunctiva and the tenon's capsule to confirm the presence of the mobile conjunctiva. Almost the entire conjunctiva was immobile due to adhesion (Figure 2A), but fortunately, some spared mobile conjunctiva was noted (Figure 2B) in the superonasal quadrant. A 0.05 mL mix of 2% lidocaine with epinephrine (1:10,000, 0.1 mL) was injected using a 30 G needle into the superior subconjunctival space located approximately 6 mm apart from the region that the XEN tip is expected to occupy. After an injection of viscoelastics to maintain the anterior chamber using a 1 mm side port, the XEN injector was advanced through a 1.5 mm clear corneal incision at the inferotemporal limbus toward the opposite superonasal target angle The injector was approached to the angle into the subconjunctival space 2 mm apart from the limbus. After confirming the allocation of the XEN gel stent in the mobile conjunctiva by the dissection described earlier, the injector was moved backwards and removed gently out of the corneal incision. The proper location and length (approximately 1 mm) of the stent in the anterior chamber were checked using a surgical gonioscope, and the mobility and length (approximately 3 mm) of the subconjunctivally located part of the stent were confirmed (Figure 2C,D). Irrigation and aspiration were carried out to remove the viscoelastics. The corneal wounds were secured by hydrosealing using a balanced salt solution. A quantity of 0.05 mL mitomycin C (MMC) 0.4 mg/mL was injected into the superonasal subconjunctival space using a 30 G needle [4].

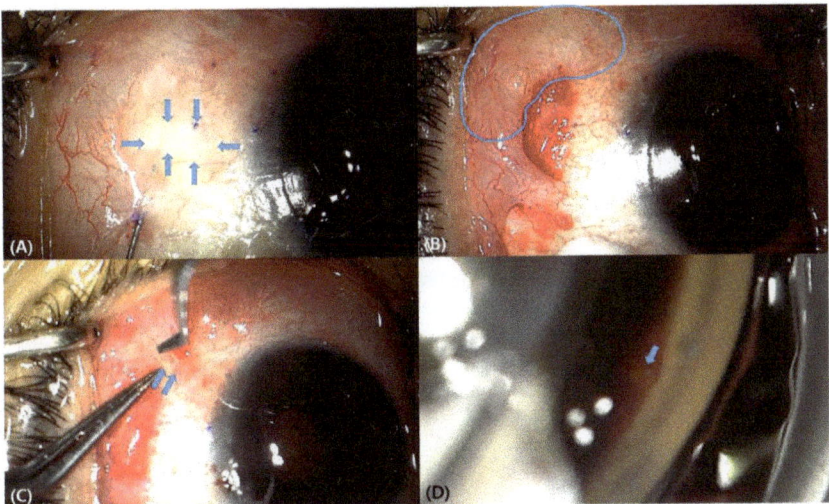

Figure 2. Intraoperative findings for XEN gel stent under a surgical microscope. (**A**) Blue arrows indicate immobile conjunctiva due to adhesion. (**B**) Blue line indicates spared conjunctiva. (**C**) Blue arrows indicate XEN gel stent. (**D**) Blue arrow indicates XEN gel stent during gonioscopy examination.

On the first day following surgery, the IOP was 10 mmHg, and moxifloxacin, prednisolone, and mydriatic eye drops were administered 4 times a day. On the 4th day after surgery, the IOP was 14 mmHg, and the vision had fully recovered to the preoperative level of 20/20. On the 11th day after surgery, the IOP was 21 mmHg, so once-daily use of preservative-free timolol/dorzolamide eye drops was initiated, and the IOP was maintained at 16 → 14 → 12 mmHg (1 → 3 → 6 months after surgery, Figure 3). Using slit-lamp examination of the bleb morphology, a localized avascular bleb was observed. Checking the morphology of blebs using OCT, a high, sparse wall was observed during the all follow-ups (Figure 4). The lengths of the fluid-filled cavity parallel and perpendicular to the section line at 6 months were 3.065 mm and 3.555 mm. The estimated size of the bleb was 34.21 mm^2.

This study adhered to the principles of the Declaration of Helsinki. Written informed consent for the report and photographs was obtained from the patient. Postoperative blebs were imaged using slit-lamp photography and a Spectralis OCT (Heidelberg Engineering GmbH, Heidelberg, Germany) on postoperative day 1, week 1, week 2, and months 1, 2, 3, and 6, as described elsewhere. Briefly, a total of 41 section scans were aligned along with the parallel line at the point where the XEN tip was located. Images with quality scores higher than 25 were included in the final qualitative analysis. The maximum bleb height was selected and measured within the 41 sections that were obtained at each visit [4].

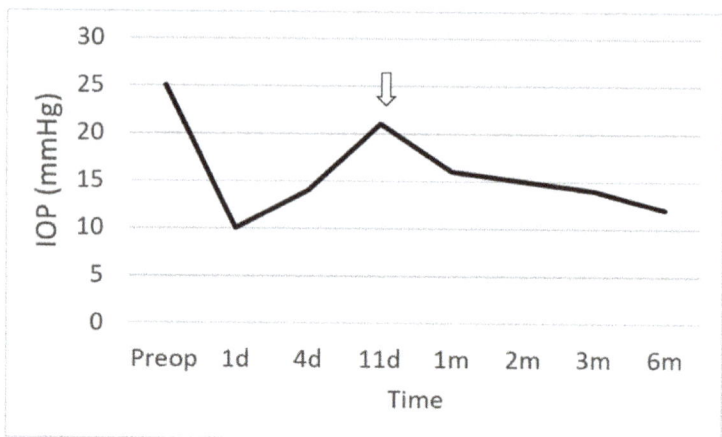

Figure 3. The change in intraocular pressure (IOP). Note that the IOP rose to 21 mmHg on postoperative day 11 (*white arrow*). The IOP was controlled after the readministration of timolol/dorzolamide eye drops once daily.

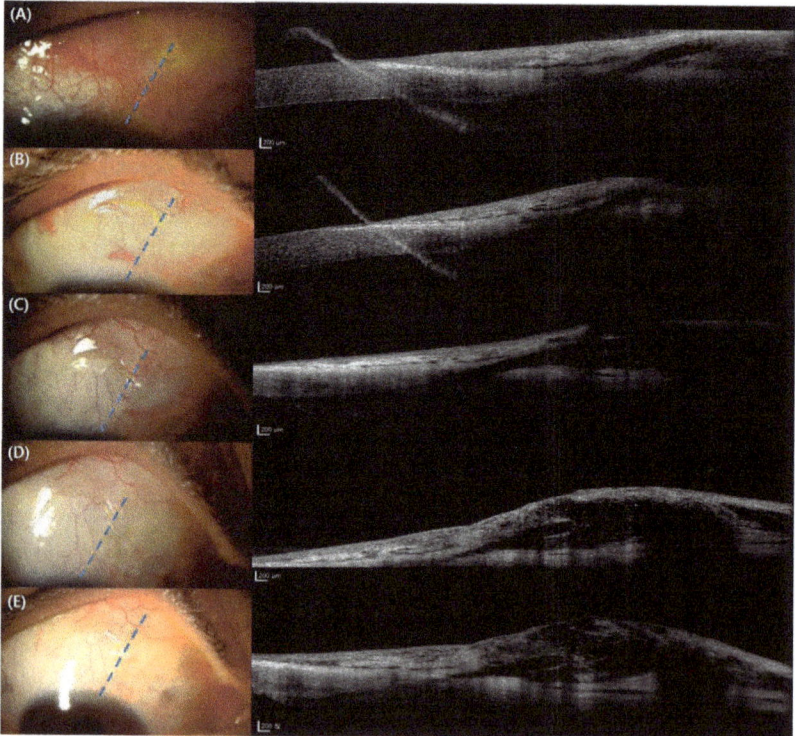

Figure 4. Bleb morphology using slit-lamp photos and AS-OCT imaging at postoperative day 1 (**A**), day 4 (**B**), day 14 (**C**), month 1 (**D**), month 3 (**E**), respectively. Note that the bleb morphology observed using slit-lamp photography exhibits characteristics of a localized avascular nature, while the bleb morphology observed using anterior segment optical coherence tomography (AS-OCT) demonstrates characteristics of a high sparse wall type. Please note that blue dashed lines represent the same location of each OCT section.

3. Discussion

The XEN gel stent is recognized as a safe and effective MIGS procedure compared to conventional trabeculectomy [5]. Both filtration surgeries are considered bleb-forming surgery, which depends on the size of their blebs. A healthy conjunctiva is required for both bleb-forming glaucoma operations. Watanabe-Kitamura et al. reported that, at 12 months post-trabeculectomy, the volume ratio correlated with the IOP and the number of eye drops needed using a 3D investigation of bleb volume after trabeculectomy. [6] Kawana et al. evaluated that the IOP showed a significant negative correlation with the horizontal and vertical lengths of the fluid-filled cavity, the height of the cavity, and the volume of the internal fluid-filled cavity [7]. The mean horizontal and vertical lengths of the cavity of successful blebs were longer than those of failed blebs (3.86 ± 2.16 mm and 4.23 ± 2.06 mm vs. 1.21 ± 1.05 mm and 1.39 ± 1.16 mm, respectively). The length of the internal cavity, in our case, also lies in this range (3.065 mm), which could imply the existence of a minimum level of bleb size. Although the IOP control after glaucoma filtration surgery is known to be influenced by the morphology and the size of the bleb after trabeculectomy [8], the minimum size of the bleb for the proper IOP control is expected. In this vein, the addition of our report can offer possible inspiration for further research on this matter.

Other quantitative parameters of the bleb associated with internal bleb morphology are also related to the IOP control. The IOP showed a negative correlation with the number of microcysts and with the volume of the hyporeflective area [7]. The bleb vascularity score at 12 months was related to the volume ratio of the bleb wall [6]. In a previous study, we compared the mean IOPs according to the bleb classifications in AS-OCT and slit-lamp images using post hoc analysis. A diffuse avascular bleb showed a lower mean IOP compared with a localized vascular bleb with statistical significance. Moreover, a localized avascular bleb showed a relatively lower mean IOP compared with a localized vascular bleb, although it did not reach statistical significance [5]. The bleb in our study can be classified as a localized avascular type, which implies that the IOP control could be better than vascular blebs.

Scleral buckling procedures can challenge IOP control in glaucoma eyes by compressing vortex veins, causing increased episcleral venous pressure [9]. Moreover, dissection of the conjunctiva inevitably induces conjunctival scarring, which could limit the feasibility of glaucoma filtration surgery. Since trabeculectomy necessitates enough healthy conjunctiva, glaucoma drainage device implantation has traditionally been preferred over trabeculectomy in glaucoma eyes with previous scleral buckling history. Therefore, it is important to preserve mobile conjunctiva as much as possible to minimize conjunctival scarring for these eyes. Vu and Junk reported that ab externo XEN gel stent implantation may successfully reduce IOP without interfering with the previous scleral buckle for three months postoperation [9]. However, the ab externo approach needs additional conjunctival dissection, which causes more fibrosis, reducing the chance of further manipulation of the surgical area in the future. In contrast, the ab interno approach method is generally considered the best way to achieve minimal invasiveness.

Surgical options for managing glaucoma eyes with minimally mobile conjunctiva are limited and challenging. Due to the previous history of encircling, superotemporal and superonasal quadrants for conjunctival dissections in both a trabeculectomy and a tube were not feasible in our cases. The original definition of MIGS tends to encompass any procedure that avoids conjunctival dissection and is approached using an ab interno clear corneal incision [1]. If the superonasal bleb created by the first XEN fails, the inferonasal quadrant can be considered the next target. Moreover, endoscopic cyclophotocoagulation (ECP) is one of the few MIGS procedures that aim to lower IOP in glaucoma eyes with minimally mobile conjunctiva where other MIGS procedures are all contraindicated. Rodrigues et al. reported that ECP can be safely and successfully performed to control IOP in an eye with severe scleromalacia [10]. However, ECP is not available in the South Korean market. Ab interno XEN gel stent implantation and endoscopic cyclophotocoagulation have the benefit of offering an exit strategy by not precluding any further glaucoma surgery, which is supposed to be one of the major advantages of MIGS.

4. Conclusions

We reported a case of refractory glaucoma with minimally mobile conjunctiva, which was successfully managed using one of the widely performed MIGS procedures, XEN gel stent implantation. A XEN gel stent is a good option for controlling IOP in glaucoma following scleral buckling surgery, especially using the ab interno approach. This is the first case in which a XEN gel stent was implanted using an ab interno approach and is feasible for controlling IOP where there is limited healthy mobile conjunctiva space.

Author Contributions: Conceptualization, S.R.; methodology, Y.K. and S.R.; validation Y.K. and S.R.; resources, Y.K. and S.R.; data curation, Y.K., M.K. and S.R.; writing—original draft preparation, Y.K.; writing—review and editing, Y.K., M.K., D.W.K. and S.R.; visualization, Y.K.; supervision, D.W.K. and S.R.; project administration, S.R. All authors have read and agreed to the published version of the manuscript.

Funding: This research received no external funding.

Institutional Review Board Statement: This study was conducted in accordance with the Declaration of Helsinki and approved by the Institutional Review Board of Bundang CHA Medical Center (IRB number: 2018-12-016) for studies involving humans.

Informed Consent Statement: Patient consent was waived because this study reported on the results of an observational study and complied with the STROBE guidelines.

Data Availability Statement: The data presented in this study are available on request from the corresponding author. The data are not publicly available due to privacy.

Conflicts of Interest: The authors declare no conflict of interest.

References

1. Richter, G.M.; Coleman, A.L. Minimally invasive glaucoma surgery: Current status and future prospects. *Clin. Ophthalmol.* **2016**, *10*, 189–206. [PubMed]
2. Feltgen, N.; Walter, P. Rhegmatogenous retinal detachment—An ophthalmologic emergency. *Dtsch. Arztebl. Int.* **2014**, *111*, 12–21, quiz 22. [PubMed]
3. Weinreb, R.N.; Aung, T.; Medeiros, F.A. The pathophysiology and treatment of glaucoma: A review. *JAMA* **2014**, *311*, 1901–1911. [CrossRef] [PubMed]
4. Kim, Y.; Lim, S.; Rho, S. Bleb Analysis Using Anterior Segment Optical Coherence Tomography and Surgical Predictors of XEN Gel Stent. *Trans. Vis. Sci. Tech.* **2022**, *11*, 26. [CrossRef] [PubMed]
5. Schlenker, M.B.; Gulamhusein, H.; Conrad-Hengerer, I.; Somers, A.; Lenzhofer, M.; Stalmans, I.; Reitsamer, H.; Hengerer, F.H.; Ahmed, I.I.K. Efficacy, Safety, and Risk Factors for Failure of Standalone Ab Interno Gelatin Microstent Implantation versus Standalone Trabeculectomy. *Ophthalmology* **2017**, *124*, 1579–1588. [CrossRef] [PubMed]
6. Watanabe-Kitamura, F.; Inoue, T.; Kojima, S.; Nakashima, K.; Fukushima, A.; Tanihara, H. Prospective 3D Investigation of Bleb Wall after Trabeculectomy Using Anterior-Segment OCT. *J. Ophthalmol.* **2017**, *2017*, 8261364. [CrossRef] [PubMed]
7. Kawana, K.; Kiuchi, T.; Yasuno, Y.; Oshika, T. Evaluation of Trabeculectomy Blebs Using 3-Dimensional Cornea and Anterior Segment Optical Coherence Tomography. *Ophthalmology* **2009**, *116*, 848–855. [CrossRef]
8. Jang, Y.K.; Choi, E.J.; Son, D.O.; Ahn, B.H.; Han, J.C. Filtering Bleb Size in the Early Postoperative Period Affects the Long-term Surgical Outcome after Trabeculectomy. *Korean J. Ophthalmol.* **2023**, *37*, 53–61. [CrossRef]
9. Vu, D.M.; Junk, A.K. XEN Gel Stent Implantation Following Encircling Scleral Buckle Surgery. *Ophthalmic Surg. Lasers Imaging Retin.* **2020**, *51*, 289–292. [CrossRef] [PubMed]
10. Rodrigues, I.A.; Lindfield, D.; Stanford, M.R.; Goyal, S. Glaucoma Surgery in Scleromalacia: Using Endoscopic Cyclophotocoagulation where Conventional Filtration Surgery or Angle Procedures are contraindicated. *J. Curr. Glaucoma* **2017**, *11*, 73–75.

Disclaimer/Publisher's Note: The statements, opinions and data contained in all publications are solely those of the individual author(s) and contributor(s) and not of MDPI and/or the editor(s). MDPI and/or the editor(s) disclaim responsibility for any injury to people or property resulting from any ideas, methods, instructions or products referred to in the content.

Article

Clinical Outcomes of XEN45®-Stent Implantation after Failed Trabeculectomy: A Retrospective Single-Center Study

Constance Weber [1,*], Sarah Hundertmark [1], Michael Petrak [1], Elisabeth Ludwig [1], Christian Karl Brinkmann [1,2], Frank G. Holz [1] and Karl Mercieca [1]

1 Department of Ophthalmology, University of Bonn, 53127 Bonn, Germany
2 Department of Ophthalmology, Dietrich-Bonhoeffer Hospital, 17022 Neubrandenburg, Germany
* Correspondence: constance.weber@ukbonn.de; Tel.: +49-228-2871-5505

Abstract: Background: The implantation of a collagen gel micro-stent (XEN45®) as a minimally invasive form of glaucoma surgery (MIGS) after a failed trabeculectomy (TE) may be an effective option with few risks. This study investigated the clinical outcome of XEN45® implantation after a failed TE, with follow-up data of up to 30 months. Materials and Methods: In this paper, we present a retrospective review of patients undergoing XEN45® implantation after a failed TE at the University Eye Hospital Bonn, Germany, from 2012 to 2020. Results: In total, 14 eyes from 14 patients were included. The mean follow-up time was 20.4 months. The mean time duration between the failed TE and XEN45® implantation was 110 months. The mean intraocular pressure (IOP) decreased from 17.93 mmHg to 12.08 mmHg after one year. This value increased again to 17.63 mmHg at 24 months and 16.00 mmHg at 30 months. The number of glaucoma medications decreased from 3.2 to 0.71, 2.0, and 2.71 at 12, 24, and 30 months, respectively. Conclusions: XEN45® stent implantation after a failed TE did not lead to an effective long-term decrease in IOP and glaucoma medications in many patients in our cohort. Nevertheless, there were cases without the development of a failure event and complications, and others in whom further, more invasive surgery was delayed. XEN45® implantation in some failed trabeculectomy cases may, therefore, be a good option, especially in older patients with multiple comorbidities.

Keywords: glaucoma surgery; MIGS; trabeculectomy; XEN; fibrosis

1. Introduction

Trabeculectomy (TE), a technique that was first developed in 1968, is still considered by many as the gold standard filtration surgery for glaucoma [1]. Although very effective, it may become necessary to perform a needling procedure or a formal revision when bleb filtration fails over the course of time [2–7]. Minimally invasive glaucoma surgeries (MIGS) were developed as an alternative to more extensive procedures, such as trabeculectomy. The term encompasses a wide group of less invasive MIGS surgeries, which are more particularly defined by an ab interno intracameral micro-incisional approach [8–10]. The XEN45® Gel Stent (Allergan Inc., Irvine, CA, USA) can be considered a type of MIGS device, albeit with the added invasiveness of sub-conjunctival filtration and the need for antimetabolite administration [11,12]. This hydrophilic stent has been shown to be quite effective in IOP reduction while having a lower complication rate compared with more aggressive surgeries, such as trabeculectomy [13,14].

In cases with failed trabeculectomy, glaucoma drainage devices or revision surgery of the failed trabeculectomy site can lead to the further lowering of IOP [15–17]. However, these interventions are associated with risks such as postoperative hypotony, postoperative wound leakage, and corneal decompensation [18]. A few studies have described the outcomes of XEN45® gel stent implantation as a therapy modality after a failed trabeculectomy, showing that it can be an effective option for certain patients [19–21]. However, there are no current studies showing long-term follow-up data beyond 12 months.

2. Materials and Methods

2.1. Patients

All the medical records of patients who underwent XEN45®implantation for chronic open-angle glaucoma, pseudo-exfoliation glaucoma, and neovascular glaucoma at the Department of Ophthalmology at the University Hospital of Bonn, Germany, from 2012 until 2020 were reviewed retrospectively. All patients received standalone XEN45® implantation without combined cataract surgery. Only those patients who had received a XEN45® implantation after a failed trabeculectomy and with complete follow-up data over 12 months were included for further analysis. Patients who had undergone surgery without an earlier trabeculectomy and those with incomplete follow-up data were subsequently excluded.

All patients underwent a full ophthalmic examination upon presentation, including an assessment of best-corrected visual acuity (BCVA) using Snellen charts (converted to logMAR for statistical evaluation), IOP measurement via Goldmann applanation tonometry, slit-lamp biomicroscopy, fundus biomicroscopy, and a visual field test, using the Humphrey 24-2 (Carl Zeiss Meditec, Inc., Dublin, CA, USA) for a visual field test. The documented data included gender, age, glaucoma type, BCVA, preoperative clinical features (such as IOP and visual field test results), and detailed follow-up information regarding BCVA, IOP, visual fields, complications, and postoperative glaucoma medication. Patients were censored for further analyses from the point of any additional glaucoma surgery. Patients received an additional glaucoma operation if the IOP was insufficiently controlled after XEN45®implantation, despite maximal therapy and visual field progression.

The failure of XEN45® implantation surgery was defined as an IOP either below 6 mmHg or over 21 mmHg, measured over two visits paid at least 3 months after surgery; the need for additional glaucoma surgery was established for persistently raised IOP and/or in cases resulting in the loss of light perception. All analyses were conducted on a de-identified data set. A waiver from the local Ethics Committee was granted, due to the retrospective nature of the study. The study protocol conformed to the ethical guidelines of the 2000 Declaration of Helsinki, as reflected in the a priori approval granted by the institution's Human Research Committee.

2.2. Statistical Analysis

Statistical analysis was performed with SPSS Statistics version 27.0.0 (IBM Corporation, New York, NY, USA). Time-dependent survival probabilities were estimated with the Kaplan–Meier method.

3. Results

In total, 14 patients were included in this study. The mean age was 71 years. After exclusions, 5 women (35.7%) and 9 men (64.3%) were included. The mean BCVA, measured preoperatively, was 0.47 logMAR. Thirteen patients (92.9%) were pseudophakic. Further characteristics of our patient cohort are described in Table 1.

The mean follow-up time was 20.4 months, with a maximum follow-up time of 34 months (12–34 months). Eight patients (57.1%) had a diagnosis of primary open-angle glaucoma (POAG), while 5 patients (35.7%) had pseudo-exfoliative (PEX) glaucoma. The preoperative mean IOP was 17.93 mmHg, with a maximum of 25 mmHg and a minimum of 11 mmHg. The mean maximum IOP obtained from each patient's medical history was 22.27 mmHg (16–35). Preoperatively, patients were on a mean number of 3.2 topical glaucoma medications. The majority of patients (7; 50%) were taking 4 pressure-lowering agents. Almost all patients (13; 92.9%) were not on additional systemic acetazolamide therapy. The mean vertical cup-to-disc ratio was 0.78. The mean deviation (MD), measured preoperatively with a Humphrey visual field analysis (24-2), was −13.75 dB and the pattern standard deviation (PSD) was 8.6 dB.

Table 1. Demographics and clinical characteristics of patients undergoing XEN stent implantation after a failed trabeculectomy.

Patient Characteristics	n = 14 (%)
Gender	
Male/Female	9 (64.3)/5 (35.7)
Age	
Mean, median (range, SD)	71.14, 74.50 (51–84; 9.51)
Glaucoma type	
Primary open-angle glaucoma	8 (57.1)
Pseudoexfoliation glaucoma	5 (35.7)
Secondary neovascular glaucoma	1 (7.1)
Follow-up time (months)	
Mean, median (range, SD)	20.36, 20.50 (12–34; 8.43)
Time between TE and XEN (months)	
Mean, median (range, SD)	110.54, 100.00 (36–270; 10.33)
Acetazolamide	
Yes/no	1 (7.1)/13 (92.9)
Number of glaucoma medications	
0	0
1	2 (14.3)
2	3 (21.4)
3	2 (14.3)
4	7 (50.0)
5	0
BCVA, measured preoperatively (logMAR)	
Mean, median (range, SD)	0.52, 0.35 (0–2.3; 0.62)
IOP preoperatively	
Mean, median (range, SD)	17.93, 18.00 (11–25; 4.45)
Maximum IOP without drops in the past	
Mean, median (range, SD)	22.27, 21.00 (16–35; 4.40)
Mean deviation (MD) (Humphrey 24-2)	
Mean, median (range, SD)	−13.75, −15,50 (−1.96−−25.25; 8.13)
Pattern standard deviation (PSD)	
Mean, median (range, SD)	8.6, 9.53 (3.1–14.54; 3.79)
Cup-to-disc ratio (CDR)	
Mean, median (range, SD)	0.78, 0.80 (0.50–0.99; 0.17)

The mean duration between the operative date of the failed trabeculectomy and the XEN45® implantation surgery was 110 months, with a maximum of 270 months and a minimum of 36 months. During the postoperative course, 3 patients (21.4%) underwent an additional glaucoma procedure. Of these 3 patients, one patient underwent trans-scleral cyclo-diode laser treatment, one patient underwent trabectome surgery, and one patient underwent *PreserFlo*® Microshunt implantation. The mean time period between XEN45® gel implantation and additional glaucoma surgery was 10.33 months (range: 1–22 months; SD: 10.69).

Of all 14 patients, 4 patients (28.6%) developed a failure event (Figure 1).

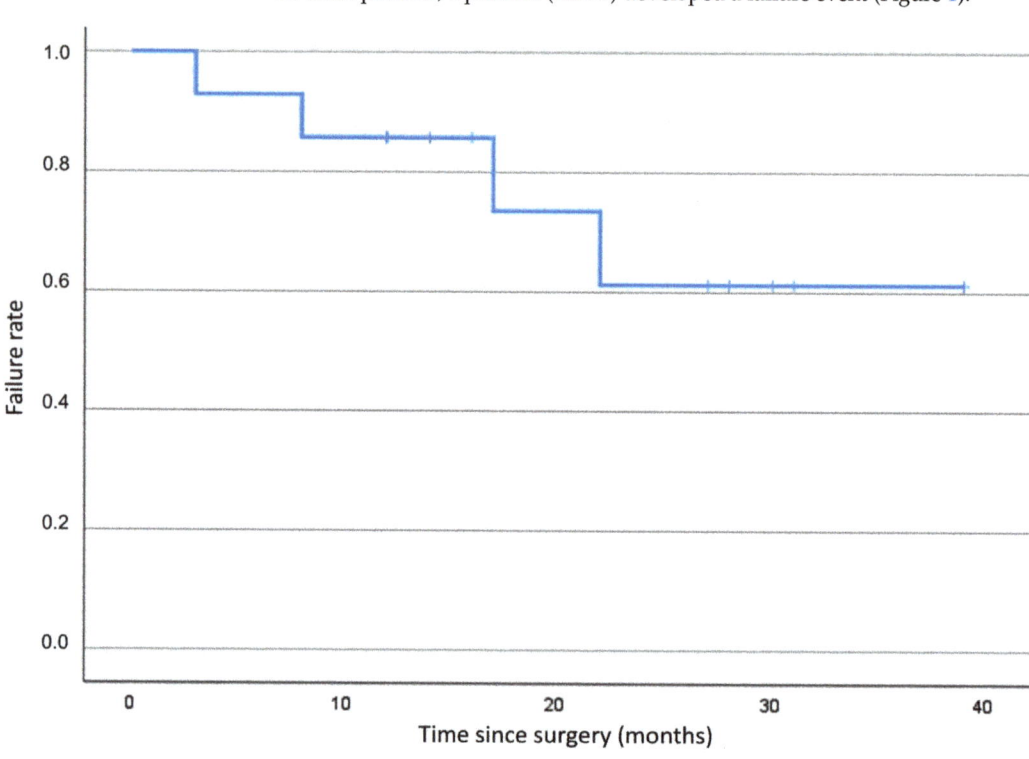

Figure 1. Kaplan–Meier curve depicting the failure rate after XEN45® implantation surgery.

Failure criteria were applied, as explained above. As aforementioned, 3 patients of the 4 (75.0%) failed due to additional glaucoma surgery, and 1 patient (25%) failed due to persistent high IOP levels over 21 mmHg, recorded over two visits (Table 2).

Five patients (35.7%) developed complications during the postoperative course; two of these had more than one complication. One patient experienced a hyphema immediately after surgery and one patient exhibited corneal oedema. These complications eventually resolved without the need for additional interventions.

One patient showed a numerical hypotony during the first days after surgery (IOP < 6 mmHg, with no sign of choroidal detachment).

Two patients underwent revision surgery of the XEN45® implant, with the repeated application of Mitomycin C; one patient underwent partial removal of the XEN45® implant (Table 2). Both patients were revised two weeks after surgery. These patients had an IOP of 5 mmHg and 10 mmHg, respectively, during the week after the revision. These IOP values went up to 12 and 14 mmHg, respectively, 10 months post revision, and 16 and 17 mmHg, respectively, 22 months post revision. Both patients were started off with pressure-lowering drops at 3 months after revision with one and three glaucoma agents, respectively.

On the first day after surgery ($n = 14$), the IOP decreased to a mean IOP of 9.86 mmHg, with an IOP drop of 40% in comparison to the preoperative IOP. The number of IOP-lowering drops was considerably lower than before surgery (0.29). One week after surgery, the results were comparable to the first day after surgery ($n = 14$). The IOP was 10.63 mmHg and the mean number of pressure-lowering eye drops was 0.5. During both time periods, the BCVA had decreased.

Table 2. Complications and failure after XEN45 stent implantation.

Complications	
Yes/no	5 (35.7)/9 (64.3)
Complications (3 patients with more than 1 complication)	
Hyphema	1 (7.1)
XEN-Revision + Mitomycin C	2 (14.2)
Needling	1 (7.1)
Partial XEN removal	1 (7.1)
Corneal oedema	1 (7.1)
Numerical hypotony	1 (7.1)
Failure yes/no	
Yes/no	4 (28.6)/10 (71.4)
Failure reason	
Loss of visual acuity to levels below light perception	0
Hypotony < 6 mmHg over two consecutive visits	0
Persistent high pressure > 21 mmHg over two consecutive visits	1 (25.0)
Additional glaucoma surgery needed	3 (75.0)
Time interval since XEN operation (months)	
Mean (range)	10.33 (1–22)

During the postoperative course, the IOP showed an increase in IOP values between 12 and 17 mmHg. One month after surgery ($n = 14$), the IOP was 15.41 mmHg; 3 months after surgery, it was 12.67 mmHg ($n = 14$), and six months after surgery, it was 12.08 mmHg ($n = 14$). One year after surgery, the follow-up data were complete for all 14 patients and showed a mean IOP of 12.08 mmHg. In comparison to the preoperative value, the mean IOP had decreased by 4 mmHg. However, the mean IOP had further increased to 17.63 mmHg at 18 months ($n = 9$), then changed to 14.25 mmHg at 24 months ($n = 7$), and to 16.00 mmHg at 30 months after surgery ($n = 7$) (Figure 2).

When only the 7 patients with a follow-up time of 24 months were included in the analysis, the mean preoperative IOP was 19.25 mmHg at month 6, 13.63 mmHg at month 12, 17.63 mmHg at month 24, and 16 mmHg at month 30.

The amount of pressure-lowering eye drops was 1.0 at one month ($n = 14$), 1.0 at 3 months ($n = 14$), 0.75 at 6 months ($n = 14$), and 0.71 at one year after surgery ($n = 14$). Compared with the preoperative amount of 3.2 drops, the number was considerably lower at one year after surgery (Figure 3).

Nevertheless, the amount increased again, with a mean of 2.0 drops at two years ($n = 7$) and 2.71 drops at 30 months after surgery ($n = 7$).

Overall, the BCVA showed some deterioration during the time period after surgery, from 0.52 logMAR, preoperatively, to 0.84 logMAR one week after surgery ($n = 14$), 0.69 logMAR after 6 months ($n = 14$), 0.72 logMAR after 12 months ($n = 14$), 0.82 logMAR after 24 months ($n = 7$), and 0.84 logMAR 30 months ($n = 7$) after surgery.

The mean preoperative cup-to-disc-ratio (CDR) was 0.78 (0.5–0.99) and showed a slight deterioration during the postoperative course, with 0.81 (0.5–0.99) after 24 months ($n = 7$) and 0.81 (0.5–0.99) after 30 months ($n = 7$).

The visual field test results showed a mean deviation of -15.75 dB at six months ($n = 14$), -16.92 dB at one year ($n = 13$), -15.46 dB at two years after surgery ($n = 6$) and -16.43 dB at 30 months ($n = 6$). In comparison to a preoperative value of -13.75 dB, these results showed a slight progression in the visual field tests. However, when comparing the pattern standard deviation with a preoperative value of 8.6 dB to 9.5 dB at 6 months (n = 14), 7.2 dB at 1 year (n = 13), 9.9 dB at 2 years (n = 6) and 10.1 dB at 30 months (n = 6), the visual field defects showed only a discrete progression.

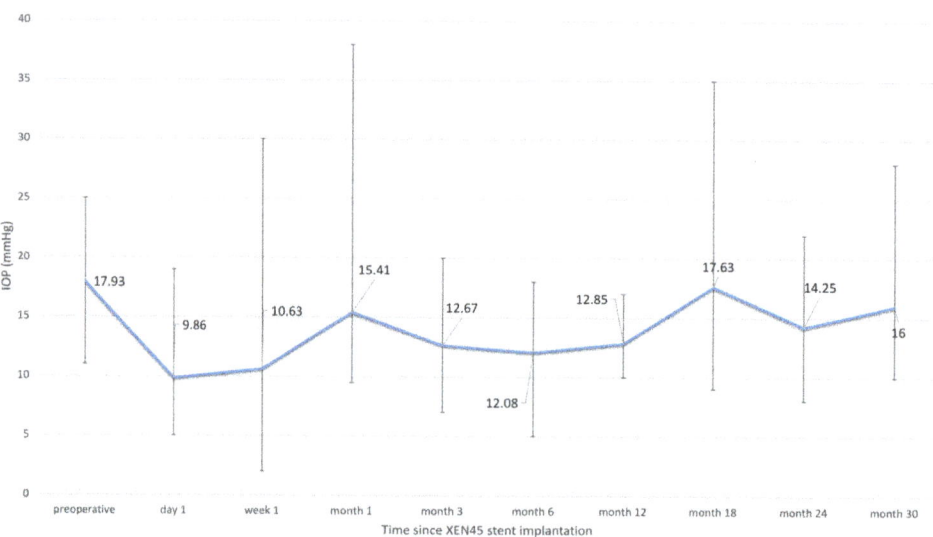

Figure 2. The IOP values (bars represent range with minimum and maximum) over time for all patients with XEN45® stent implantation after a failed trabeculectomy.

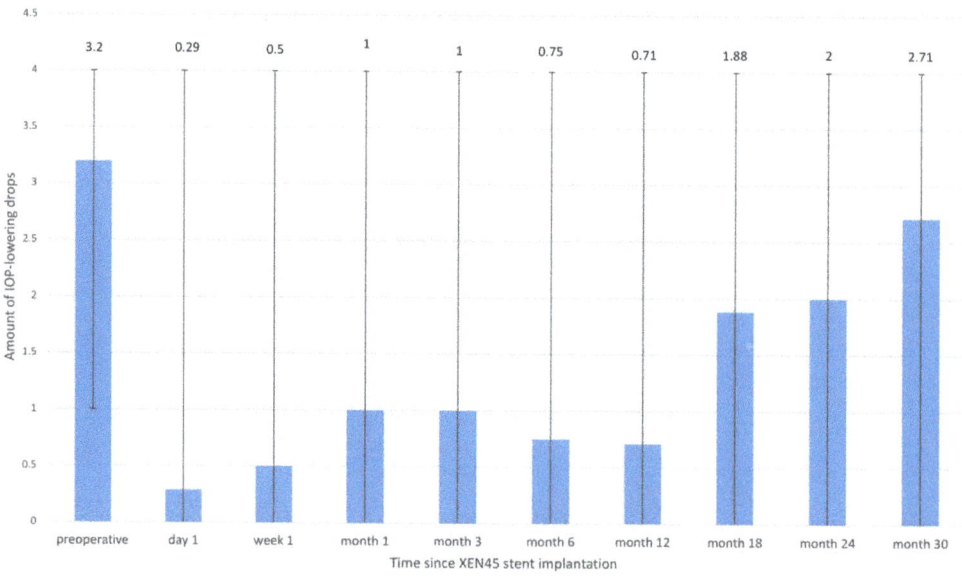

Figure 3. Number of IOP-lowering agents (bars represent a range with the minimum and maximum) over time for all patients undergoing XEN45® stent implantation after a failed trabeculectomy.

4. Discussion

To date, trabeculectomy remains the mainstay of surgical treatment for primary open-angle glaucoma for many glaucoma surgeons worldwide. Although the techniques have been refined over time, and scarring can be managed more effectively by the use of mitomycin C and 5-fluorouracil, failure is still frequent. Gedde and colleagues described a probability of failure for trabeculectomy of 28% during the first three years after surgery. Reasons for failure were inadequate IOP reduction, reoperation for glaucoma, persistent hypotony, or the loss of light perception [22]. Fontana and colleagues even state that only half of the cases achieved long-term low IOP after trabeculectomy [23].

The feasibility of using a less invasive glaucoma procedure after a failed trabeculectomy, such as a XEN45® implant, has only been described in a few studies, but, to our knowledge, these cases have only a limited follow-up.

To the best of our knowledge, our study shows the longest periods of follow-up results available until now for XEN45® stent implantation after a failed trabeculectomy. This aspect is especially important because the efficacy of a glaucoma procedure can only be fully evaluated after a long follow-up period. Our study contained a follow-up time of 20.4 months (12–34 months). Data were complete for every patient of our cohort after one year, were still complete for half of the patients after 24 months, and complete for 7 patients after 30 months. The other half were lost to follow-up or were censored due to failure events. Karimi and colleagues performed a retrospective study with 17 patients in 2018, but they only included follow-up data for 12 months [19]. Bormann and colleagues performed examinations of 31 eyes of 28 patients who received a XEN45®after an insufficient trabeculectomy and included follow-up data for up to twelve months [20]. Düzgün and colleagues demonstrated a mean follow-up period of 14.2 months [21].

We included 14 patients with a preoperative IOP of 17.93 mmHg, with a range from 11 mmHg to 25 mmHg. One patient had a preoperative IOP of 11 mmHg, which is considered quite low for listing this patient for surgery. However, this patient had been prescribed an intake of acetazolamide and the maximum amount of pressure-lowering medication, with an even lower target IOP.

In our cohort, the IOP was lowered to an IOP of 12.08 mmHg on average (preoperative measurement: 17.93 mmHg) and the usage of pressure-lowering agents decreased to a mean of 0.71 (preoperative measurement: 3.2 drops). After a time interval of one year, in comparison with our study, the aforementioned studies reported effective IOP-lowering after XEN45® stent implantation. Düzgun et al. described 14 patients who received XEN45® in the inferonasal quadrant, who showed an IOP-reduction of 49.3% (from 24.14 mmHg to 12.23 mmHg) and a reduction in eyedrops from 3.71 to 1.31, on average [21]. Karimi and colleagues performed a retrospective study with 17 patients in 2018, showing that XEN45® reduced the IOP from 21.5 to 13.6 mmHg and the number of pressure-lowering medications from 2.8 to 1.0 after 12 months [19]. Bormann and colleagues stated that XEN45® reduced the IOP from 23.5 to 18.0 at 12 months, postoperatively [20]. All these studies, including our own, demonstrate an efficient reduction in IOP and in the number of pressure-lowering eyedrops at one year post-XEN45® stent implantation after a failed trabeculectomy, and concluded that XEN45® could be a good method to overcome failed trabeculectomies with minimally invasive surgery.

The above-referenced studies did not report further outcomes from other time points. To the best of our knowledge, there are no other studies presenting data on 2-year results for XEN45® implantation after a failed trabeculectomy. Karimi and colleagues even conclude in their list of study limitations that a follow-up beyond 12 months would have been better to evaluate the procedure's true efficacy after a failed TE.

In our study, we were able to maintain a connection with half of our patients for follow-up data after 30 months. The outcome after two years and 30 months showed that, unfortunately, the IOP-lowering and drug-reducing effect decreased, and, in some patients, had even reached a similar level as preoperatively. The mean IOP increased from 12.08 mmHg at month 12 to 17.63 mmHg at month 18, 14.25 mmHg at month 24, and 16.00 mmHg at month 30 after surgery. The IOP drop between month 18 ($n = 9$) and month 24 ($n = 7$) might be due to the exclusion of one patient who had higher IOP values and was subsequently excluded from analysis because of a failure event, while the other patient with rather high IOP values did not have further follow-up appointments. However, it must be taken into account that follow-up data at 24 and 30 months after surgery were not available for every patient and that the results can be affected by selection bias. To rule this out, we compared the IOP when only including those seven patients with an available follow-up time of 24 months (preop: 19.25, month 12: 13.63 mmHg, month 24: 17.63 mmHg). This subgroup analysis showed that these patients had a higher preoperative IOP than the average group and, thus, the IOP remained lower at month 24 than preoperatively, but was still considerably higher than after a year. The long-term follow-up data included in our study shows that XEN45® stent implantation first leads to an IOP reduction during the first year, with an increasing IOP during the second year. This is most probably due to fibrosis formation around the subconjunctival portion of the stent.

Since one of the main reasons for failure in TE is bleb fibrosis, and since the XEN45® follows the same principle of subconjunctival filtration, it seems logical that a XEN45® stent would suffer from the same problem and, thus, would not be effective after a longer time period. Furthermore, one assumes that a failed trabeculectomy would mean that that particular patient would also be at higher risk of subconjunctival scarring and bleb failure, both pre-trabeculectomy and also even more so after having already undergone a bleb-modifying operation. In these cases, a glaucoma drainage device (GDD), where a tube drains into the untouched post-equatorial subconjunctival space, is considered by many to be the preferred therapy option after a failed TE, especially if post-TE interventions, such as bleb needling and/or repeated antimetabolite application, have been unsuccessful in restoring bleb function. However, tube surgeries can also pose certain risks, which a XEN45® stent avoids to a significant degree. A GDD procedure is usually more complex and time-consuming and will more often result in major complications, especially with regard to persistent postoperative hypotony, corneal endothelial cell loss, and transconjunctival erosions. In addition, general anesthesia is more often necessary for GDD than it is for XEN45®.

In concordance with the other studies described earlier, XEN45® stent implantation is a safe procedure with mostly minor complications. In our study, 5 patients (35.7%) developed complications; however, most of these were resolved without the need for additional interventions. One patient (7.1%) had a hyphema immediately after surgery, one patient (7.1%) developed numerical hypotony, and one patient (7.1%) exhibited corneal oedema, all of these complications resolving themselves without further interventions. Bormann and colleagues reported that 4 eyes (13%) developed choroidal detachment, due to postoperative hypotony, and 4 eyes (13%) developed a subconjunctival hemorrhage. Düzgün and colleagues reported that 5 eyes (35.7%) developed intracameral hemorrhage and 3 eyes (21.4%) developed postoperative numerical hypotony [21]. Both complications were resolved without additional procedures. The authors did not report any severe complications and there were no cases of vision loss, bleb infection, or stent exposure in their study. The most frequent complication described in the study published by Karimi et al. [19] was the occurrence of numerical hypotony (IOP < 6 mmHg), which resolved itself, as in our patients, without intervention within a week. All the above-mentioned studies, including ours, demonstrate that XEN45® stent implantation is a safe procedure with a small risk of major complications.

However, XEN45® stent implantation may quite often be followed by small postoperative interventions and revision procedures to maintain its IOP-lowering effect. In our study, two patients (14.2%) had to undergo revision surgery of the implant with the repeated administration of Mitomycin C, one patient (7.1%) underwent needling, and one patient (7.1%) underwent a partial removal of the XEN45® implant. Bormann and colleagues reported similar results, with 10% needing an open revision of the conjunctiva, while 9 eyes (29%) received postoperative needling. Düzgün and colleagues reported that six eyes (42.8%) required postoperative bleb needling during the postoperative course. Karimi et al. reported that postoperative bleb intervention was performed in 9 eyes (52.9%), with a mean of 2.4 postoperative bleb needling/injections. Most patients required one of these interventions after one month.

This relative lack of risk is why XEN45® stent implantation should still be considered in selected cases after a failed trabeculectomy, especially in older people with multiple co-morbidities, as it offers a less invasive and quicker approach to lowering IOP for a period of time, albeit with the risk of an increase during the postoperative course. Additionally, failed XEN45® rescue surgery does not preclude GDD surgery in the future, which continues to be a treatment option later in due course.

To the best of our knowledge, our study is the only one that includes data on visual field progression. Our 2-year results showed a slight progression of the mean deviation. The visual field test results showed a mean deviation of −13.75 dB, preoperatively, and −15.46 dB at two years after surgery. The pattern standard deviation showed a similar development from 8.6 dB, preoperatively, to 9.9 dB at 2 years. One must consider that these results are partially biased due to the selection bias inherent in the retrospective nature of this study. On top of that, in the German healthcare system, patients are usually referred to tertiary care centers in the case of insufficient pressure control or the progression of their visual fields, whereas adequately controlled patients are followed up by their respective local ophthalmologists.

The slight progression in visual field results shows that there might be another downside to performing a XEN45® implantation after a failed TE. In these patients, after another rescue operation is performed, an ophthalmologist might feel safer about visual fields and IOP control and may be rather conservative toward more extensive surgeries in cases where the XEN45® fails as well. Eventually, ineffective treatment with XEN45® might impede or delay other, more appropriate, treatment options in the longer term. In addition to that, patients might be hesitant to have another operation since they have only just been operated upon and would not be able to comprehend the relative implications of less and more invasive surgery. It is therefore imperative that after a failed trabeculectomy, one must consider which patients might truly benefit from XEN45® stent implantation. It seems that younger patients with a high risk of scarring might benefit more from alternative procedures, such as GDD surgery.

Author Contributions: Conceptualization: C.W. and K.M.; methodology: K.M.; software: C.W.; validation: M.P. and F.G.H.; formal analysis: C.W.; investigation: S.H.; resources: C.K.B. and M.P.; data curation: C.W., S.H. and E.L., writing—original draft: C.W., writing—review and editing: M.P., F.G.H. and K.M., visualization: C.W.; supervision: K.M.; project administration: K.M.; funding: none. All authors have read and agreed to the published version of the manuscript.

Funding: This research received no external funding.

Institutional Review Board Statement: A waiver from the local Ethics Committee was granted, due to the retrospective nature of the study. The study protocol conformed to the ethical guidelines of the 2000 Declaration of Helsinki, as reflected in the a priori approval granted by the institution's Human Research Committee.

Informed Consent Statement: Patient consent was waived due to the retrospective nature of the study.

Data Availability Statement: All datasets generated during and/or analyzed during the current study are available from the corresponding author on reasonable request.

Conflicts of Interest: The authors declare no conflict of interest.

References

1. Cairns, J.E. Trabeculectomy. Preliminary report of a new method. *Am. J. Ophthalmol.* **1968**, *66*, 673–679. [CrossRef] [PubMed]
2. Kwong, A.; Law, S.K.; Kule, R.R.; Nouri-Mahdavi, K.; Coleman, A.L.; Caprioli, J.; Giaconi, J.A. Long-term outcomes of resident-versus attending-performed primary trabeculectomy with mitomycin C in a United States residency program. *Am. J. Ophthalmol.* **2014**, *157*, 1190–1201. [CrossRef] [PubMed]
3. Klink, T.; Kann, G.; Ellinger, P.; Klink, J.; Grehn, F.; Guthoff, R. The prognostic value of the wuerzburg bleb classification score for the outcome of trabeculectomy. *Ophthalmologica* **2011**, *225*, 55–60. [CrossRef] [PubMed]
4. Landers, J.; Martin, K.; Sarkies, N.; Bourne, R.; Watson, P. A twenty-year follow-up study of trabeculectomy: Risk factors and outcomes. *Ophthalmology* **2012**, *119*, 694–702. [CrossRef] [PubMed]

5. Vesti, E.; Raitta, C. A review of the outcome of trabeculectomy in open-angle glaucoma. *Ophthalmic Surg Lasers* **1997**, *28*, 128–132. [CrossRef] [PubMed]
6. Romero, P.; Hirunpatravong, P.; Alizadeh, R.; Kim, E.A.; Nouri-Mahdavi, K.; Morales, E.; Law, S.K.; Caprioli, J. Trabeculectomy with Mitomycin-C: Outcomes and Risk Factors for Failure in Primary Angle-closure Glaucoma. *J. Glaucoma* **2018**, *27*, 101–107. [CrossRef]
7. Mittal, D.; Bhoot, M.; Dubey, S. Trabeculectomy with Mitomycin-C: Outcomes and Risk Factors for Failure in Primary Angle-closure Glaucoma. *J. Glaucoma* **2018**, *27*, e186. [CrossRef]
8. Saheb, H.; Ahmed, I.I.K. Micro-invasive glaucoma surgery: Current perspectives and future directions. *Curr. Opin. Ophthalmol.* **2012**, *23*, 96–104. [CrossRef]
9. Nichani, P.; Popovic, M.M.; Schlenker, M.B.; Park, J.; Ahmed, I.I.K. Microinvasive glaucoma surgery: A review of 3476 eyes. *Surv. Ophthalmol.* **2021**, *66*, 714–742. [CrossRef]
10. SooHoo, J.R.; Seibold, L.K.; Radcliffe, N.; Kahook, M.Y. Minimally invasive glaucoma surgery: Current implants and future innovations. *Can. J. Ophthalmol.* **2014**, *49*, 528–533. [CrossRef]
11. Lewis, R.A. Ab interno approach to the subconjunctival space using a collagen glaucoma stent. *J. Cataract. Refract. Surg.* **2014**, *40*, 1301–1306. [CrossRef]
12. Galal, A.; Bilgic, A.; Eltanamly, R.; Osman, A. XEN Glaucoma Implant with Mitomycin C 1-Year Follow-Up: Result and Complications. *J. Ophthalmol.* **2017**, *2017*, 5457246. [CrossRef]
13. Lenzhofer, M.; Kersten-Gomez, I.; Sheybani, A.; Gulamhusein, H.; Strohmaier, C.; Hohensinn, M.; Dick, H.B.; Hitzl, W.; Eisenkopf, L.; Sedarous, F.; et al. Four-year results of a minimally invasive transscleral glaucoma gel stent implantation in a prospective multi-centre study. *Clin. Exp. Ophthalmol.* **2019**, *47*, 581–587. [CrossRef]
14. Rauchegger, T.; Angermann, R.; Willeit, P.; Schmid, E.; Teuchner, B. Two-year outcomes of minimally invasive XEN Gel Stent implantation in primary open-angle and pseudoexfoliation glaucoma. *Acta Ophthalmol.* **2021**, *99*, 369–375. [CrossRef]
15. Lee, N.; Ma, K.T.; Bae, H.W.; Hong, S.; Seong, G.J.; Hong, Y.J.; Kim, C.Y. Surgical results of trabeculectomy and Ahmed valve implantation following a previous failed trabeculectomy in primary congenital glaucoma patients. *Korean J. Ophthalmol.* **2015**, *29*, 109–114. [CrossRef]
16. Hirunpatravong, P.; Reza, A.; Romero, P.; Kim, E.A.; Nouri-Mahdavi, K.; Law, S.K.; Morales, E.; Caprioli, J. Same-site Trabeculectomy Revision for Failed Trabeculectomy: Outcomes and Risk Factors for Failure. *Am. J. Ophthalmol.* **2016**, *170*, 110–118. [CrossRef]
17. Dubey, S.; Rajurkar, K. Same-site Trabeculectomy Revision for Failed Trabeculectomy: Outcomes and Risk Factors for Failure. *Am. J. Ophthalmol.* **2017**, *177*, 239–240. [CrossRef]
18. Khaw, P.T.; Chiang, M.; Shah, P.; Sii, F.; Lockwood, A.; Khalili, A. Enhanced Trabeculectomy: The Moorfields Safer Surgery System. *Dev. Ophthalmol.* **2017**, *59*, 15–35.
19. Karimi, A.; Hopes, M.; Martin, K.R.; Lindfield, D. Efficacy and Safety of the Ab-interno Xen Gel Stent After Failed Trabeculectomy. *J. Glaucoma* **2018**, *27*, 864–868. [CrossRef]
20. Bormann, C.; Schmidt, M.; Busch, C.; Rehak, M.; Scharenberg, C.T.; Unterlauft, J.D. Implantation of XEN After Failed Trabeculectomy: An Efficient Therapy? *Klin. Monbl. Augenheilkd.* **2021**, *239*, 86–93. [CrossRef]
21. Düzgün, E.; Olgun, A.; Karapapak, M.; Alkan, A.A.; Ustaoğlu, M. Outcomes of XEN Gel Stent Implantation in the Inferonasal Quadrant after Failed Trabeculectomy. *J. Curr. Glaucoma Pract.* **2021**, *15*, 64–69. [CrossRef] [PubMed]
22. Gedde, S.J.; Feuer, W.; Lim, K.; Barton, K.; Goyal, K.; Ahmed, I.; Brandt, J. Treatment Outcomes in the Primary Tube Versus Trabeculectomy Study after 3 Years of Follow-u. *Ophthalmology* **2020**, *127*, 333–345. [CrossRef] [PubMed]
23. Fontana, H.; Nouri-Mahdavi, K.; Lumba, J.; Ralli, M.; Caprioli, J. Trabeculectomy with mitomycin C: Outcomes and risk factors for failure in phakic open-angle glaucoma. *Ophthalmology* **2006**, *113*, 930–936. [CrossRef] [PubMed]

Disclaimer/Publisher's Note: The statements, opinions and data contained in all publications are solely those of the individual author(s) and contributor(s) and not of MDPI and/or the editor(s). MDPI and/or the editor(s) disclaim responsibility for any injury to people or property resulting from any ideas, methods, instructions or products referred to in the content.

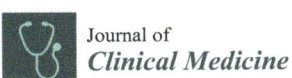

Article

Outcomes of Deep Sclerectomy following Failed XEN Gel Stent Implantation in Open-Angle Glaucoma: A Prospective Study

Giorgio Enrico Bravetti [1,*], Kevin Gillmann [1], Harsha L. Rao [2], André Mermoud [1] and Kaweh Mansouri [1,3]

1 Glaucoma Research Center, Montchoisi Clinic, Swiss Visio, 1006 Lausanne, Switzerland
2 Narayana Nethralaya, 63, Bannerghatta Road, Hulimavu, Bangalore 560099, India
3 Department of Ophthalmology, University of Denver, Denver, CO 80208, USA
* Correspondence: giorgioenrico.bravetti@gmail.com; Tel.: +41-(21)-619-37-42

Abstract: Background: The purpose of this study is to evaluate the outcome of deep sclerectomy (DS) as a secondary procedure following failed ab-interno XEN gel stent implantation in patients with open-angle glaucoma. Methods: Prospective, single-center, non-randomized, interventional study. Consecutive eyes that underwent mitomycin C (MMC) augmented XEN gel stent surgery, with uncontrolled intraocular pressure (IOP) or signs of disease progression, were included to undergo MMC-augmented DS. Primary efficacy outcome was surgical success, defined as complete when the unmedicated IOP was 12 mmHg or less, or 15 mmHg or less and 20% lower than at the timing of XEN failure and defined as qualified when the IOP fulfilled the same conditions with fewer medications than before deep sclerectomy. Secondary measures were mean reduction in IOP and in the number of medications, and the rates of complications. Results: Seventeen eyes were enrolled with a mean age of 72.1 ± 8.2 years (66.7% women). The mean follow-up was 20.1 ± 4.9 months, with more than 12-month data available from 15 eyes. Following DS, IOP decreased significantly from 22.6 ± 5.3 mmHg to 12.3 ± 5.5 (45.6%; $p < 0.001$). Antiglaucoma medications dropped from 1.1 ± 0.9 to 0.3 ± 0.7. Complete success was obtained in 40% of eyes using the threshold of 12 mmHg or less and a 20% decrease of IOP, and in 60% using the 15 mmHg or less threshold. Adverse events were observed in 20% of eyes (bleb leakage (13.3%); hypotony (6.7%)). No cases of choroidal detachment or hypotony maculopathy were reported. Conclusions: Failed XEN gel stent implantation does not seem to negatively affect the safety and efficacy of subsequent deep sclerectomy surgery.

Keywords: glaucoma; open-angle glaucoma; minimally invasive glaucoma surgery; MIGS; XEN gel stent; non-penetrating glaucoma surgery; deep sclerectomy; safety; secondary procedure

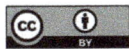

1. Introduction

Glaucoma management is currently based on lowering intraocular pressure (IOP) in order to prevent the progressive loss of retinal ganglion cells [1]. In recent years, the development of alternative approaches to traditional filtering surgery has caused a shift in glaucoma management. Minimally invasive glaucoma surgery (MIGS) techniques provide clinicians with a safe, effective, and minimally-invasive surgical alternative, encouraging an early transition from topical therapies to surgery, while delaying, or avoiding, more invasive procedures, such as filtering techniques [2]. The popularity of MIGS is based on the assumption that these procedures have little or no effect on the outcome of subsequent glaucoma surgery. Scarce data, however, are available to support this assumption.

The XEN gel stent (Allergan, Dublin, CA, USA) is one of these surgical options that targets the subconjunctival outflow pathway through an ab-interno placement [3]. It has demonstrated safety and efficacy in lowering IOP in a wide array of situations: as a standalone first-line procedure [4], in eyes with failed prior surgery [5], in combination with cataract surgery [6–8], and in eyes with primary open-angle glaucoma (POAG) and pseudo-exfoliative glaucoma (PEXG) [9,10]. In view of these findings, the XEN gel stent is being increasingly used as a surgical approach in early-to-moderate glaucoma. Nevertheless, as a bleb-creating procedure, a failure of the procedure may impair the efficacy of subsequent filtering surgeries that rely on conjunctival integrity. Despite a recent study demonstrating that mitomycin C (MMC)-augmented trabeculectomy following failed XEN gel stent surgery is technically feasible, and a case report wherein XEN-augmented Baerveldt surgery was used to rescue a failed XEN, data on surgeries following failed XEN gel stents remain scarce [11,12].

The aim of this study was to assess the safety and efficacy of secondary non-penetrating deep sclerectomy (DS) after failed XEN gel stent implantation.

2. Materials and Methods

2.1. Study Design

This was an investigator-initiated, prospective, interventional study, conducted at a single tertiary glaucoma center. The study complies with the tenets of the Declaration of Helsinki and was approved by the local ethical committee (Institutional Review Board). Written informed consent was obtained from all included patients. The study was registered in the National Library of Medicine database (ClinicalTrials.gov identifier, NCT04381611).

2.2. Study Population

Consecutive eyes that underwent secondary DS with MMC following failed XEN gel stent implantation at the same institution (Glaucoma Research Centre, Montchoisi Clinic, Swiss Visio, Lausanne, Switzerland) between October 2015 and April 2018 were prospectively enrolled. Every effort was made to enroll all suitable patients as per the inclusion and exclusion criteria. Inclusion criteria were as follows: a diagnosis of primary or secondary open-angle glaucoma, previous XEN gel stent implantation carried out at the investigation center, uncontrolled glaucoma despite needling revisions and medical therapy. Glaucoma was defined as the association of repeatable visual field defects (persistent scotoma on at least two consecutive standard automated perimetry tests (Octopus, Haag Streit, Koeniz, Switzerland) with a test reliability index $\geq 15\%$) and an abnormal optic disc appearance (presence of neuroretinal rim thinning or localized or diffuse retinal nerve fiber layer defects) indicative of glaucoma, as observed under slit-lamp examination or on spectral-domain optical coherence tomography (SD-OCT) imaging (Spectralis OCT, Heidelberg Engineering AG, Heidelberg, Germany). Systematic gonioscopic examination was carried out to confirm angle opening. Glaucoma was considered as uncontrolled when functional and/or structural tests identified persistent signs of progression, or when IOP was persistently above the eye-specific target set by the treating ophthalmologist. The choice of the secondary procedure was left at the discretion of the treating surgeon. In addition, eyes with a post-operative follow-up shorter than 12 months were excluded from this analysis.

2.3. Primary Procedure: XEN Gel Stent

The XEN gel stent has a length of 6 mm, a 150-µm external diameter, and an inner lumen of 45 µm that was calculated using Hagen-Poiseuille law in order to avoid post-operative hypotony and achieve a resistance of 6–8 mmHg under physiological conditions of an aqueous production rate of 2 to 2.5 µL/min [13,14]. The aim of the device is to create an artificial pathway through the trabecular meshwork and the sclera, allowing aqueous flow from the anterior chamber (AC) to the subconjunctival space.

All surgeries were conducted at the investigation center by one of two experienced surgeons (A.M. and K.M.), as either standalone or combined procedures, using a standardized ab interno technique previously detailed [7]. In all cases, intraoperative 0.1 mL MMC at a concentration of 0.02% was injected under Tenon's capsule and spread with a microsponge applied to conjunctiva before the implant was injected. The MMC was not washed out.

During the postoperative follow-up, if the treatment target IOP was not achieved after the first post-operative month, or if disease progression was noted, interventional treatment was performed as follows: If obstruction of the AC-tip of XEN Gel Stents was suspected, it was relieved by YAG fibrinolysis [15]; flat blebs were treated by needling revision procedures up to three times; and in other cases, IOP-lowering medications were re-introduced. In cases that were refractory to those measures, non-penetrating DS or glaucoma drainage device surgery was considered on an individual basis.

2.4. Secondary Procedure: Deep Sclerectomy

Enrolled patients all underwent secondary DS following failed primary XEN gel stent implantation.

Since the 1990s, DS has been recognized as a safer alternative to trabeculectomy, offering comparable success rates and minimizing the risk of postoperative complications [16–20]. The essential difference with trabeculectomy is the non-penetrating nature of DS, through the creation of a filtration membrane, the trabeculo-Descemet's membrane (TDM). Moreover, in DS, the excision of the inner scleral flap creates an intrascleral lake, potentially increasing aqueous flow through intrascleral and suprachoroidal pathways, in addition to subconjunctival filtration [21–24].

All the surgical procedures were performed by one of the same glaucoma surgeons who initially performed XEN gel stent implantation (A.M. or K.M.) [25]. When a different site could be selected, the XEN gel stent was left in place. Otherwise, when it was not possible to avoid the old surgical site, the device was removed following conjunctival opening. Three surgical sponges soaked with 0.2 mg/mL MMC were inserted under the conjunctiva for 2–3 min before the scleral dissection. After the sponges were removed, washout was performed. No case had to be converted to a trabeculectomy because of perforation of the TDM.

Beyond the first post-operative month, when the filtration through the TDM was considered to be insufficient because of elevated IOP, a laser goniopuncture (LGPT) was performed with the neodymium (Nd):YAG laser in the anterior thinnest portion of the TDM. After the LGPT opening of the TDM, if the treatment target IOP was not achieved, needling revisions were performed. After the needling revision, IOP-lowering medications were reintroduced postoperatively if the patient's target IOP was not reached.

2.5. Outcome Measures

Success of the secondary procedure was defined either as complete, if the unmedicated IOP at last follow-up visit was $\leq$12 mmHg, $\leq$15 mmHg, or $\leq$18 mmHg, both with and without a relative IOP reduction $\geq$20% or more, compared to the last IOP prior to reoperation (DS), or as qualified if the IOP met the same thresholds with fewer medications than immediately before DS. Loss of light perception, serious irreversible complications, IOP over 18 mmHg, or any subsequent glaucoma surgical intervention following DS were considered surgical failures. Further drainage or filtering surgery, surgical revisions, and cyclodestruction were all considered reoperations, and as such, failure of the procedure. LGPTs and needling procedures were not considered reoperations. Secondary efficacy and safety outcome measures included the mean reduction in IOP and topical hypotensive medications, the number of LGPTs and needling revisions required to maintain IOP within individual target ranges, and the rate of surgical failure. Safety endpoints included the rate of intraoperative complications and post-operative AEs during the entire follow-up.

2.6. Statistical Analysis

Descriptive statistics included mean and standard deviation (SD) for normally distributed variables, and median and interquartile range (IQR) for non-normally distributed variables. Kaplan–Meier survival curves were used to assess the cumulative probability of success and failure. Baseline IOP was defined as the mean of the last two preoperative measures. Associations between failure and demographic or clinical variables such as age, gender, ethnicity, diagnosis, or number of preoperative treatments or surgeries were assessed. All tests were two-tailed and a *p*-value less than 0.05 was considered statistically significant. Statistical analyses were performed with commercially available software (StataCorp, College Station, TX, USA).

3. Results

3.1. Baseline Characteristics of Study Population

Out of a total of 149 eyes that underwent XEN standalone or XEN plus phacoemulsification surgery between January 2015 and June 2016, 24 eyes needed subsequent glaucoma interventions because of clinical evidence of failing bleb with elevated IOP, above the individual target range. Out of those, 17 (70.8%) were deemed suitable to undergo secondary MMC-augmented DS and were enrolled in this study. Among the others, 3 eyes (12.5%) underwent surgical bleb revision, 2 (8.3%) had a second XEN gel stent implantation, 1 (4.2%) underwent placement of a Baerveldt glaucoma drainage device (Abbot Inc., Lake Bluff, IL, USA) augmented with the XEN gel stent, and 1 (4.2%) underwent surgical reposition of the XEN gel stent. Two patients were lost to follow-up before their 12-month appointment. Sufficient clinical data were thus available from 15 eyes (62.5%) of 14 patients. These patients were considered eligible for analysis. As only one subject (7.14% of the entire cohort population) had both eyes eligible for the analysis, a statistical correction was not applied for the presence of two eyes from the same patient.

The mean ± SD follow-up was 20.1 ± 4.9 months (range 12 to 24). The mean age of the study population at enrolment was 72.1 ± 8.2 years, 66.7% ($n = 10$) were female, and 80% ($n = 12$) were Caucasians. In all, 33.3% had a diagnosis of POAG, followed by PEXG (26.6%). The primary XEN gel stent implantation had been a standalone procedure for 5 eyes (33.3%); the remainder were combined with phacoemulsification (10 eyes, 66.7%). The average time of failure for primary XEN gel stent was 11.1 ± 7.6 months (range, 1 to 28 months). Glaucoma severity as per Hodapp–Parrish–Anderson criteria ranged from mild-to-moderate, with a mean visual field MD of 5.3 ± 2.9 dB at enrolment. Baseline characteristics of the study patients are summarized in Table 1.

Table 1. Baseline demographics and clinical characteristics of study population.

Demographic and Clinical Data	Mean ± SD (%)
Age (years)	72.1 ± 8.2
Range	53–89
Female gender	10 (66.7%)
Study eye	
Right	8 (53.3%)
Left	7 (46.6%)
Ethnicity	
Caucasian	12 (80%)
Black	2 (13.3%)
Asian	1 (6.7%)
Bilateral cases	1
Diagnosis	
POAG	5 (33.3%)
PEXG	4 (26.6%)
Pigmentary glaucoma	3 (20%)
Other	3 (20%)
Central corneal thickness (μm)	540.1 ± 53.7
pre-XEN Visual field (dBs)	
MD	5.3 ± 2.9
sLV	3.9 ± 1.9

Table 1. Cont.

Demographic and Clinical Data	Mean ± SD (%)
pre-XEN OCT RNFL thickness (μm)	85.6 ± 16.5
pre-XEN BCVA (decimal)	0.8 ± 0.3
Baseline BCVA (decimal)	0.9 ± 0.2
pre-XEN IOP (mmHg)	21.1 ± 3.7
Baseline IOP (mmHg)	22.6 ± 5.3
pre-XEN Medications	1.5 ± 1.1
Baseline Medications	1.1 ± 0.9

BCVA = best-corrected visual acuity; dB = decibels; IOP = intraocular pressure; MD = mean deviation; POAG = primary open-angle glaucoma; PEXG = pseudoexfoliation glaucoma; RNFL = retinal nerve fiber layer; SD = standard deviation; sLV = square of loss of variance.

3.2. Safety

No intraoperative complications were noted among the studied cohort, neither at time of primary XEN gel stent surgery nor at time of secondary DS. None of the combined procedures were associated with posterior capsule rupture or the need for anterior vitrectomy.

3.3. Intraocular Pressure, Medication Use and Visual Acuity

Mean medicated IOP before XEN gel stent surgery (pre-XEN), before DS (baseline), and at last follow-up visit after DS were 21.1 ± 3.7 mmHg, 22.6 ± 5.3 mmHg, and 12.3 ± 5.5 mmHg, respectively. Overall, we observed a reduction of 45.6% in IOP between the time of XEN failure and the last follow-up visit after DS ($p < 0.001$). The number of anti-glaucoma medications concomitantly dropped from 1.5 ± 1.1 (pre-XEN) and 1.1 ± 0.9 (baseline) to 0.3 ± 0.7, representing a reduction of 72.7% following secondary DS ($p = 0.014$). At the last follow-up visit, 13.3% of eyes ($n = 2$) required antiglaucoma medications to achieve target IOP. Antiglaucoma medications and IOP progression throughout the follow-up period are presented in Figures 1 and 2. Mean BCVA at last follow-up visit after DS remained statistically unchanged compared to BCVA at baseline (0.9 ± 0.2 decimals).

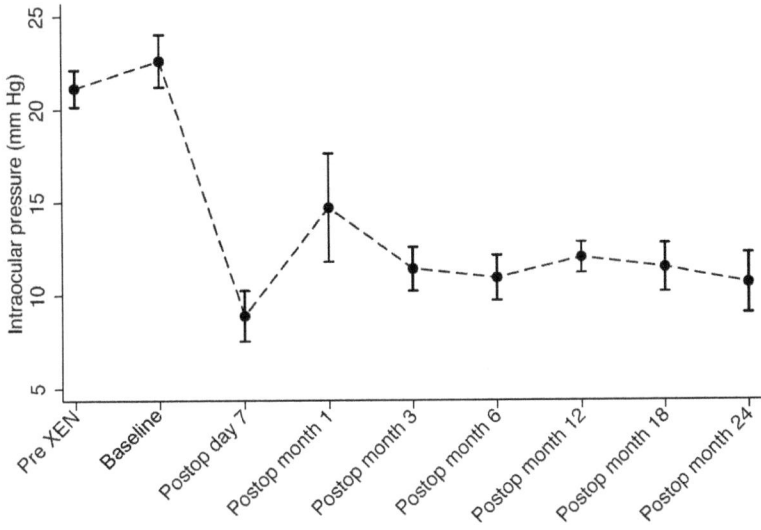

Figure 1. Graph showing mean intraocular pressure through 24 months of follow-up.

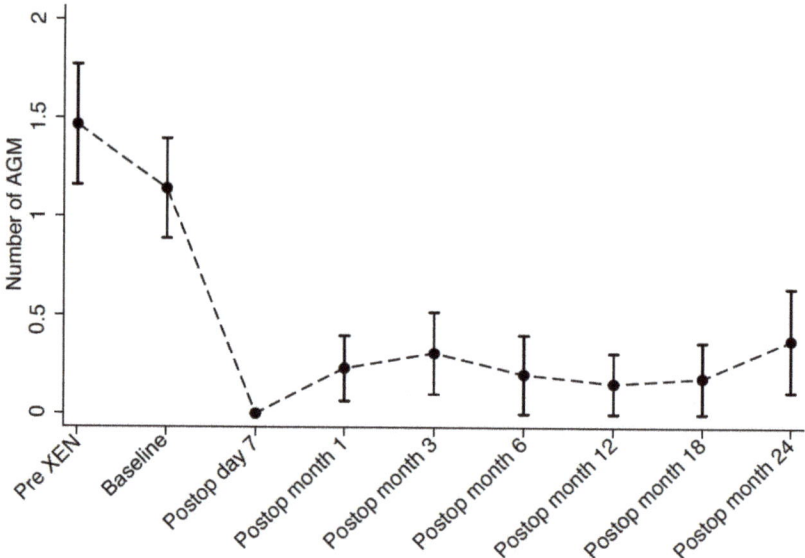

Figure 2. Graph showing the number of antiglaucoma medications (AGM) through 24 months of follow-up.

3.4. Primary Outcome: Surgical Success

Complete success at last follow-up visit was achieved in 40% of eyes using the strictest threshold of 12 mmHg or less with a concomitant 20% IOP reduction from baseline, whereas 60% of eyes achieved an unmedicated IOP of 15 mmHg or less and 66.7% achieved an unmedicated IOP of 18 mmHg or less. Qualified success was obtained in 46.7% of eyes using the 12-mmHg or less and 20% IOP reduction from baseline definition, while 66.7% and 80% of eyes reached a medicated IOP of 15 mmHg or less and 18 mmHg or less, respectively. The Kaplan–Meier survival curves are presented in Figure 3. Out of 15 eyes, 3 (20%) were classified as complete failure due to an uncontrolled intraocular hypertension above 18 mmHg, despite medical treatment and needling revisions, which required further surgical intervention. Among reoperated eyes, 2 underwent surgical bleb revision, and one underwent implantation of the eyeWatch system (Rheon Medical, Lausanne, Switzerland) [26]. The average time of complete failure was 6.3 ± 6.1 months after secondary surgery. Table 2 presents the surgical success and failure rates against all definitions. Association analysis showed no statistically significant association between surgical outcome and any of the patients' demographics or recorded clinical data.

3.5. Postoperative Interventions

After DS, needling revisions were performed in 46.7% ($n = 7$) of eyes; 85.7% of them ($n = 6$) required a single intervention to control their IOP, while 14.3% ($n = 1$) required two needling interventions over the entire follow-up period. On average, the first needling intervention was performed 6.6 ± 7.1 months after surgery. The only patient who required more than one needling treatment underwent the procedure at 6 and 24 months, postoperatively. Laser goniopuncture was performed in nine eyes (60.0%), including all eyes that subsequently required a needling intervention. Postoperative interventions are summarized ion Table 3.

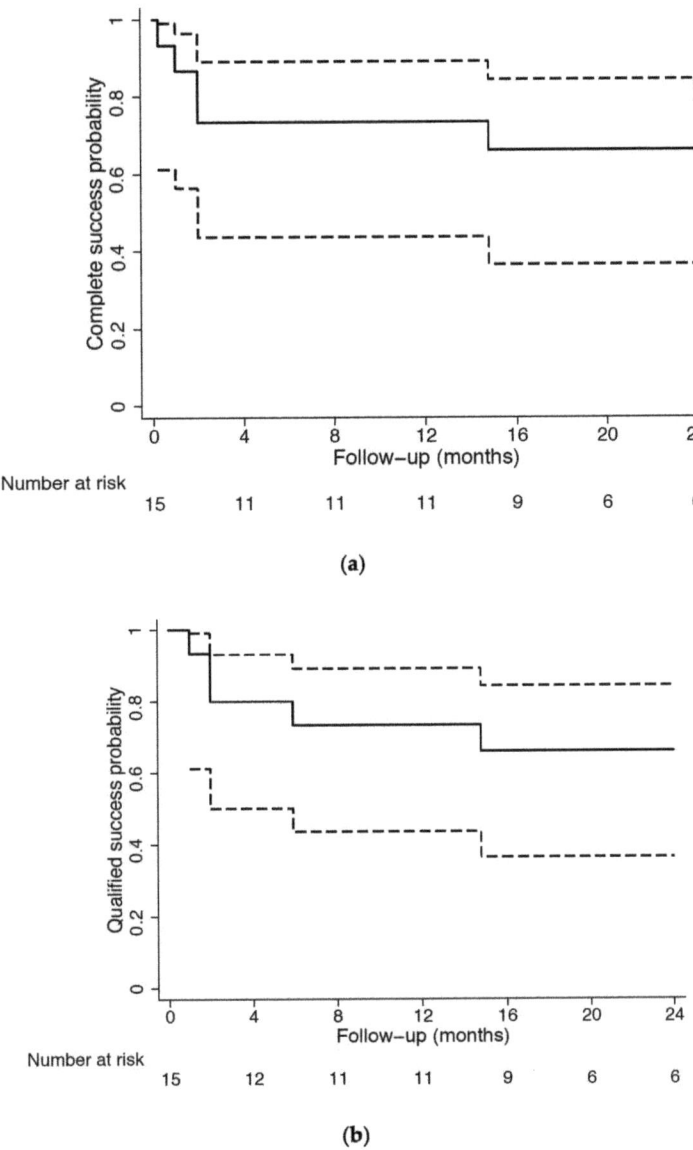

Figure 3. Cumulative probability of complete (**a**) and qualified (**b**) success (Kaplan–Meier curves) using the 15 mmHg or less intraocular pressure threshold.

Table 2. Surgical success and failure rates against all definitions.

Definition	Percentage
Complete success (unmedicated)	
Intraocular pressure ≤ 12 mmHg	40
With a reduction of more than 20% from baseline	40
Intraocular pressure ≤ 15 mmHg	60
With a reduction of more than 20% from baseline	60

Table 2. *Cont.*

Definition	Percentage
Intraocular pressure ≤ 18 mmHg	66.7
With a reduction of more than 20% from baseline	66.7
Qualified success (medicated)	
Intraocular pressure ≤ 12 mmHg	46.7
With a reduction of more than 20% from baseline	46.7
Intraocular pressure ≤ 15 mmHg	66.7
With a reduction of more than 20% from baseline	66.7
Intraocular pressure ≤ 18 mmHg	80
With a reduction of more than 20% from baseline	80
Complete failure	20

Table 3. Postoperative interventions during the follow-up.

Postoperative Interventions	Percentage
Total of needling revisions	46.7
# 1 needling revision	85.7
# 2 needling revisions	14.3
Laser Goniopuncture	60

3.6. Postoperative Complications

Three eyes (20.0%) experienced refractory intraocular hypertension, requiring further surgery, two eyes (13.3%) experienced persistent bleb leakage and required conjunctival sutures. The latter occurred at a mean post-operative time of 1.5 ± 0.5 months. One eye (6.7%) experienced persistent hypotony, defined as IOP persistently <5 mmHg without evidence of bleb leakage, choroidal detachment, folds, or loss of visual acuity. This case of hypotony resolved following a 1-month topical treatment of dexamethasone and bromhydrate scopolamine, three times a day. Postoperative complications are reported in Table 4.

Table 4. Postoperative complications during the follow-up.

Postoperative Complications	Percentage
Refractory intraocular hypertension requiring further surgery	20
Persistent bleb leakage requiring conjunctival sutures	13.3
Persistent hypotony, defined as IOP persistently <5 mmHg	6.7

4. Discussion

The current study represents, to the best of our knowledge, the first prospective study describing the outcomes of DS with MMC following failed XEN gel stent with MMC surgery, with a long-term postoperative follow-up. Its results suggest that failed primary XEN implantation may not affect the safety or efficacy outcomes of secondary filtering surgery. Although, in our experience, performing secondary DS was marginally more challenging than a primary procedure, there was a relatively low rate of postoperative AEs following the reoperation. Moreover, no serious sight-treating complications were observed. In terms of efficacy, a good long-term IOP-lowering effect was achieved, with a mean IOP reduction of 45.6% from the medicated IOP levels at the timing of XEN failure. Meanwhile, a concomitant and significant decrease (−72.7%) in antiglaucoma medications was observed. The number of antiglaucoma medications prior to DS seems to be very low (1.1 ± 0.9). The reason behind that probably reflects the Swiss Medical Care System and the real-life environment of the present study. Indeed, the time the patient had to wait from the moment a diagnosis of a failed XEN had been made and the subsequent reoperation is very low (sometimes only days or weeks), so in most of the cases it was not even necessary to give extra antiglaucoma medications to the patient. Furthermore, the rates of surgical failure due to uncontrolled IOP requiring subsequent glaucoma procedures within 24 months (20%) was within the reported rates for primary DS [27–29].

In recent years, studies have demonstrated that, although the success rates of XEN gel stents remain reasonably high at 24 months, its success rates gradually decrease over time. Mansouri et al. [6,7] observed a complete success rate of 62.4% at 1 year versus 51.9% at 2 years, using an 18 mmHg IOP threshold. Our group has identified increasing rates of reoperation (6% at 1 year vs. 11.4% at 2 years) rates that were also observed by other research groups [4,6,7]. These rates were shown to be even higher in Black and Afro-Latino populations, with up to 40% requiring secondary glaucoma surgery by 12 months [30]. Moreover, several studies have found that stent-related complications such as blockage of the internal lumen [15,31], device degradation [32], or device movements [33] can occur months to years after implantation, with a subsequent need of surgical reintervention.

Despite ample data on the frequency and causes of failure of the XEN gel stent, there is a paucity of evidence on how to manage glaucoma patients once this technique fails. Gizzi et al. [11] demonstrated that MMC-augmented trabeculectomy following failed XEN gel stent surgery is technically feasible and effective in lowering IOP. Nevertheless, they observed a significant incidence of early-onset bleb leaks (37.5%), a high rate of hypotony (25%) leading to frequent shallow choroidal detachment (12.5%), and chorioretinal macular folds (12.5%) with resulting visual loss (50% losing two Snellen lines). In comparison, the present study suggests that secondary DS is safer than secondary trabeculectomy following failed XEN gel stent implantation. These conclusions are in keeping with the results of studies and meta-analyses comparing primary DS and primary trabeculectomy [34,35]. Moreover, the results of the present study are similar in terms of IOP reduction, medication reduction, and complication rate to the reported outcomes of primary DS, supporting the assumption that XEN gel stent implantation as a primary procedure has little to no effect on the outcome of subsequent DS [25,36–39].

However, analyses of secondary procedures are required due to the prolonged and cumulative tissue exposure to MMC during the XEN implantation and the subsequent procedures, which might increase the long-term rates of bleb-related complications and altered ciliary body function. For these reasons, it may be advisable that secondary procedures use lower MMC concentrations or exposure time, or less potent antimetabolites such as 5-fluorouracil. Nevertheless, the present study reports low rates of bleb complications despite the use of intraoperative MMC in similar doses to those generally used in trabeculectomy. As a result, we hypothesize that the difference in safety lies in the nature of the two filtering techniques used. Indeed, it has been widely shown that DS is associated with a lower rate of postoperative complications compared to trabeculectomy [16–20], and may have some advantages in high-risk-of-failure eyes. The main technical differences are the non-penetration of the anterior chamber intraoperatively, and the removal of the deeper scleral flap during the DS. The creation of a filtration membrane, the TDM, is responsible for the gradual reduction of the IOP, intra- and postoperatively. Excessive flow in the early postoperative period was suspected to contribute to a number of complications of trabeculectomy. The preservation of the TDM in DS acts as a protective mechanism with this regard. In addition, it was shown that the non-penetrative nature of DS reduces the amount of intraocular inflammation, which is known to contribute to the failure of filtering surgery and may compromise bleb survival [40–42]. After primary DS, shallow AC, hypotony maculopathy, and AC inflammation are infrequent. Furthermore, the excision of the deeper scleral flap creates an additional outflow pathway by forming an intrascleral lake, which is believed to potentiate suprachoroidal flow and reduce pressure on the subconjunctival bleb [21–24]. These mechanisms are thought to further contribute to creating a more diffuse and posterior bleb morphology compared to that achieved through trabeculectomy. All those features are probably responsible for the lower rate of bleb leakage found in the present study (13.3% vs 37.5% after secondary trabeculectomy) [11].

Previously, Laroche et al. [12] used a Baerveldt tube in order to rescue a failed XEN gel stent via a technique previously described for refractory glaucoma [43]. In a patient with a failed XEN gel stent, a 250-Baerveldt tube was inserted in the superonasal quadrant and positioned to be connected with the present XEN implant. The double lumen was then sutured to secure the position. The follow-up of this case report reached only one month postoperatively, reporting an unmedicated IOP of 5 mmHg. Although the XEN-augmented Baerveldt technique constitutes a new and innovative variation of a standard glaucoma drainage device (GDD), by lowering the risks of complications traditionally associated with tube surgeries, such as early postoperative hypotony or long term corneal endothelial cell loss, its relevance to rescuing failed XEN devices appears less relevant. Indeed, patients selected for XEN gel stent implantation generally suffer from early-to-moderate glaucoma and are unlikely to require a device usually reserved for more advanced or refractory cases for a number of years, which may be beyond the XEN gel stent's lifespan. Second, GDD surgery is characterized by a high technical difficulty. In addition, prospective studies on XEN-augmented Baerveldt implantation have reported a high rate of failure and reoperation at 12 months, even if in non-refractory eyes [44,45]. On the other hand, XEN-augmented Baerveldt technique could prove useful to rescue a failed XEN gel stent in cases where conjunctiva is not deemed adequate for filtering surgery.

Study Limitations

The present study has several limitations. First, it was not a randomized controlled comparative study and there was no control group. In particular, the absence of a control group with other filtering or cyclophotoablative surgical procedures seems to be a strong limitation for the value of the results and can be partially explained by the design of the study and by the treatment algorithm used by the surgeons, who generally apply a non-penetrating glaucoma surgery after a failed MIGS. Another limitation was the absence of a preoperative medication washout. This can be explained by the uncontrollable nature of glaucoma in the enrolled cohort, associated with the risk of disease progression over the washout period. Furthermore, the nature of the studied indication implies that only a relatively small number of patients met the inclusion criteria, leading to a potential size bias. The fact that all cases were operated by the same two surgeons, in a single tertiary glaucoma center, may be considered both a limitation and a strength. Finally, another limitation of our study is that it was conducted in a predominantly homogenous (Caucasian) population. More research is needed to evaluate the success of secondary procedures in the longer term and in other ethnicities.

5. Conclusions

The present study suggested that failed MMC-augmented XEN gel stent implantation does not affect the outcomes of subsequent filtering surgery. Furthermore, it demonstrated that secondary deep sclerectomy with MMC following failed MMC-augmented XEN gel stent implantation produced a significant and sustained IOP reduction over 24 months postoperatively. Moreover, this surgical approach remains relatively safe in high-risk-of-failure eyes and seems to display higher success rates and lower rates of AEs compared to MMC-augmented trabeculectomy and XEN-augmented Baerveldt techniques used for the same indication.

Author Contributions: All authors contributed to the study conception and design. Material preparation, data collection, and analysis were performed by A.M., K.M., H.L.R., K.G. and G.E.B. The first draft of the manuscript was written by G.E.B., K.M. and K.G. commented on previous versions of the manuscript. All authors have read and agreed to the published version of the manuscript.

Funding: This research received no external funding.

Institutional Review Board Statement: The study was conducted in accordance with the Declaration of Helsinki and approved by the local ethical committee (Institutional Review Board), (protocol code CER-VD NCT04381611).

Informed Consent Statement: Informed consent was obtained from all subjects involved in the study.

Data Availability Statement: The datasets used and/or analyzed during the current study are available from the corresponding author on reasonable request.

Acknowledgments: Supported in part by the Swiss Glaucoma Research Foundation, Lausanne, Switzerland.

Conflicts of Interest: G.E.B. and K.G. declare that they have no competing interests. H.L.R. acts as a consultant for Santen, Carl-Zeiss Meditec, Allergan. A.M. acts as a consultant for Alcon, Allergan, Santen, Swiss Advanced Vision, Rheon Medical, Glaukos, Diopsys Inc., DeepCube. K.M. acts as a consultant for Santen, Alcon, Allergan, ImplanData, Sensimed, Topcon, Optovue.

Abbreviations

DS	deep sclerectomy
MMC	mitomycin-C
IOP	intraocular pressure
MIGS	minimally invasive glaucoma surgery
POAG	primary open angle glaucoma
PEXG	pseudoexfoliative glaucoma
SD-OCT	spectral-domain optical coherence tomography
AC	anterior chamber
TDM	trabeculo-Descemet's membrane
LGPT	laser goniopuncture
SD	standard deviation
IRQ	interquartile range
MD	mean deviation
sLV	square of loss of variance
RNFL	retinal nerve fiber layer
BCVA	best corrected visual acuity
AGM	antiglaucoma medications
dB	decibel
AE	adverse event
GDD	glaucoma drainage device

References

1. Weinreb, R.N.; Aung, T.; Medeiros, F.A. The pathophysiology and treatment of glaucoma: A review. *JAMA* **2014**, *311*, 1901–1911. [CrossRef]
2. Lavia, C.; Dallorto, L.; Maule, M.; Ceccarelli, M.; Fea, A.M. Minimally-invasive glaucoma surgeries (MIGS) for open angle glaucoma: A systematic review and meta-analysis. *PLoS ONE* **2017**, *12*, e0183142. [CrossRef] [PubMed]
3. Chaudhary, A.; Salinas, L.; Guidotti, J.; Mermoud, A.; Mansouri, K. XEN Gel Implant: A new surgical approach in glaucoma. *Expert Rev. Med. Devices* **2018**, *15*, 47–59. [CrossRef] [PubMed]
4. Schlenker, M.B.; Gulamhusein, H.; Conrad-Hengerer, I.; Somers, A.; Lenzhofer, M.; Stalmans, I.; Reitsamer, H.; Hengerer, F.H.; Ahmed, I.I.K. Efficacy, Safety, and Risk Factors for Failure of Standalone Ab Interno Gelatin Microstent Implantation versus Standalone Trabeculectomy. *Ophthalmology* **2017**, *124*, 1579–1588. [CrossRef] [PubMed]
5. Grover, D.S.; Flynn, W.J.; Bashford, K.P.; Lewis, R.A.; Duh, Y.J.; Nangia, R.S.; Niksch, B. Performance and Safety of a New Ab Interno Gelatin Stent in Refractory Glaucoma at 12 Months. *Am. J. Ophthalmol.* **2017**, *183*, 25–36. [CrossRef] [PubMed]
6. Mansouri, K.; Guidotti, J.; Rao, H.L.; Ouabas, A.; D'Alessandro, E.; Roy, S.; Mermoud, A. Prospective Evaluation of Standalone XEN Gel Implant and Combined Phacoemulsification-XEN Gel Implant Surgery: 1-Year Results. *J. Glaucoma* **2018**, *27*, 140–147. [CrossRef]
7. Mansouri, K.; Bravetti, G.E.; Gillmann, K.; Rao, H.L.; Ch'ng, T.W.; Mermoud, A. Two-Year Outcomes of XEN Gel Stent Surgery in Patients with Open-Angle Glaucoma. *Ophthalmol. Glacoma* **2019**, *2*, 309–318. [CrossRef]
8. Gillmann, K.; Bravetti, G.E.; Rao, H.L.; Mermoud, A.; Mansouri, K. Impact of Phacoemulsification Combined with XEN Gel Stent Implantation on Corneal Endothelial Cell Density: 2-Year Results. *J. Glaucoma* **2020**, *29*, 155–160. [CrossRef]
9. Mansouri, K.; Gillmann, K.; Rao, H.L.; Guidotti, J.; Mermoud, A. Prospective Evaluation of XEN Gel Implant in Eyes With Pseudoexfoliative Glaucoma. *J. Glaucoma* **2018**, *27*, 869–873. [CrossRef]
10. Gillmann, K.; Bravetti, G.E.; Mermoud, A.; Rao, H.L.; Mansouri, K. XEN Gel Stent in Pseudoexfoliative Glaucoma: 2-Year Results of a Prospective Evaluation. *J. Glaucoma* **2019**, *28*, 676–684. [CrossRef]

11. Gizzi, C.; Mohamed-Noriega, J.; Elkarmouty, A.; Scott, A. Trabeculectomy Following Failed Ab Interno Gelatin Microstent: Case Series. *J. Glaucoma* **2018**, *27*, e168–e173. [CrossRef] [PubMed]
12. Laroche, D.; Ng, C.; Lynch, G. Baerveldt Attached to XEN: A New Technique to Manage Failed XEN Glaucoma Surgery. *J. Glaucoma* **2018**, *27*, 382–384. [CrossRef] [PubMed]
13. Sheybani, A.; Reitsamer, H.; Ahmed, I.I. Fluid Dynamics of a Novel Micro-Fistula Implant for the Surgical Treatment of Glaucoma. *Investig. Ophthalmol. Vis. Sci.* **2015**, *56*, 4789–4795. [CrossRef] [PubMed]
14. Lewis, R.A. Ab interno approach to the subconjunctival space using a collagen glaucoma stent. *J. Cataract. Refract. Surg.* **2014**, *40*, 1301–1306. [CrossRef]
15. Gillmann, K.; Mansouri, K.; Bravetti, G.E.; Mermoud, A. Chronic Intraocular Inflammation as a Risk Factor for XEN Gel Stent Occlusion: A Case of Microscopic Examination of a Fibrin-obstructed XEN Stent. *J. Glaucoma* **2018**, *27*, 739–741. [CrossRef]
16. Ambresin, A.; Shaarawy, T.; Mermoud, A. Deep sclerectomy with collagen implant in one eye compared with trabeculectomy in the other eye of the same patient. *J. Glaucoma* **2002**, *11*, 214–220. [CrossRef]
17. Shaarawy, T.; Mansouri, K.; Schnyder, C.; Ravinet, E.; Achache, F.; Mermoud, A. Long-term results of deep sclerectomy with collagen implant. *J. Cataract. Refract. Surg.* **2004**, *30*, 1225–1231. [CrossRef]
18. El Sayyad, F.; Helal, M.; El-Kholify, H.; Khalil, M.; El-Maghraby, A. Nonpenetrating deep sclerectomy versus trabeculectomy in bilateral primary open-angle glaucoma. *Ophthalmology* **2000**, *107*, 1671–1674. [CrossRef]
19. Schwenn, O.; Springer, C.; Troost, A.; Yun, S.H.; Pfeiffer, N. Deep sclerectomy using a hyaluronate implant versus trabeculectomy. A comparison of two glaucoma operations using mitomycin C. *Ophthalmologe* **2004**, *101*, 696–704. [CrossRef]
20. Mermoud, A.; Schnyder, C.C.; Sickenberg, M.; Chiou, A.G.; Hediguer, S.E.; Faggioni, R. Comparison of deep sclerectomy with collagen implant and trabeculectomy in open-angle glaucoma. *J. Cataract Refract. Surg.* **1999**, *25*, 323–331. [CrossRef]
21. Delarive, T.; Rossier, A.; Rossier, S.; Ravinet, E.; Shaarawy, T.; Mermoud, A. Aqueous dynamic and histological findings after deep sclerectomy with collagen implant in an animal model. *Br. J. Ophthalmol.* **2003**, *87*, 1340–1344. [CrossRef] [PubMed]
22. Aptel, F.; Dumas, S.; Denis, P. Ultrasound biomicroscopy and optical coherence tomography imaging of filtering blebs after deep sclerectomy with new collagen implant. *Eur. J. Ophthalmol.* **2009**, *19*, 223–230. [CrossRef] [PubMed]
23. Johnson, D.H.; Johnson, M. How does nonpenetrating glaucoma surgery work? Aqueous outflow resistance and glaucoma surgery. *J. Glaucoma* **2001**, *10*, 55–67. [CrossRef] [PubMed]
24. Kazakova, D.; Roters, S.; Schnyder, C.C.; Achache, F.; Jonescu-Cuypers, C.; Mermoud, A.; Krieglstein, G. Ultrasound biomicroscopy images: Long-term results after deep sclerectomy with collagen implant. *Graefes Arch. Clin. Exp. Ophthalmol.* **2002**, *240*, 918–923. [CrossRef]
25. Roy, S.; Mermoud, A. Deep Sclerectomy. *Dev. Ophthalmol.* **2017**, *59*, 36–42. [CrossRef]
26. Villamarin, A.; Roy, S.; Bigler, S.; Stergiopulos, N. A new adjustable glaucoma drainage device. *Investig. Ophthalmol. Vis. Sci.* **2014**, *55*, 1848–1852. [CrossRef]
27. Anand, N.; Kumar, A.; Gupta, A. Primary phakic deep sclerectomy augmented with mitomycin C: Long-term outcomes. *J. Glaucoma* **2011**, *20*, 21–27. [CrossRef]
28. Sangtam, T.; Roy, S.; Mermoud, A. Outcome and Complications of Combined Modified Deep Sclerectomy and Trabeculectomy for Surgical Management of Glaucoma: A Pilot Study. *Clin. Ophthalmol.* **2020**, *14*, 795–803. [CrossRef]
29. Harju, M.; Suominen, S.; Allinen, P.; Vesti, E. Long-term results of deep sclerectomy in normal-tension glaucoma. *Acta Ophthalmol.* **2018**, *96*, 154–160. [CrossRef]
30. Laroche, D.; Nkrumah, G.; Ng, C. Real-World Retrospective Consecutive Study of Ab Interno XEN 45 Gel Stent Implant with Mitomycin C in Black and Afro-Latino Patients with Glaucoma: 40% Required Secondary Glaucoma Surgery at 1 Year. *Middle East Afr. J. Ophthalmol.* **2019**, *26*, 229–234. [CrossRef]
31. Gillmann, K.; Bravetti, G.E.; Mansouri, K. Delayed Obstruction of XEN Gel Stent by Cell Debris in Primary Open-angle Glaucoma: A New Insight into the Pathophysiology of Filtration Device Failure. *J. Curr. Glaucoma Pract.* **2019**, *13*, 113–115. [CrossRef] [PubMed]
32. Widder, R.A.; Kuhnrich, P.; Hild, M.; Rennings, C.; Szumniak, I.; Rossler, G.F. Intraocular Degradation of XEN45 Gel Stent 3 Years After its Implantation. *J. Glaucoma* **2019**, *28*, e171–e173. [CrossRef] [PubMed]
33. Gillmann, K.; Bravetti, G.E.; Mermoud, A.; Mansouri, K. Anterior Chamber XEN Gel Stent Movements: The Impact on Corneal Endothelial Cell Density. *J. Glaucoma* **2019**, *28*, e93–e95. [CrossRef]
34. Rulli, E.; Biagioli, E.; Riva, I.; Gambirasio, G.; De Simone, I.; Floriani, I.; Quaranta, L. Efficacy and safety of trabeculectomy vs nonpenetrating surgical procedures: A systematic review and meta-analysis. *JAMA Ophthalmol.* **2013**, *131*, 1573–1582. [CrossRef]
35. Eldaly, M.A.; Bunce, C.; Elsheikha, O.Z.; Wormald, R. Non-penetrating filtration surgery versus trabeculectomy for open-angle glaucoma. *Cochrane Database Syst. Rev.* **2014**, *15*, 2. [CrossRef]
36. Roy, S.; Mermoud, A. Deep sclerectomy. *Dev. Ophthalmol.* **2012**, *50*, 29–36. [CrossRef]
37. Mostafaei, A.; Taheri, N.; Ghojazadeh, M.; Latifi, A.; Moghaddam, N. Comparison of the effect of mitomycin C and bevacizumab-methylcellulose mixture on combined phacoemulsification and non-penetrating deep sclerectomy surgery on the intraocular pressure (a clinical trial study). *Int. Ophthalmol.* **2019**, *39*, 2341–2351. [CrossRef]
38. Paletta Guedes, R.A.; Gravina, D.M.; Paletta Guedes, V.M.; Chaoubah, A. Use of a Collagen Matrix Implant as an Adjuvant in Combined Surgery Involving Phacoemulsification and Nonpenetrating Deep Sclerectomy. *J. Glaucoma* **2019**, *28*, 363–366. [CrossRef] [PubMed]

39. Bhartiya, S.; Dhingra, D.; Shaarawy, T. Revisiting Results of Conventional Surgery: Trabeculectomy, Glaucoma Drainage Devices, and Deep Sclerectomy in the Era of MIGS. *J. Curr. Glaucoma Pract.* **2019**, *13*, 45–49. [CrossRef]
40. Chiou, A.G.; Mermoud, A.; Jewelewicz, D.A. Post-operative inflammation following deep sclerectomy with collagen implant versus standard trabeculectomy. *Graefes Arch. Clin. Exp. Ophthalmol.* **1998**, *236*, 593–596. [CrossRef]
41. Dupas, B.; Fardeau, C.; Cassoux, N.; Bodaghi, B.; LeHoang, P. Deep sclerectomy and trabeculectomy in uveitic glaucoma. *Eye* **2010**, *24*, 310–314. [CrossRef] [PubMed]
42. Siriwardena, D.; Kotecha, A.; Minassian, D.; Dart, J.K.; Khaw, P.T. Anterior chamber flare after trabeculectomy and after phacoemulsification. *Br. J. Ophthalmol.* **2000**, *84*, 1056–1057. [CrossRef] [PubMed]
43. D'Alessandro, E.; Guidotti, J.M.; Mansouri, K.; Mermoud, A. XEN-augmented Baerveldt: A New Surgical Technique for Refractory Glaucoma. *J. Glaucoma* **2017**, *26*, e90–e92. [CrossRef] [PubMed]
44. Teixeira, F.J.; Sousa, D.C.; Machado, N.M.; Caiado, F.; Barao, R.; Sens, P.; Abegao Pinto, L. XEN-augmented Baerveldt surgical success rate and comparison with the Ahmed Valve. *Acta Ophthalmol.* **2020**, *98*, e870–e875. [CrossRef]
45. Bravetti, G.E.; Mansouri, K.; Gillmann, K.; Rao, H.L.; Mermoud, A. XEN-augmented Baerveldt drainage device implantation in refractory glaucoma: 1-year outcomes. *Graefes Arch. Clin. Exp. Ophthalmol.* **2020**, *258*, 1787–1794. [CrossRef]

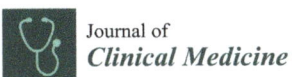

Review

Effectiveness and Safety of Xen Gel Stent in Glaucoma Surgery: A Systematic Review of the Literature

Carlo Enrico Traverso [1,2], Roberto G. Carassa [3], Antonio Maria Fea [4], Michele Figus [5,*], Carlo Astarita [6], Benedetta Piergentili [6], Vanessa Vera [7] and Stefano Gandolfi [8]

1. Eye Clinic, IRCCS San Martino Polyclinic Hospital, 16132 Genoa, Italy; mc8620@mclink.it
2. Department of Neurosciences, Rehabilitation, Ophthalmology, Genetics, Maternal and Child Health (DiNOGMI), University of Genoa, 16126 Genoa, Italy
3. Centro Italiano Glaucoma, 20124 Milan, Italy; carassa@glaucoma.it
4. Department of Surgical Sciences, University of Turin, 10122 Turin, Italy; antoniomfea@gmail.com
5. Department of Surgical, Medical and Molecular Pathology and Critical Care Medicine, University of Pisa, 56126 Pisa, Italy
6. AbbVie S.r.l., 04011 Campoverde, LT, Italy; carlo.astarita@abbvie.com (C.A.); benedetta.piergentili@hotmail.it (B.P.)
7. AbbVie Inc., North Chicago, IL 60064, USA; vanessa.vera@abbvie.com
8. Department of Medicine and Surgery, University of Parma, 43121 Parma, Italy; s.gandolfi@rsadvnet.it
* Correspondence: michele.figus@unipi.it

Abstract: Although topical medical therapy and selective-laser-trabeculoplasty represent the treatments of choice to reduce intraocular pressure, many patients do not achieve adequate glaucoma control; therefore, they require further options and eventually surgery. Trabeculectomy is still considered the gold standard, but the surgical management of glaucoma has undergone continuous advances in recent years, XEN-gel-stent has been introduced as a safer and less traumatic means of lowering intraocular pressure (IOP) in patients with open-angle glaucoma (OAG). This study aimed to review the effectiveness and safety of clinical data on XEN-stent in OAG patients with a Synthesis-Without-Meta-analysis (SWiM) methodology. A total of 339 studies were identified following a literature search adhering to PRISMA guidelines and, after evaluation, 96 studies are discussed. XEN63 and XEN45 device data were collected both short and long term. In addition, this document has evaluated different aspects related to the XEN implant, including: its role compared to trabeculectomy; the impact of mitomycin-C dose on clinical outcomes; postoperative management of the device; and the identification of potential factors that might predict its clinical outcomes. Finally, current challenges and future perspectives of XEN stent, such as its use in fragile or high myopia patients, were discussed.

Keywords: glaucoma; XEN; microinvasive filtering-surgery; trabeculectomy

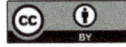

1. Introduction

The term open-angle glaucoma covers a wide range of chronic and progressive optic neuropathies which have the loss of retinal ganglion cells and their axons in common, as well as the subsequent loss of the visual field [1].

Lowering intraocular pressure (IOP) is currently considered as the main known modifiable risk factor [2]. Topical hypotensive medication and selective laser trabeculoplasty are currently considered as the first treatment approaches in most patients [3]. However, some patients do not achieve adequate glaucoma control; therefore, they require further therapies and eventually surgery [3–5], such as trabeculectomy [6], which unfortunately may lead to potential vision-threatening complications [7].

Glaucoma surgery has experienced important advances over the last several years.

One of the most important advances in glaucoma surgery in recent years was the development of the minimally or microinvasive glaucoma surgery (MIGS) devices [8]. They have been developed as safer and less traumatic means of lowering IOP in patients with glaucoma [8,9].

The definition of the term MIGS has been evolving since its introduction [9,10], and the generally accepted definition of MIGS has been changing over the years [11].

Among the different MIGS devices, XEN gel stents obtained the CE mark in December 2015 and were approved by the Food and Drug Administration (FDA) in November 2016 [12].

According to the classical definition, XEN is not defined as a MIGS because it is a bleb-forming device [9]; therefore, minimally invasive or micro-incisional filtration surgery have been suggested as more appropriate terms.

The aim of the current paper is to review the effectiveness and safety clinical data of XEN stent in open-angle glaucoma (OAG) patients.

XEN Gel Stent

The XEN gel stent (AbbVie Inc., Chicago, IL, USA) was originally developed as an ab interno procedure that reduces IOP by draining aqueous fluid from the anterior chamber into the subconjunctival space [13–15]. Unlike other MIGS devices that target Schlemm's canal and the supraciliary space to lower IOP, XEN gel stent was the first micro-incisional filtration surgical procedure to drain aqueous to subconjunctival space [14,15].

The stent is a hydrophilic tube that is 6 mm long, and it is composed of porcine gelatine crosslinked with glutaraldehyde to prevent degradation when implanted [13,16].

The XEN device is based on the Hagen–Poiseuille law of laminar flow, where the length and the inner diameter of the tube determine the flow resistance and, consequently, the flow rate. Three different devices with different inner diameters, namely 45, 63, and 140 µm, were investigated [13].

The 140 µm XEN device has not been commercialized to date and the evidence is limited to a single paper [17]. The evidence evaluating the clinical outcomes of the XEN63 device is very limited [18–23] and most studies were performed with an earlier version of the device injector that was never marketed [18–21]. The new XEN63 device uses the same needle injector as the XEN45 for preventing early sideflow and hypotony [22].

Although the XEN45 device was originally designed for ab interno implantation [13–15], surgeons have been gaining experience with the device, and different changes aiming to provide better clinical outcomes have been introduced in the implantation technique [24–26].

Systematic reviews are currently considered as an essential source of evidence when making decisions in the clinical management of patients [27]. However, there are some limitations in relation to the method used (Preferred Reporting Items for Systematic Reviews and Meta-Analyses [PRISMA]; http://www.prisma-statement.org/, accessed on 1 July 2023) [28,29]. Pooling data is not possible in all cases due to high levels of heterogeneity or lack of data [12,29]. In addition, there is a growing clinical demand to respond to complex questions or situations that incorporate various data sources due to their characteristics [30,31]. These facts have opened the door to a growing number of narrative syntheses of quantitative data. However, a major concern about such papers is lack of transparency and the consequent introduction of bias [32,33].

Synthesis Without Meta-analysis (SWiM) has emerged as a systematic review to address questions that meta-analysis may not be able to provide an adequate answer for [34].

This SWiM aims to examine the currently available scientific evidence to answer different clinical questions about the XEN device.

2. Materials and Methods

2.1. Information Sources and Search Strategy

This SWiM was carried out according to the guidelines of the of the PRISMA statement [35], although the current systematic review was not registered.

A group of Italian glaucoma specialists convened to review the currently available evidence about the efficacy and safety of XEN devices in patients with glaucoma. Searches of MEDLINE, the Cochrane Database, EMBASE, and Google Scholar were conducted using the search terms "Glaucoma", "Open-angle glaucoma", "XEN", "MIGS", "Combined surgery", and "Gel implant". References cited in selected articles were also reviewed to identify additional relevant reports.

In addition, abstracts from the American Glaucoma Society, American Academy of Ophthalmology, European Glaucoma Society, and Association of Research in Vision and Ophthalmology were manually searched for relevant publications.

2.2. Study Selection, Data Extraction, and Synthesis Method

The authors independently generated the queries for the literature search and selected the articles fulfilling the criteria established for each subject and solved any disagreement through discussion and consensus.

Limits were set for articles written in English, French, Spanish, Portuguese, and Italian with human subjects. The studies were published between August 2014 and April 2023.

Additionally, the following exclusion criteria were applied: (1) the study did not examine clinical outcomes or response to treatment of XEN device (any device); (2) the study was on subjects other than human adults; (3) the publication was a review article, an editorial, or an opinion piece.

To synthesize the results, we applied the SWiM guidelines [34].

3. Results

3.1. Results of the PRISMA Procedure

The steps of the literature search are summarized in the PRISMA 2009 flow diagram (Figure 1). A total of 339 records were identified after the initial search. After the removal of duplicates, 187 scientific papers remained. After careful review, 96 papers met all the requirements of the inclusion/exclusion criteria and were included for qualitative synthesis (Figure 1).

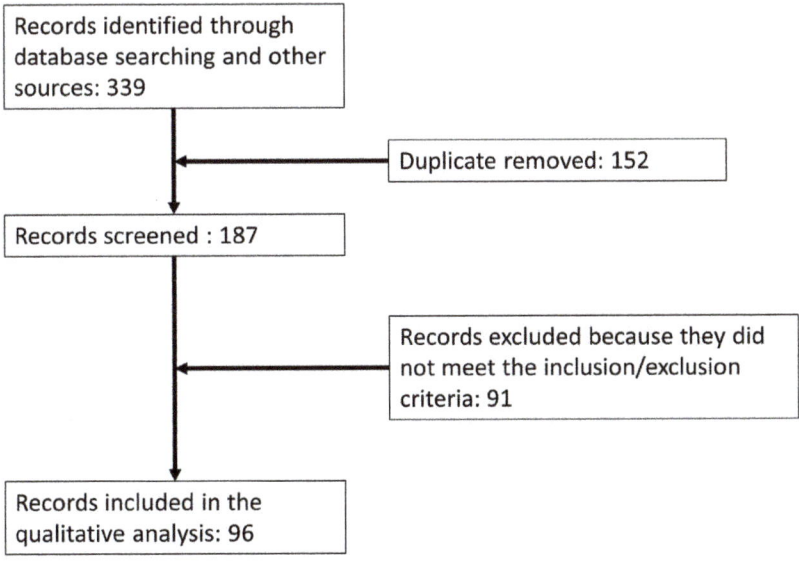

Figure 1. PRISMA 2009 flow diagram.

3.2. XEN63

The currently available scientific evidence evaluating the clinical outcomes of XEN63 is very limited [18–23] (See Table 1), and most of the evidence was generated from a former device that was never commercialized; therefore, we will not go into detail analysing the results of those articles [18–21].

Table 1. An overview of currently available scientific evidence with the XEN63 device.

Study	Follow-Up	Preop IOP, mmHg	Final IOP, mmHg	IOP Lowering	Mean Preoperative NOHM	Mean NOHM, Last Visit	Success Rates, (%) [1]
Fea et al. [22]	3 months	27.0 ± 7.8 *	12.2 ± 3.4 *	−14.8 (−20.1 to −9.5) **	2.3 ± 0.9 *	0.1 ± 0.4 *	69.6
Fea et al. [23]	18 months	27.0 ± 7.8 *	14.1 ± 3.4 *	−12.9 (−16.9 to −8.9) **	2.3 ± 0.9 *	1.0 ± 1.4 *	77.8

* Mean (Standard deviation). ** Mean (95% confidence interval). [1] Complete success. Preop: preoperative; IOP: intraocular pressure; NOHM: number of ocular hypotensive medications.

To date, there are two papers evaluating the efficacy and safety of the XEN63 device. Fea et al. [22] evaluated the new XEN63 device and found a mean (95% confidence interval, 95% CI) IOP lowering effect of −14.8 (−20.1 to −9.5) mmHg, $p < 0.0001$ at month-3, reporting that the mean IOP achieved with XEN63 was consistently lower than that obtained with XEN45. This may be an important point because the larger calibre of the Xen 63 device could by clinically meaningful for patients with high preoperative IOP.

Additionally, Fea et al. [23] evaluated the effectiveness and safety of the new XEN63 device over a follow-up period of 18 months in patients with glaucoma in a real clinical setting. They reported significant IOP lowering and a reduction in the number of ocular hypotensive drugs during a follow-up period of 18 months. Moreover, the incidence rate of adverse events was relatively low and most of them were mild in severity [23].

Table 1 summarizes the main outcomes of XEN63 according to the current evidence.

3.3. XEN45

3.3.1. Effect on Intraocular Pressure Lowering and Reduction in the Number of IOP-Lowering Medications

Multiple studies have evaluated the IOP lowering effect of the XEN device, either alone or in combination with cataract surgery, in patients with glaucoma [36–101]. Although most of the studies were performed in patients with primary open-angle glaucoma (POAG), other studies were performed in patients with pseudoexfoliative glaucoma (PXG) [40,42,54,72,98] or glaucoma secondary to uveitis [47].

The results of a systematic review and meta-analysis published recently, which used a pooled analysis with a random effects model, have shown a mean (95% CI) IOP lowering from baseline of −7.8 (−7.4 to −8.2) mmHg and −8.4 (−6.9 to −9.8) mmHg in the eyes of patients who underwent XEN-solo and XEN + Phaco, respectively. All patients were treated and followed up as routine clinical practice between May 2013 and February 2020. The mean sample size was 79 ± 67 and the average follow-up time was 17.0 ± 8.1 months [12].

Similarly, Yang et al. [102] did not find significant differences in IOP lowering between XEN-solo and XEN + Phaco (standardized mean difference: −0.01, 95% CI −0.09 to 0.08, p value 0.894). Moreover, Panarelli et al. [103] reported that, on average, successful gel stent surgery achieved a postoperative IOP of approximately 14.0 mm Hg and reduction to fewer than 1 ocular hypotensive medication.

Regarding the number of ocular hypotensive medications (See Tables 2–4), Chen et al. [12] reported a significant reduction in the number of ocular hypotensive drugs in both XEN-solo procedures (Mean: −1.97 drugs; 95% CI: −2.19 to −1.75 drugs, $p < 0.001$) and in the XEN + Phaco ones (Mean: −1.86 drugs; 95% CI: −2.11 to −1.60 drugs, $p < 0.001$).

Table 2. A comparison of the clinical outcomes of XEN45 after 12 months of follow-up.

Study	Type of Study	N	Preop IOP, mm Hg	M12 IOP, mm Hg	M12 IOP Lowering	Mean Preoperative NOHM	Mean NOHM, Last Visit	Needling Rates at Last Follow-Up Visit, n (%)
Ozal et al. [37] [1]	Retrospective	15	36.1 ± 3.7 *	16.7 ± 3.6 *	−19.3 ± 5.0 *	3.6 ± 0.5 *	0.3 ± 0.9 *	Not reported
Galal et al. [38]	Prospective	13	16.0 ± 4.0 *	12.0 ± 3.0	23 *,†	1.9 ± 1.0 *	0.13 ± 0.11 *	4 (30.7)
Grover et al. [39]	Prospective	65	25.1 ± 3.7 *	15.9 ± 5.2 *	−9.1 (−10.7 to 7.5) **	3.5 ± 1.0 *	1.7 †	21 (32.3)
Hengerer et al. [40]	Retrospective	242	32.2 ± 9.1 *	14.2 ± 4.0	32.2 *,†	3.1 ± 1.0 *	0.3 ± 0.7 *	67 (27.7) ***
De Gregorio et al. [41]	Prospective	33	22.5 ± 3.7 *	13.1 ± 2.4 *	−9.4 ± 3.1 *	2.5 ± 0.9 *	0.4 ± 0.8 *	Not reported
Mansouri et al. [42]	Prospective	149	20.0 ± 7.1 *	13.9 ± 4.3	−31 *,†	1.9 ± 1.3 *	0.5 ± 0.8 *	55 (36.9)
Widder et al. [44]	Retrospective	261	24.3 ± 6.6 *	16.8 ± 7.6 *	−7.5 ± 7.1 *	2.6 ± 1.1 *	0.2 ± 0.7 *	80 (34)
Reitsamer et al. [45]	Prospective	202	21.4 ± 3.6 *	14.9 ± 4.5 *	−6.5 ± 5.3 *	2.7 ± 0.9 *	1.1 ± 1.2 *	83 (41.1)
Kalina et al. [47]	Prospective	47	22.3 ± 7.3 *	13.4 ± 3.6 *	−8.9 ± 5.8 *	3.0 ± 1.2 *	0.8 ± 1.3 *	14 (29.8)
Marcos-Parra et al. [48]	Retrospective	65	19.1 ± 5.4 *	N.A.	−6.7 (−12.9 to −0.5) **	2.5 ± 0.8 *	0.2 ± 0.6 *	13 (20.0)
Sng et al. [50]	Prospective	31	15.6 ± 2.7 *	12.1 ± 2.6 *	−3.5 ± 2.7 *	1.4 ± 0.6 *	0.1 ± 0.4 *	Not reported
Gabbay et al. [51]	Retrospective	151	22.1 ± 6.5 *	15.4 ± 5.9 *	−6.7 ± 6.2 *	2.77 ± 1.1 *	0.5 ± 1.0 *	57 (37.7)
Laborda-Guirao et al. [52]	Retrospective	80	21.0 ± 5.2 *	14.7 (13.9 to 15.4) **	−6.3 (−8.8 to −4.4) **	2.8 (2.7 to 3.0) **	1.1 (0.8 to 1.3) **	7 (8.8)
Heidinger et al. [53]	Retrospective	199	22.8 ± 6.9 *	17.1 ± 5.9 *	−5.7 ± 6.6 *	2.9 ± 1.0 *	1.8 ± 1.4 *	44 (22.1)
Ibáñez-Muñoz et al. [54]	Retrospective	21	22.3 (21.0–23.5) **	15.3 (14.3–16.3) **	−7.3 (−9.7 to −5.0) **	3.0 ± 1.0 *	1.2 ± 1.2 *	19 (26.0)
Karimi et al. [55]	Retrospective	259	19.3 ± 6.0 *	14.3 ± 4.4 *	−5.1 ± 5.6 *	2.6 ± 0.1 *	1.6 ± 0.5 *	106 (40.9) [2]
Laroche et al. [56]	Retrospective	20	15.3 ± 6.2 *	12.9 ± 4.5 *	−2.4 ± 5.4 *	3.6 ± 0.7 *	1.8 ± 1.5	0 (0.0)
Smith et al. [57]	Retrospective	68	22.1 ± 6.4 *	14.8 ± 5.1 *	−7.3 ± 5.8 *	2.9 ± 0.8 *	1.1 ± 1.1 *	30 (44.1)
Mansouri et al. [59]	Prospective	109	20.0 ± 7.5 *	N.A.	N.A.	2.0 ± 1.3 *	0.6 ± 0.9 *	58 (45)
Post et al. [61]	Prospective	20	21.6 ± 2.3 *	17.7 ± 2.1 *	−3.9 ± 2.2 *	3.2 ± 0.8 *	1.6 ± 1.0 *	5 (25.0)
Chao et al. [64]	Retrospective	37	21.7 ± 7.7 *	15.0 ± 2.0 *	−6.7 ± 5.6 *	3.4 ± 0.9 *	1.3 ± 1.5 *	17 (45.9)
Schargus et al. [66]	Retrospective	153	23.9 ± 7.4 *	15.4 ± 5.1 *	−8.5 ± 6.4 *	2.6 ± 1.2 *	0.8 ± 1.3 *	64 (35.3)
Theilig et al. [67]	Retrospective	100	24.5 ± 6.7 *	16.6 ± 4.8 *	N.A.	3.0 ± 1.1 *	1.4 ± 1.5 *	42 (42.0)
Subaşı et al. [69]	Retrospective	30	20.4 ± 4.8 *	15.0 ± 1.9 *	−6.2 ± 0.9 *	3.1 ± 1.0 *	0.9 ± 1.1 *	13 (43.3)

Table 2. Cont.

Study	Type of Study	N	Preop IOP, mm Hg	M12 IOP, mm Hg	M12 IOP Lowering	Mean Preoperative NOHM	Mean NOHM, Last Visit	Needling Rates at Last Follow-Up Visit, n (%)
Fea et al. [70]	Prospective	171	23.9 ± 7.6 *	15.5 ± 3.9 *	−7.4 ± 7.9	3.0 ± 1.0 *	0.5 ± 1.0 *	79 (46.2)
Rauchegger et al. [71]	Retrospective	79	23.4 ± 7.9 *	14.6 ± 3.6 *	31(20–42) *, ‡	2.7 ± 1.1 *	1.0 ± 1.2 *	37 (62)
Eraslam et al. [81]	Retrospective	26	23.9 ± 6.8 *	16.4 ± 2.6 *	−7.5 ± 5.2 *	2.9 ± 0.7	0.9 ± 0.9	21 (36.2)
Lewczuk et al. [83] [3]	Retrospective	86	25.0 ± 7.5 *	16.8 ± 5.1 *	−8.2 ± 6.4 *	Not reported	Not reported	30 (69.8)
Wanichwecharungruang and Ratprasatporn [84]	Retrospective	57	21.6 ± 4.0	15 †	−30.6 *,†	2.1 ± 1.4 *	0.5 ± 0.7 *	10 (17.5)
Reitsamer et al. [86]	Retrospective	212	20.7 ± 5.1	14.8 †	−5.6 †	2.5 ± 1.0 *	0.7 ± 1.0 *	78 (36.8)
Nicolau et al. [89]	Retrospective	186	18.1 ± 5.1 *	13.7 ± 5.6 *	−4.4 ± 5.3 *	2.5 ± 1.1 *	0.8 ± 1.0	25 (13%)
Monja-Alarcón et al. [95]	Retrospective	63	17.6 (0.7) **	12.6 (0.3) **	21.9 ± 27.6 *,‡	2.1 (1.9 to 2.3) ‡	0.2 (0.04 to 0.3) ‡	19 (30.2)
Buenasmañanas-Maeso et al. [96]	Retrospective	63	17.6 ± 5.3 *	12.6 (12.0 to 13.3) ‡	−21.9 ± 27.4 *	2.1 (1.9 to 2.3) ‡	0.2 (0.04 to 0.3) ‡	8 (12.7)
Almendral et al. [99]	Retrospective	63	17.6 ± 5.3 *	12.6 ± 2.6 *	−22.0 ± 27.5 *	2.1 ± 0.7 *	0.2 ± 0.5 *	7 (11.1)

† Data about standard deviation was not provided. * Mean (Standard deviation). ** Mean (95% confidence interval). *** Percentage. ‡ 95% Confidence interval. *** All the needling procedures were done between week 1 and month 3. [1] Data calculated from Table 2 of the paper. [2] Postoperative bleb needling or antimetabolite injection. [3] Data from naive patients. Abbreviations: IOP: intraocular pressure; N: number of eyes; NOHM: number of ocular hypotensive medications.

Table 3. A comparison of the clinical outcomes of XEN45 after 24 months of follow-up.

Study	Type of Study	N	Preop IOP, mm Hg	M 24 IOP, mm Hg	M 24 IOP Lowering, mm Hg	Mean Preoperative NOHM	Mean NOHM, Last Visit	Needling Rates at Last Follow-Up Visit, n (%)
Reitsamer et al. [45]	Prospective	202	21.4 (3.6) *	15.2 ± 4.2 *	−6.2 ± 4.9 *	2.7 ± 0.9 *	1.1 ± 1.2 *	83 (41.1)
Gabbay et al. [51]	Retrospective	151	22.1 ± 6.5 *	14.5 ± 3.3 *	−7.6 ± 5.2 *	2.77 ± 1.1 *	0.5 ± 1.0 *	57 (37.7)
Karimi et al. [55]	Retrospective	259	19.3 ± 6.0 *	13.5 ± 3.3 *,[1]	−5.8 ± 4.8 *	2.6 ± 0.1 *	1.1 ± 1.3 *,[1]	106 (40.9) [2]
Mansouri et al. [59]	Prospective	113	20.0 ± 7.5 *	14.1 ± 3.7 *	−6.4 ± 5.9 *	2.0 ± 1.3 *	0.6 ± 0.9 *	58 (45)
Scheres et al. [63]	Retrospective	41	19.2 ± 4.4 *	13.8 ± 3.8 *	−5.4 ± 4.1 *	2.5 ± 1.4 *	0.9 ± 1.2 *	8 (20)
Subaşı et al. [69]	Retrospective	30	20.4 ± 4.8 *	14.8 ± 1.9 *	−6.4 ± 1.2 *	3.1 ± 1.0 *	0.9 ± 1.1 *	13 (43.3)

Table 3. Cont.

Study	Type of Study	N	Preop IOP, mm Hg	M 24 IOP, mm Hg	M 24 IOP Lowering, mm Hg	Mean Preoperative NOHM	Mean NOHM, Last Visit	Needling Rates at Last Follow-Up Visit, n (%)
Rauchegger et al. [71]	Retrospective	79	23.4 ± 7.9 *	14.8 ± 4.4	29(30–41) *	2.7 ± 1.1 *	1.0 ± 1.2 *	37 (62)
Wanichwecharungruang and Ratprasatporn [84]	Retrospective	77	21.6 ± 4.0	14.6 ± 3.5 *	32.4 *,†	2.1 ± 1.4	0.5 ± 0.7 *	10 (17.5)
Lewczuk et al. [85]	Retrospective	72	24.8 ± 8.0 *	17.5 ± 5.8 *,³	−7.3 ± 7.0 *	Not reported	Not reported	43 (67.2)
Nicolau et al. [89]	Retrospective	186	18.1 ± 5.1 *	12.6 ± 3.1 *	−5.5 ± 4.2 *	2.5 ± 1.1 *	1.7 ± 1.7 *	25 (13%)
Szigiato et al. [94]	Retrospective	141	23.3 ± 7.0 *	13.3 ± 4.7 *	−10.0 ± 6.0 *	3.4 ± 0.8 *	1.9 ± 1.5 *	54 (38.3)
Gillmann et al. [98] POAG PEX	Prospective	57 53	19.8 ± 5.8 * 19.8 ± 8.2 *	14.5 ± 3.6 * 14.2 ± 3.8 *	−5.3 ± 4.8 * −5.6 ± 6.4 *	1.9 ± 1.6 * 2.0 ± 1.3 *	0.6 ± 0.9 * 0.4 ± 0.7 *	42.8 43.2
Vukmirovic et al. [101]	Retrsopective	262	20.40 ± 6.31 *	Not reported	Not reported	2.70 ± 1.01 *	0.6 ± 0.9	111 (42.4)

[1] Month-18 IOP. [2] Postoperative bleb needling or antimetabolite injection. [3] IOP at the last study visit (mean follow-up period was 26.87 ± 15.33 months). [†] Data about standard deviation was not provided. [*] Mean ± Standard deviation. [**] Percentage. Abbreviations: IOP: intraocular pressure; N: number of eyes; NOHM: number of ocular hypotensive medications; PEX: Pseudoexfoliative glaucoma.

Table 4. A comparison of the long-term follow-up clinical outcomes of XEN45.

Study	Type of Study	N	Length of Study (months)	Preoperative IOP (mmHg)	Final IOP	IOP Lowering (%)	Mean Reduction in Ocular Hypotensive Medication
Lenzhofer et al. [19]	Prospective	34	48	22.5 ± 4.2 *	13.4 ± 3.1 *	40.4	1.2
Gillmann et al. [60] XEN alone	Prospective	26	36	21.0 ± 7.4 *	12.9 ± 2.9 *	38.6	2.1
XEN + Phaco	Prospective	76	36	20.0 ± 6.9 *	12.9 ± 3.4 *	35.5	1.4
Nuzzi et al. [80]	Retrospective	23	36	24.9 ± 6.1 *	19.6 ± 2.1 *	21.3	Not reported
Reitsamer et al. [86]	Retrospective	76	36	20.7 ± 5.1 *	13.9 ± 4.3 *	32.9	1.4
Gabbay et al. [87]	Retrospective	205	36	22.6 ± 7.0 *	14.0 ± 2.9 *	38.1	2.0
Capelli et al. [93]	Retrospective	34	36	23 (19–28) **	Not reported	Not reported	Not reported
Marcos-Parra et al. [100]	Retrospective	63	36	19.1 ± 5.0 *	14.9 ± 3.8 *	−4.2 ± 4.7 *	−1.9 ± 0.8 *

Abbreviations: IOP: intraocular pressure; N: number of eyes. * Mean ± Standard deviation. ** Median (Interquartile range).

Similar results have been published by Yan et al. [102], who found a statistically significant reduction in ocular hypotensive medications (standardized mean difference: 2.11, 95% CI 1.84 to 2.38, p value < 0.001). Furthermore, after adjusting for different covariates, the reduction in the number of ocular hypotensive drugs was significantly lower in the XEN + Phaco group than in the XEN-solo group (Risk ratio: 1.45, 95% CI 1.06 to 1.99, p value 0.019) [102].

IOP Lowering at 12 Months

Thirty-four studies have evaluated the IOP lowering effect of the XEN device over 12 months of follow-up (see Table 2). On average, the results of the different studies pointed in the same general direction, mostly indicating that XEN45 provided IOPs below 15 mmHg after one year of follow-up (Table 2), which is consistent with the most recent meta-analysis published [12,101,102].

IOP Lowering at 24 Months

Twelve studies have evaluated the IOP lowering effect of XEN45 after 24 months of follow-up (See Table 3). The results of the different studies included in this SWiM paper have shown that, after 2 years of follow-up, XEN45 provided a good IOP lowering, with final IOPs ≤15 mmHg and an IOP lowering that ranged between −5 and −10 mmHg (Table 3).

IOP Lowering at 36-Months

Six papers have evaluated the longer-term efficacy of XEN45 in terms of IOP lowering and reducing the number of ocular hypotensive medications, (See Table 4). With the exception of one paper (n = 23 eyes), which reported an IOP of 19.6 ± 2.1 mmHg at 36 months [78], currently available evidence shows good hypotensive effects for XEN45, with IOPs at 36–48 months in the range of 13–14 mmHg, as well as a significant reduction in the number of ocular hypotensive medications [45,61,81,87,88,94,101]. In addition, compared to preoperative values, the reduction in IOP was greater than 30% (Table 4).

Current evidence has demonstrated the efficacy and safety of the XEN45 device in the short, medium, and long term.

3.3.2. Can XEN45 Be Safely and Effectively Implanted in Myopic Patients?

Evidence surrounding the use of XEN45 in myopic OAG patients is limited [52,64,104–106]. In fact, there are currently only two studies that specifically evaluated the efficacy and safety of XEN45 in patients with high myopia.

Laborda-Guirao et al. did not find significant differences between OAG eyes with or without high myopia in intraocular pressure (IOP) lowering, success rate, reduction in the number of ocular hypotensive medications, or postoperative complications, which clearly suggested that XEN45 may be safely and effectively used in glaucomatous eyes with high myopia [52].

Chao et al. [64], have retrospectively evaluated the effectiveness and safety of the XEN45 in East Asian patients with primary open angle glaucoma (POAG). Although this study did not specifically evaluate the efficacy and safety of XEN45 in patients with high myopia, the mean spherical equivalent was -5.13 ± 4.44 diopters, with a range of -13.63 to -2.88 diopters and mean axial length of 26.67 ± 1.65 mm (up to 29.34 mm). According to the results of this study, axial length was not significantly associated with success, either complete (odds ratio: 0.082, $p = 0.559$) or qualified (odds ratio: 0.659; $p = 0.186$); need of subsequent intervention (odds ratio: 0.959, $p = 0.803$); or need of additional surgery (odds ratio: 1.382, $p = 0.382$). Additionally, no major complications were observed [64]. These results suggested that axial length did not have any influence on XEN45 outcomes.

Sacchi et al. [105], in a retrospective study (which included seven eyes followed for 2 years) evaluated the effectiveness and safety of Xen 45 in patients with medically uncontrolled glaucoma and concomitant high myopia (>6 Diopters). Preoperative mean IOP was significantly lowered from 22.1 ± 4.9 mmHg to 14.8 ± 4.0 mmHg at month-24, $p < 0.0001$. Regarding safety, two eyes had hypotony (without maculopathy) and one eye had choroidal detachment [106]. According to the results of this study, the XEN implant had a better safety profile than trabeculectomy, with a similar hypotensive profile [105].

Additionally, Fea et al. assessed the effectiveness and safety of XEN in 31 glaucomatous eyes with a refractive error higher than -6 D and an axial length ≥ 26 mm [106]. Mean preoperative IOP (95% CI) was significantly lowered from 23.5 (20.5–26.4) mm Hg to 13.0 (12.2–13.8) mm Hg, $p < 0.0001$. Regarding safety, hypotony (an IOP <6 mm Hg) was reported in eight eyes (28.6%) during the first postoperative day and remained for a week [106].

Conversely, one publication described the clinical outcomes of XEN45 in a high myopic eye. The patient required a XEN removal to control IOP, which resulted in loss of the remaining visual field in the eye [104].

Currently available scientific evidence suggests that XEN45 may be effectively and safely implanted in myopic eyes. However, there is a need for a prospective study specifically evaluating the clinical outcomes of XEN45 in eyes with OAG and high myopia.

3.3.3. XEN-Solo Versus XEN + Phaco: Is There a Difference in Terms of IOP Lowering?

This question has brought an increasing interest among glaucoma specialists.

Fifteen papers have compared the efficacy of XEN45 solo or in combination with cataract surgery (phacoemulsification). After reviewing the literature, the most plausible conclusion is that there is no agreement regarding the superiority of the solo procedure over the combined procedure with cataract surgery (See Table 5).

Table 5. A comparison of the clinical outcomes of XEN45 solo and in combination with cataract surgery (Phacoemulsification).

Study	N	Follow-Up (months)	Preop IOP, mm Hg	Final IOP, mm Hg	Final IOP Lowering	Mean Preoperative NOHM	Mean NOHM, Last Visit
Ozal et al. [37] [1] XEN XEN + Phaco	9 6	12	36.7 ± 4.1 * 35.2 ± 3.2 *	17.0 ± 4.2 * 15.5 ± 2.3 *	−19.7 ± 4.2 * −19.7 ± 2.8 *	3.7 ± 0.5 * Not estimable	0.3 ± 0.9 * Not estimable

Table 5. Cont.

Study	N	Follow-Up (months)	Preop IOP, mm Hg	Final IOP, mm Hg	Final IOP Lowering	Mean Preoperative NOHM	Mean NOHM, Last Visit
Lenzhofer et al. [19] XEN XEN + Phaco	35 29	48	22.5 ± 6.5 * 23.4 ± 6.3 *	13.2 ± 5.2 * 12.7 ± 6.9 *	−9.5 ± 5.9 * −13.7 ± 6.6 *	3.0 ± 0.9 * 1.4 ± 0.6	0.8 ± 0.9 * 0.1 ± 0.4
Reitsamer et al. [45] XEN XEN + Phaco	106 79	24	21.7 ± 3.8 * 21.0 ± 3.4 *	15.4 ± 4.2 * 14.9 ± 4.5 *	−6.3 ± 4.0 * −6.1 ± 4.0 *	2.7 ± 0.9 * 2.9 ± 1.0	1.2 ± 1.2 * 1.4 ± 1.3 *
Kalina et al. [47] XEN XEN + Phaco	20 27	12	24.2 ± 8.2 * 21.0 ± 6.5 *	13.0 ± 4.5 * 13.6 ± 2.9 *	−11.2 ± 6.6 * −7.4 ± 5.0 *	Not reported	Not reported
Parra et al. [48] XEN XEN + Phaco	17 48	12	22.2 ± 6.8 * 18.0 ± 4.5 *	N.A.	−6.7 (−10.4 to −3.0) ** −3.5 (−5.0 to −2.0) **	2.5 ± 0.8 * 2.1 ± 0.9 *	0.2 ± 0.6 * 0.1 ± 0.3 *
Laborda-Guirao et al. [52] XEN XEN + Phaco	40 40	12	21.8 ± 5.3 * 20.1 ± 5.1 *	−14.4 (−15.7 to −13.2) ** −14.9 (−15.8 to −14.1) **	−6.8 ± 0.9) ‡ −5.9 ± 0.9) ‡	Not reported	Not reported
Karimi et al. [55] XEN XEN + Phaco	187 72	18	19.6 (18.8–20.5) ** 18.3 (17.0–19.7) **	13.5 (12.3–14.7) ** 14.0 †	Not reported	Not reported	Not reported
Gillmann et al. [60] XEN XEN + Phaco	26 66	36	21.0 ± 7.4 * 20.0 ± 6.9 *	12.9 ± 2.9 * 12.9 ± 3.4 *	−8.1 ± 5.6 * −7.1 ± 5.4 *	2.4 ± 1.5 * 1.9 ± 1.2 *	0.3 ± 0.8 * 0.5 ± 0.9 *
Olgun et al. [65] XEN XEN + Phaco	51 45	24	24.4 ± 4.3 * 24.8 ± 3.5 *	14.2 ± 2.2 * 13.4 ± 1.4 *	−10.2 ± 3.5 * −11.4 ± 2.7 *	3.4 ± 0.5 * 3.4 ± 0.4 *	2.2 ± 2.0 * 1.8 ± 1.7 *
Theilig et al. [67] XEN XEN + Phaco	48 52	12	24.4 ± 6.6 * 24.8 ± 6.9 *	16.9 ± 5.9 * 16.4 ± 4.2 *	−7.5 ± 6.2 * −8.6 ± 5.3 *	3.1 ± 1.2 * 2.8 ± 1.1 *	1.5 ± 1.4 * 0.9 ± 1.4 *
Fea et al. [70] XEN XEN + Phaco	115 56	12	25.0 † 21.4 †	15.8 † 15.4 †	−8.8 ± 7.5 * −4.5 ± 8.4 *	3.0 ± 1.0 * 2.5 ± 1.0 *	0.5 † 0.5 †
Schargus et al. [79] XEN XEN + Phaco	38 42	24	24.1 ± 4.7 * 25.4 ± 5.6 *	15.7 ± 3.0 * 14.7 ± 3.2 *	−8.4 ± 3.9 * −10.7 ± 4.6 *	3.3 ± 0.8 * 2.9 ± 0.6 *	1.2 ± 0.8 * 1.0 ± 0.4 *
Eraslam et al. [81] XEN XEN + Phaco	26 32	12	23.7 ± 6.0 * 24.4 ± 7.2 *	16.3 ± 3.0 * 16.4 ± 2.3 *	−7.4 ± 4.7 * −8.0 ± 5.3 *	2.9 ± 0.7 * 2.9 ± 0.6 *	1.0 ± 0.9 * 0.8 ± 0.8 *
Reitsamer et al. [86] XEN XEN + Phaco	98 76	36	20.4 ± 4.7 * 20.4 ± 5.5 *	14.2 † 13.6 †	−6.4 † −6.7 †	2.6 ± 1.0 * 2.4 ± 1.0 *	1.1 ± 1.3 * 1.2 ± 1.1 *
Marcos-Parra et al. [100] XEN XEN + Phaco	37 117	36	21.2 ± 6.2 * 18.4 ± 4.3 *	14.5 ± 4.0 * 14.9 ± 3.1 *	−3.1 ± 0.8 ‡ −3.8 ± 0.4 ‡	2.6 ± 0.7 * 1.9 ± 0.8 *	0.4 ± 0.8 *,1 0.2 ± 0.5 *

† Data about standard deviation was not provided. * Mean ± Standard deviation. ** Mean (95% confidence interval). ‡ Mean ± Standard error of the mean. [1] Greater reduction in the XEN-alone than in the XEN + Phaco group (mean difference: 0.4 drugs; 95% CI: 0.1 to 0.7; $p = 0.0134$). Abbreviations: IOP: intraocular pressure; NOHM: number of ocular hypotensive medications.

According to the results of Chen et al. [12], both XEN alone (mean difference: −7.8 mmHg; 95% CI: −8.21 to −7.38 mmHg, $p < 0.001$) and XEN + Phaco (mean difference: −8.35 mmHg; 95% CI: −9.82 to −6.88 mmHg, $p < 0.001$) significantly lowered the IOP.

Similarly, Yang et al. [103], in a systematic review and metanalysis, did not find significant differences between XEN and phaco-XEN surgery in terms of IOP after surgery (standardized mean difference: −0.01, 95% CI −0.09 to 0.08, p value 0.894). Nevertheless, the reduction in the number of ocular hypotensive medications was greater in the XEN solo group ($p = 0.019$) [102].

However, another systematic review and meta-analysis published by Wang et al. [107] has shown different results. They found better results for XEN alone compared to XEN + Phaco procedures in IOP lowering, but not in reducing ocular hypotensive medications [107].

In light of the available scientific evidence and based on our own experience, the XEN45 device, either alone or in combination with cataract surgery (phacoemulsification), significantly lowers IOP and reduces the number of ocular hypotensive medications. Similar to trabeculectomy, there are no data to support the superiority of the combined surgery over the solo surgery, and vice versa.

3.3.4. XEN Versus Trabeculectomy: Is There a Difference in Terms of IOP Lowering?

Due mainly to its well-stablished IOP lowering effect, trabeculectomy is currently considered as the gold standard in glaucoma surgery [5]. However, it may lead to potential vision-threatening complications [6].

The Gold-Standard Pathway Study (GPS) [108] was the first multicenter, prospective, and randomized study comparing the effectiveness and safety of XEN45 versus trabeculectomy in glaucoma that was poorly controlled with topical IOP-lowering therapy. The results of this study showed that the mean IOP change from baseline was significantly greater at month 12 in the trabeculectomy group (0.024), although both treatments significantly lowered IOP from preoperative values ($p < 0.001$). XEN and trabeculectomy significantly reduced the preoperative mean number of ocular hypotensive medications, without significant differences between them ($p = 0.068$).

In addition, XEN was noninferior to trabeculectomy, regarding the prespecified primary endpoint (62.1% and 68.2% achieved the primary endpoint, respectively; $p = 0.487$), namely the percentage of patients achieving ≥20% IOP reduction from baseline at Month 12 without medication increase, clinical hypotony, vision loss to counting fingers, or secondary surgical intervention. Finally, XEN resulted in less need for in-office postoperative interventions ($p = 0.024$ after excluding laser suture lysis), faster visual recovery ($p < 0.05$), and greater 6-month improvements in visual function problems ($p \leq 0.022$) [108].

Similarly, Marcos-Parra et al. [48] compared the IOP lowering effect and the reduction in ocular hypotensive medications between the XEN device and trabeculectomy in OAG patients. They reported a significantly greater IOP lowering in the trabeculectomy group than in the XEN group ($p = 0.001$), with a similar reduction in the ocular hypotensive drugs [48]. However, this difference was mainly due to the combined surgery (glaucoma + cataract). When comparing the IOP lowering effect between XEN + Phaco and Trabeculectomy + Phaco, IOP lowering from preoperative values was found to be significantly greater in the Trabeculectomy + Phaco group at day 1, week 1, and months 1 and 3. While comparing XEN alone versus trabeculectomy alone, the only significant differences were observed in month 6. Moreover, in terms of success rates, there were no differences in the proportion of eyes who achieved a final IOP ≥6 and ≤16 mmHg ($p = 0.1317$), although it was slightly lower in the XEN (66.2%) than in the trabeculectomy group (78.6%) [48].

Additionally, Schlenker et al. [109] observed similar rates of complete and qualified success for both interventions.

Wang et al. [102], in a systematic review and meta-analysis, reported no significant differences between XEN gel implant and trabeculectomy on lowering IOP, although the analysis showed a high heterogeneity (I2:60%). However, after a sensitive analysis that excluded the Schenkler et al. study [109] and reduced the heterogeneity (I2:0%), the results showed that trabeculectomy was more effective in lowering IOP, without significant differences in terms of the reduction in ocular hypotensive medications [102].

Table 6 shows a comparison of the clinical outcomes of XEN45 and Trabeculectomy.

Table 6. A comparison of the clinical outcomes of XEN45 and trabeculectomy. Adapted from Chen et al. [12], Wang et al. [107], and Sheybani et al. [108].

Study	XEN		Trabeculectomy		MD (95% CI) between Surgeries [1]
	MD	SD	MD	SD	
Parra et al. [48]	−4.34	9.3	−7.73	8.97	0.37 (0.01 to 0.73)
Teus et al. [58] Chen et al. [12] Wang et al. [107]	−7.2 −8.8	9.2 5.2	−10.5 −8.5	9.2 5.3	−3.30 (−6.08 to −0.52) −0.06 (−0.86 to 0.75)
Olgun et al. [65]	−11	6.4	−16	9.7	0.63 (0.17 to 1.09)
Wagner et al. [72]	−8.5	5.3	−8.8	5.2	−0.30 (−4.51 to 3.91)
Wanichwecharungruang and Ratprasatporn [84]	−7	3.8	−10	5	−3.0 (−4.65 to −1.35)
Sheybani et al. [108]	−8.7 *	5	−10.8	4.7	−2.1 (−3.9 to −0.3)
Schlenker et al. [109]	−11	0.74	−11	7.29	0.0 (−0.21 to 0.21)
Sacchi et al. [110]	−13.38	2.76	−15.17	3.2	0.59 (0.04 to 1.15)
Olgun et al. [111]	−11	6.4	−16	9.7	−5.00 (−8.86 to −1.14)

[1] Random effect model. * Extracted directly from the study. NP: not provided.

Compared to trabeculectomy, XEN45 has been associated with several advantages, including less conjunctival manipulation, less postoperative inflammation, and lower incidence of postoperative adverse events. Moreover, the rates of postoperative interventions seem to be lower with XEN45 than with trabeculectomy. Therefore, XEN45 could be considered as the first-choice surgery in certain types of patients.

3.3.5. XEN Implant: What Dose of Mitomycin-c Is the Most Effective?

Mitomycin-c (MMC) and 5-fluorouracil (5-FU) have been commonly used in traditional glaucoma filtration surgery, with good evidence suggesting a significant increase in surgery success; however, there is also an increase in the risk of complications [112].

Although MMC was not initially used in all studies [17,19,21], the use of intraoperative MMC has become a common practice of the XEN implant surgical technique [36–101].

Regarding XEN45, MMC concentration may influence clinical outcomes. It has been suggested that the success rate may be related to the MMC dose, although other studies have shown a lack of correlation between MMC dosage and the surgical outcomes [113]. In general terms, the use of MMC seemed to increase the therapeutic success rate after XEN45 gel stent implantation, although the ideal dose has not been stablished yet.

Selection of MMC concentration is based on a patient-tailored approach. This may entail an important bias because surgeons will use higher concentrations of MMC in more complicated cases in which they anticipate that the possibility of surgical failure is greater.

A study comparing the efficacy and safety of two MMC doses (0.01% versus 0.02%) in eyes who underwent a XEN45 device implant, either alone or in combination with phacoemulsification, was recently published [95]. The results of this study found that IOP lowering, number of hypotensive medication reduction, or incidence of adverse events were not related to MMC concentration [95]. The lack of significant differences, in terms of IOP lowering or reducing hypotensive medications, between MMC 0.01% and MMC 0.02% raises the possibility of using lower doses of MMC. However, it should be mentioned that MMC 0.01% was not associated with lower incidence rates of adverse events [95].

So far, there is no evidence to recommend the use of a specific MMC concentration. It seems that MMC dose does not significantly impact either the IOP lowering or the reduction in the number of ocular hypotensive medications, so it would seem prudent to recommend "the lowest dose of MMC that, in the surgeon's opinion, may be effective in that patient". However, new studies will be necessary to clarify this issue.

3.3.6. XEN 45 Device Implant: Postoperative Bleb Management

Bleb fibrosis is a common complication that may occur after a XEN implant, with rates as high as 45% [114]. Needling is a minimally invasive procedure that is commonly used for restoring the functionality of failed filtering blebs [115].

The most frequently reported postoperative intervention in eyes who underwent a XEN device is needling of the conjunctival bleb, which ranges from 5% to 62% [12] (Tables 2–4 show the needling rates reported in the different studies).

Needling is not currently considered as an additional procedure, but rather as part of the normal bleb management in XEN implant surgery (similarly to laser suture lysis in trabeculectomy). In most cases, needling is required within the first month postoperatively.

However, in most studies, needling has been used as a rescue strategy once bleb failure has occurred.

Primary needling, at the time of ab interno XEN implantation, has been recently proposed as a technique that may reduce the number of postoperative interventions [96,116].

In a retrospective study, Kerr et al. [116] reported that primary needling at the time of XEN insertion was associated with a significant reduction in the number of bleb interventions ($p = 0.003$) and, consequently, the subsequent postoperative visits ($p = 0.043$). Additionally, compared to preoperative values, this technique has provided a significant reduction in both IOP and ocular hypotensive medication [116].

More recently, Buenasmañanas-Maeso et al. [96] performed a retrospective study that assessed the efficacy and safety of primary needling in eyes who underwent a XEN45 implant, either alone or in combination with phacoemulsification. According to the results of this study, primary needling was associated with fewer postoperative interventions. Nevertheless, these eyes were not associated with greater IOP lowering or a greater reduction in ocular hypotensive therapy [96].

Regarding the use of primary needling, there is not enough evidence to recommend its use on a routine basis. Therefore, from a clinical point of view, its use was reserved for those cases in which the XEN implant was twisted, trapped, or did not appear free and mobile in the subconjunctival space. Additionally, it may eventually be used in eyes with previously failed glaucoma surgery or in eyes with pathologies that may be associated with an increased risk of conjunctival fibrosis.

3.3.7. Can XEN45 Device Be Considered a Safe Procedure?

Although XEN has emerged as a safer and less traumatic approach for lowering IOP in patients with glaucoma, it is not free of complications.

According to the currently available scientific evidence, transient hypotony (defined as IOP <6 mmHg) is the most commonly reported complication of XEN45, with an incidence rate of 9.59%. In the vast majority of patients, hypotony is successfully resolved without additional surgery interventions and the rate of chronic hypotony is very low [12].

The second most common adverse event is hyphema (5.53%). Most of patients have grade I hyphema (less than 1/3 of anterior chamber), which had resolved spontaneously by the first week after surgery [12]. The third most commonly reported adverse event is the incidence of transient IOP spikes, which have been reported in 2.11% of eyes (in most cases associated with hyphema) [12].

Figure 2 shows an overview of the incidence of different adverse events reported after XEN implantation. Regarding the number of corneal endothelial cells, trabeculectomy and glaucoma drainage device implantation can damage corneal endothelial cells [117–120]. With regards to the impact of XEN on the corneal endothelial cells' loss, there were no significant differences between XEN + phacoemulsification and phacoemulsification alone [121–123]. Additionally, the corneal endothelial cell density reduction after XEN implantation as a solo procedure was low [122].

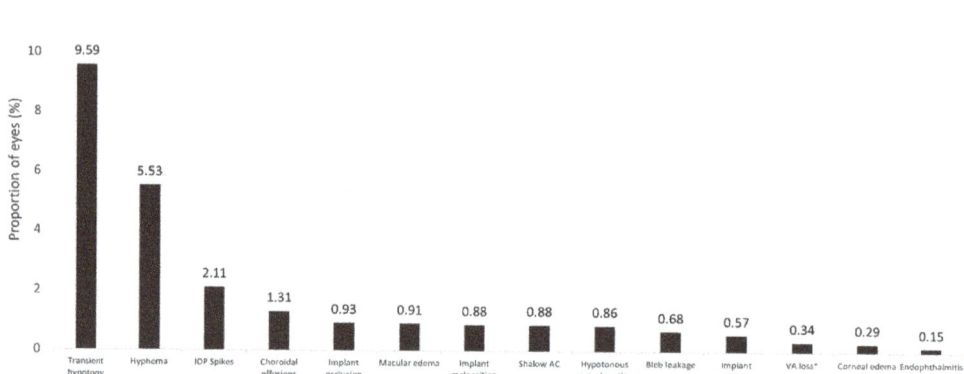

Figure 2. Incidence rate of adverse events reported after XEN implantation (*n* = 4410). Adapted from Chen et al. [12]. * ≥2 Snellen lines vison loss lasting >1 month. IOP: intraocular pressure; AC: anterior chamber; VA: visual acuity.

The results of a prospective, cross-sectional, and non-randomized clinical trial suggested that, in eyes who underwent a XEN standalone procedure, there were no significant changes in endothelial cell counts over the follow-up period (5 years). However, a statistically significant reduction in the central endothelial cell count was observed in the eyes who underwent a combined procedure (XEN + phacoemulsification) at different timepoints. This clearly suggests that the loss of corneal endothelial cells seems to be related with the cataract surgery, rather than with the XEN implant [123].

Both the experience of the panel and the scientific evidence have shown an acceptable safety profile of the XEN implant. The rate of serious complications (endophthalmitis, hypotonus maculopathy, corneal or macular edema) is low. Moreover, compared to trabeculectomy, the XEN implant has provided a better safety profile [93].

3.3.8. XEN45 Device: Is It Possible to Predict Its Clinical Outcomes?

Different studies have evaluated potential predictive factors for failure [19,42,50,70,98] or for success [52,64,116].

Three studies [42,50,70] found that none of the evaluated factors were significantly associated with surgery failure, whereas two studies reported that the risk of failure is greater in men than in women [19,98]. However, Gabbay et al. [87] reported that women were more likely to fail. Gillmann et al. [98] observed that eyes with a primary OAG diagnosis and those requiring needling are more likely to fail.

Fea et al. [70] suggested that patients with lower IOP at day 1 and month 1 had a higher chance of success. The same was true if the difference between month 1 and week 1 IOP was lower than 6 mmHg.

Regarding surgery success, each mmHg increase in preoperative IOP was positively associated with surgery success (Odds ratio: 1.33; 95% CI: 1.13 to 1.55, *p* = 0.0004) [52].

Chao et al. [64] reported that surgical success was more likely for eyes with a better preoperative visual field mean deviation and lower IOP at day 1, week 2, and month 1.

Conversely, Ibáñez-Muñoz et al. [116] found that none of the analysed factors were statistically associated with success.

The question of whether patient ethnicity impacts the XEN clinical outcomes has not been fully elucidated. Success rates appear to be lower in Black and Afro-Latino patients than in Caucasian populations [12,51,56]. Similarly, it has been observed that the ethnic Chinese group presents a reoperation rate as high as 45.9% [64]. However, other studies have suggested that there is no relationship between the ethnic origin of the patients and the clinical outcomes of XEN [39,62].

4. Discussion

The objective of this article was to address, in the most practical way possible, different aspects related to the XEN device that may generate doubts, mainly for specialists who are beginning to use this technique.

Based on currently available evidence, the XEN45 device, either alone or in combination with cataract surgery, significantly lowers IOP and reduces the number of ocular hypotensive medications in patients with glaucoma [12,36–101,108,110,111,116]. There are promising results with the new XEN63, but the evidence is very limited [22,23].

Compared to trabeculectomy [12,48,58,65,72,84,108–111], XEN seems not to be comparable in terms of IOP lowering, although XEN has similar efficacy in reducing the number of ocular hypotensive medications and provided a better safety profile.

Regarding its implantation technique, XEN has usually been delivered using an ab interno approach through a corneal incision [36–101]. However, as surgeons have been gaining experience with the device, different changes that aim to provide better clinical outcomes have been introduced in the implantation technique [24–26].

High myopia represents a challenging scenario in glaucoma patients who need surgical treatment. There are two studies that assessed the efficacy and safety of XEN in patients with high myopia. The results of both studies have pointed in the same direction, clearly indicating that the XEN device is an effective and safe option in patients with high myopia [105,106].

Trabeculectomy is still considered as the gold standard in glaucoma surgery [5]. It effectively lowers IOP and reduced the need of ocular hypotensive medications [6]. However, it requires a close postoperative follow-up to prevent potential complications that may lead to severe vision loss [7,124–126].

Nevertheless, XEN has been associated with lower conjunctival manipulation and incidence of postoperative complications and adverse effects [12,48,93,100].

For precisely this reason, this need for postoperative conjunctival manipulation has been one of the main points of discussion of XEN. The vast majority of the studies show a rate of needling which ranges from approximately 20 to 40% (See Tables 2 and 3).

Primary needling (at the time of ab interno XEN implantation) has emerged as a valuable option to reduce the number of postoperative interventions [96,116].

Regarding the existence of predictive factors of the XEN clinical outcomes, current evidence does not show conclusive results.

Finally, regarding the impact of the XEN device on the corneal endothelium, current evidence suggests that XEN does not have a significant impact on corneal endothelial cell loss [121–123], unlike what occurs with trabeculectomy or other drainage devices [117–120].

5. Conclusions

According to published evidence, the XEN45 device lowers IOP by approximately 35% from preoperative values, obtaining a mean IOP value of ≤ 15 mmHg, as far as 4 years after surgery. In addition, XEN significantly reduced the need for ocular hypotensive medication, with a mean number of postoperative hypotensive medications ≤ 1 drug.

Based on the evidence and panel's opinion, the XEN device may be considered as the first surgical option in patients who require a target IOP in the mid to low teens. Even though trabeculectomy seems to have a better IOP-lowering effect, the XEN device has been shown to have a better safety profile.

Although XEN device implantation is a relatively new procedure, a large number of studies have been published in recent years, pointing to its long-term potential in the treatment of glaucoma.

Several issues related to XEN clinical outcomes remain to be clarified, such as the role of ethnicity, factors influencing the outcomes, needling rates and the role of primary needling, the impact of high myopia, and the use of XEN in different types of glaucoma, including narrow-angle and angle-closure glaucoma.

Data from randomized and multicentre clinical trials will help surgeons develop patient-tailored management strategies.

Author Contributions: Conceptualization, C.E.T. and S.G.; methodology, R.G.C. and A.M.F.; software, C.A. and B.P.; validation, M.F. and A.M.F.; formal analysis, C.A.; investigation, Not Applicable; resources, R.G.C. and S.G.; data curation, V.V.; writing—original draft preparation, V.V. and M.F.; writing—review and editing, S.G. and C.E.T.; visualization, M.F.; supervision, M.F.; project administration, C.A. and B.P.; funding acquisition, C.E.T. and M.F. All authors have read and agreed to the published version of the manuscript.

Funding: The medical writer and editorial assistance for this manuscript was supported by AbbVie with no input into the preparation, review, approval, and writing of the manuscript. The authors maintained complete control over the manuscript content, and it reflects their opinions.

Institutional Review Board Statement: Not applicable.

Informed Consent Statement: Not applicable.

Data Availability Statement: Not applicable.

Acknowledgments: The authors wish to thank Antonio Martinez from Ciencia y Deporte SL, for medical writing and editorial assistance.

Conflicts of Interest: This manuscript was funded by AbbVie S.r.l. AbbVie participated in writing, reviewing, and approving the publication. No honoraria or payments were made for authorship. C. Astarita and V. Vera are AbbVie employees and may own AbbVie stocks/options. B. Piergentili was a former AbbVie employee. She is now affiliated with Alnylam Italia Srl. She has nothing else to declare. A.M. Fea is consultant for Glaukos, EliosVision, Ivantis, Oculus, EyeD, iSTAR, Santen, Abbvie. S. Gandolfi research contracts and/or unrestricted research Grants from Ivantis, Glaukos, AERIE and Allergan/AbbVie, Advisory Board of Santen, Novartis, Baush and Lomb, Allergan/AbbVie, Fidia, Visufarma and AERIE, Speakers' bureau of Allergan/AbbVie, Santen, Omikron, Visufarma, Baush and Lomb and Novartis. C. E. Traverso: support to the Department from Novartis, Bausch and Lomb, Alcon, Santen. Occasional travel support/speaker fee from Abbvie, Alcon, Santen, Omikron. R. Carassa and M. Figus have no conflicts of interest to declare.

References

1. Weinreb, R.N.; Leung, C.K.; Crowston, J.G.; Medeiros, F.A.; Friedman, D.S.; Wiggs, J.L.; Martin, K.R. Primary open-angle glaucoma. *Nat. Rev. Dis. Prim.* **2016**, *2*, 16067. [CrossRef] [PubMed]
2. Heijl, A.; Leske, M.C.; Bengtsson, B.; Hyman, L.; Bengtsson, B.; Hussein, M.; Early Manifest Glaucoma Trial Group. Reduction of intraocular pressure and glaucoma progression: Results from the Early Manifest Glaucoma Trial. *Arch. Ophthalmol.* **2002**, *120*, 1268–1279. [CrossRef] [PubMed]
3. European Glaucoma Society Terminology and Guidelines for Glaucoma, 5th Edition. *Br. J. Ophthalmol.* **2021**, *105* (Suppl. S1), 1–169. [CrossRef]
4. Lichter, P.R.; Musch, D.C.; Gillespie, B.W.; Guire, K.E.; Janz, N.K.; Wren, P.A.; CIGTS Study Group. Interim clinical outcomes in the Collaborative Initial Glaucoma Treatment Study comparing initial treatment randomized to medications or surgery. *Ophthalmology* **2001**, *108*, 1943–1953. [CrossRef] [PubMed]
5. Newman-Casey, P.A.; Robin, A.L.; Blachley, T.; Farris, K.; Heisler, M.; Resnicow, K.; Lee, P.P. The Most Common Barriers to Glaucoma Medication Adherence: A Cross-Sectional Survey. *Ophthalmology* **2015**, *122*, 1308–1316. [CrossRef]
6. Landers, J.; Martin, K.; Sarkies, N.; Bourne, R.; Watson, P. A twenty-year follow-up study of trabeculectomy: Risk factors and outcomes. *Ophthalmology* **2012**, *119*, 694–702. [CrossRef]
7. Jampel, H.D.; Musch, D.C.; Gillespie, B.W.; Lichter, P.R.; Wright, M.M.; Guire, K.E.; Collaborative Initial Glaucoma Treatment Study Group. Perioperative complications of trabeculectomy in the collaborative initial glaucoma treatment study (CIGTS). *Am. J. Ophthalmol.* **2005**, *140*, 16–22. [CrossRef]
8. Bar-David, L.; Blumenthal, E.Z. Evolution of Glaucoma Surgery in the Last 25 Years. *Rambam Maimonides Med. J.* **2018**, *9*, e0024. [CrossRef]
9. Saheb, H.; Ahmed, I.I. Micro-invasive glaucoma surgery: Current perspectives and future directions. *Curr. Opin. Ophthalmol.* **2012**, *23*, 96–104. [CrossRef]

10. Ahmed, I.I. MIGS and the FDA: What's in a Name? *Ophthalmology* **2015**, *122*, 1737–1739. [CrossRef]
11. Caprioli, J.; Kim, J.H.; Friedman, D.S.; Kiang, T.; Moster, M.R.; Parrish, R.K., 2nd; Rorer, E.M.; Samuelson, T.; Tarver, M.E.; Singh, K.; et al. Special Commentary: Supporting Innovation for Safe and Effective Minimally Invasive Glaucoma Surgery: Summary of a Joint Meeting of the American Glaucoma Society and the Food and Drug Administration, Washington, DC, February 26, 2014. *Ophthalmology* **2015**, *122*, 1795–1801. [CrossRef]
12. Chen, X.Z.; Liang, Z.Q.; Yang, K.Y.; Lv, K.; Ma, Y.; Li, M.Y.; Li, M.Y.; Wu, H.J. The Outcomes of XEN Gel Stent Implantation: A Systematic Review and Meta-Analysis. *Front. Med.* **2022**, *9*, 804847. [CrossRef] [PubMed]
13. Lewis, R.A. Ab interno approach to the subconjunctival space using a collagen glaucoma stent. *J. Cataract. Refract. Surg.* **2014**, *40*, 1301–1306. [CrossRef]
14. Lavia, C.; Dallorto, L.; Maule, M.; Ceccarelli, M.; Fea, A.M. Minimally-invasive glaucoma surgeries (MIGS) for open angle glaucoma: A systematic review and meta-analysis. *PLoS ONE* **2017**, *12*, e0183142. [CrossRef] [PubMed]
15. Ansari, E. An Update on Implants for Minimally Invasive Glaucoma Surgery (MIGS). *Ophthalmol. Ther.* **2017**, *6*, 233–241. [CrossRef]
16. Shute, T.S.; Dietrich, U.M.; Baker, J.F.; Carmichael, K.P.; Wustenberg, W.; Ahmed, I.I.; Sheybani, A. Biocompatibility of a Novel Microfistula Implant in Nonprimate Mammals for the Surgical Treatment of Glaucoma. *Investig. Opthalmol. Vis. Sci.* **2016**, *57*, 3594–3600. [CrossRef]
17. Sheybani, A.; Dick, H.B.; Ahmed, I.I. Early Clinical Results of a Novel Ab Interno Gel Stent for the Surgical Treatment of Open-angle Glaucoma. *J. Glaucoma* **2016**, *25*, e691–e696. [CrossRef]
18. Sheybani, A.; Lenzhofer, M.; Hohensinn, M.; Reitsamer, H.; Ahmed, I.I. Phacoemulsification combined with a new ab interno gel stent to treat open-angle glaucoma: Pilot study. *J. Cataract. Refract. Surg.* **2015**, *41*, 1905–1909. [CrossRef] [PubMed]
19. Lenzhofer, M.; Kersten-Gomez, I.; Sheybani, A.; Gulamhusein, H.; Strohmaier, C.; Hohensinn, M.; Burkhard Dick, H.; Hitzl, W.; Eisenkopf, L.; Sedarous, F.; et al. Four-year results of a minimally invasive transscleral glaucoma gel stent implantation in a prospective multi-centre study. *Clin. Exp. Ophthalmol.* **2019**, *47*, 581–587. [CrossRef]
20. Fernández-García, A.; Zhou, Y.; García-Alonso, M.; Andrango, H.D.; Poyales, F.; Garzón, N. Comparing Medium-Term Clinical Outcomes following XEN®45 and XEN®63 Device Implantation. *J. Ophthalmol.* **2020**, *2020*, 4796548. [CrossRef] [PubMed]
21. Lavin-Dapena, C.; Cordero-Ros, R.; D'Anna, O.; Mogollón, I. XEN 63 gel stent device in glaucoma surgery: A 5-years follow-up prospective study. *Eur. J. Ophthalmol.* **2021**, *31*, 1829–1835. [CrossRef]
22. Fea, A.M.; Menchini, M.; Rossi, A.; Posarelli, C.; Malinverni, L.; Figus, M. Early Experience with the New XEN63 Implant in Primary Open-Angle Glaucoma Patients: Clinical Outcomes. *J. Clin. Med.* **2021**, *10*, 1628. [CrossRef]
23. Fea, A.M.; Menchini, M.; Rossi, A.; Posarelli, C.; Malinverni, L.; Figus, M. Outcomes of XEN 63 Device at 18-Month Follow-Up in Glaucoma Patients: A Two-Center Retrospective Study. *J. Clin. Med.* **2022**, *11*, 3801. [CrossRef]
24. Panarelli, J.F.; Yan, D.B.; Francis, B.; Craven, E.R. XEN Gel Stent Open Conjunctiva Technique: A Practical Approach Paper. *Adv. Ther.* **2020**, *37*, 2538–2549. [CrossRef]
25. Vera, V.; Gagne, S.; Myers, J.S.; Ahmed, I.I.K. Surgical Approaches for Implanting Xen Gel Stent without Conjunctival Dissection. *Clin. Ophthalmol.* **2020**, *14*, 2361–2371. [CrossRef] [PubMed]
26. Tan, N.E.; Tracer, N.; Terraciano, A.; Parikh, H.A.; Panarelli, J.F.; Radcliffe, N.M. Comparison of Safety and Efficacy Between Ab Interno and Ab Externo Approaches to XEN Gel Stent Placement. *Clin. Ophthalmol.* **2021**, *15*, 299–305. [CrossRef] [PubMed]
27. Donnelly, C.A.; Boyd, I.; Campbell, P.; Craig, C.; Vallance, P.; Walport, M.; Whitty, C.J.M.; Woods, E.; Wormald, C. Four principles to make evidence synthesis more useful for policy. *Nature* **2018**, *558*, 361–364. [CrossRef]
28. Liberati, A.; Altman, D.G.; Tetzlaff, J.; Mulrow, C.; Gøtzsche, P.C.; Ioannidis, J.P.; Clarke, M.; Devereaux, P.J.; Kleijnen, J.; Moher, D. The PRISMA statement for reporting systematic reviews and meta-analyses of studies that evaluate healthcare interventions: Explanation and elaboration. *BMJ* **2009**, *339*, b2700. [CrossRef] [PubMed]
29. Petticrew, M.; Anderson, L.; Elder, R.; Grimshaw, J.; Hopkins, D.; Hahn, R.; Krause, L.; Kristjansson, E.; Mercer, S.; Sipe, T.; et al. Complex interventions and their implications for systematic reviews: A pragmatic approach. *J. Clin. Epidemiol.* **2013**, *66*, 1209–1214. [CrossRef]
30. Cochrane Collaboration. Cochrane Strategy to 2020. 2017. Available online: https://community.cochrane.org/sites/default/files/uploads/00%20S2020%202017%20Targets%20End%20of%20Year%20Report.pdf (accessed on 21 April 2023).
31. Smith, E.A.; Cooper, N.J.; Sutton, A.J.; Abrams, K.R.; Hubbard, S.J. A review of the quantitative effectiveness evidence synthesis methods used in public health intervention guidelines. *BMC Public Health* **2021**, *21*, 278. [CrossRef]
32. Valentine, J.C.; Wilson, S.J.; Rindskopf, D.; Lau, T.S.; Tanner-Smith, E.E.; Yeide, M.; LaSota, R.; Foster, L. Synthesizing Evidence in Public Policy Contexts: The Challenge of Synthesis When There Are Only a Few Studies. *Eval. Rev.* **2017**, *41*, 3–26. [CrossRef] [PubMed]
33. Campbell, M.; Katikireddi, S.V.; Sowden, A.; Thomson, H. Lack of transparency in reporting narrative synthesis of quantitative data: A methodological assessment of systematic reviews. *J. Clin. Epidemiol.* **2019**, *105*, 1–9. [CrossRef]
34. Campbell, M.; McKenzie, J.E.; Sowden, A.; Katikireddi, S.V.; Brennan, S.E.; Ellis, S.; Hartmann-Boyce, J.; Ryan, R.; Shepperd, S.; Thomas, J.; et al. Synthesis without meta-analysis (SWiM) in systematic reviews: Reporting guideline. *BMJ* **2020**, *368*, l6890. [CrossRef] [PubMed]
35. Moher, D.; Liberati, A.; Tetzlaff, J.; Altman, D.G.; PRISMA Group. Preferred reporting items for systematic reviews and meta-analyses: The PRISMA statement. *PLoS Med.* **2009**, *6*, e1000097. [CrossRef] [PubMed]

36. Pérez-Torregrosa, V.T.; Olate-Pérez, Á.; Cerdà-Ibáñez, M.; Gargallo-Benedicto, A.; Osorio-Alayo, V.; Barreiro-Rego, A.; Duch-Samper, A. Combined phacoemulsification and XEN45 surgery from a temporal approach and 2 incisions. *Arch Soc. Esp. Oftalmol.* **2016**, *91*, 415–421. [CrossRef] [PubMed]
37. Ozal, S.A.; Kaplaner, O.; Basar, B.B.; Guclu, H.; Ozal, E. An innovation in glaucoma surgery: XEN45 gel stent implantation. *Arq. Bras. Oftalmol.* **2017**, *80*, 382–385. [CrossRef] [PubMed]
38. Galal, A.; Bilgic, A.; Eltanamly, R.; Osman, A. XEN Glaucoma Implant with Mitomycin C 1-Year Follow-Up: Result and Complications. *J. Ophthalmol.* **2017**, *2017*, 5457246. [CrossRef]
39. Grover, D.S.; Flynn, W.J.; Bashford, K.P.; Lewis, R.A.; Duh, Y.J.; Nangia, R.S.; Niksch, B. Performance and Safety of a New Ab Interno Gelatin Stent in Refractory Glaucoma at 12 Months. *Am. J. Ophthalmol.* **2017**, *183*, 25–36. [CrossRef]
40. Hengerer, F.H.; Kohnen, T.; Mueller, M.; Conrad-Hengerer, I. Ab Interno Gel Implant for the Treatment of Glaucoma Patients with or Without Prior Glaucoma Surgery: 1-Year Results. *J. Glaucoma* **2017**, *26*, 1130–1136. [CrossRef]
41. De Gregorio, A.; Pedrotti, E.; Russo, L.; Morselli, S. Minimally invasive combined glaucoma and cataract surgery: Clinical results of the smallest ab interno gel stent. *Int. Ophthalmol.* **2018**, *38*, 1129–1134. [CrossRef]
42. Mansouri, K.; Guidotti, J.; Rao, H.L.; Ouabas, A.; D'Alessandro, E.; Roy, S.; Mermoud, A. Prospective Evaluation of Standalone XEN Gel Implant and Combined Phacoemulsification-XEN Gel Implant Surgery: 1-Year Results. *J. Glaucoma* **2018**, *27*, 140–147. [CrossRef] [PubMed]
43. Tan, S.Z.; Walkden, A.; Au, L. One-year result of XEN45 implant for glaucoma: Efficacy, safety, and postoperative management. *Eye* **2018**, *32*, 324–332. [CrossRef]
44. Widder, R.A.; Dietlein, T.S.; Dinslage, S.; Kühnrich, P.; Rennings, C.; Rössler, G. The XEN45 Gel Stent as a minimally invasive procedure in glaucoma surgery: Success rates, risk profile, and rates of re-surgery after 261 surgeries. *Graefes Arch. Clin. Exp. Ophthalmol.* **2018**, *256*, 765–771. [CrossRef]
45. Reitsamer, H.; Sng, C.; Vera, V.; Lenzhofer, M.; Barton, K.; Stalmans, I.; Apex Study Group. Two-year results of a multicenter study of the ab interno gelatin implant in medically uncontrolled primary open-angle glaucoma. *Graefes Arch. Clin. Exp. Ophthalmol.* **2019**, *257*, 983–996. [CrossRef] [PubMed]
46. Qureshi, A.; Jones, N.P.; Au, L. Urgent Management of Secondary Glaucoma in Uveitis Using the Xen-45 Gel Stent. *J. Glaucoma* **2019**, *28*, 1061–1066. [CrossRef] [PubMed]
47. Kalina, A.G.; Kalina, P.H.; Brown, M.M. XEN® Gel Stent in Medically Refractory Open-Angle Glaucoma: Results and Observations After One Year of Use in the United States. *Ophthalmol. Ther.* **2019**, *8*, 435–446. [CrossRef]
48. Parra, M.T.M.; López, J.A.S.; Grau, N.S.L.; Ceausescu, A.M.; Santonja, J.J.P. XEN implant device versus trabeculectomy, either alone or in combination with phacoemulsification, in open-angle glaucoma patients. *Graefes Arch. Clin. Exp. Ophthalmol.* **2019**, *257*, 1741–1750. [CrossRef]
49. Lenzhofer, M.; Strohmaier, C.; Hohensinn, M.; Hitzl, W.; Steiner, V.; Baca, B.; Moussa, S.; Motloch, K.; Reitsamer, H.A. Change in visual acuity 12 and 24 months after transscleral ab interno glaucoma gel stent implantation with adjunctive Mitomycin C. *Graefes Arch. Clin. Exp. Ophthalmol.* **2019**, *257*, 2707–2715. [CrossRef]
50. Sng, C.C.A.; Chew, P.T.K.; Htoon, H.M.; Lun, K.; Jeyabal, P.; Ang, M. Case Series of Combined XEN Implantation and Phacoemulsification in Chinese Eyes: One-Year Outcomes. *Adv. Ther.* **2019**, *36*, 3519–3529. [CrossRef]
51. Gabbay, I.E.; Allen, F.; Morley, C.; Pearsall, T.; Bowes, O.M.; Ruben, S. Efficacy and safety data for the XEN45 implant at 2 years: A retrospective analysis. *Br. J. Ophthalmol.* **2020**, *104*, 1125–1130. [CrossRef]
52. Laborda-Guirao, T.; Cubero-Parra, J.M.; Hidalgo-Torres, A. Efficacy and safety of XEN 45 gel stent alone or in combination with phacoemulsification in advanced open angle glaucoma patients: 1-year retrospective study. *Int. J. Ophthalmol.* **2020**, *13*, 1250–1256. [CrossRef] [PubMed]
53. Heidinger, A.; Schwab, C.; Lindner, E.; Riedl, R.; Mossböck, G. A Retrospective Study of 199 Xen45 Stent Implantations from 2014 to 2016. *J. Glaucoma* **2019**, *28*, 75–79. [CrossRef] [PubMed]
54. Ibáñez-Muñoz, A.; Soto-Biforcos, V.S.; Chacón-González, M.; Rúa-Galisteo, O.; Arrieta-Los Santos, A.; Lizuain-Abadía, M.E.; Del Río Mayor, J.L. One-year follow-up of the XEN®implant with mitomycin-C in pseudoexfoliative glaucoma patients. *Eur. J. Ophthalmol.* **2019**, *29*, 309–314. [CrossRef] [PubMed]
55. Karimi, A.; Lindfield, D.; Turnbull, A.; Dimitriou, C.; Bhatia, B.; Radwan, M.; Gouws, P.; Hanifudin, A.; Amerasinghe, N.; Jacob, A. A multi-centre interventional case series of 259 ab-interno Xen gel implants for glaucoma, with and without combined cataract surgery. *Eye* **2019**, *33*, 469–477. [CrossRef]
56. Laroche, D.; Nkrumah, G.; Ng, C. Real-World Retrospective Consecutive Study of Ab Interno XEN 45 Gel Stent Implant with Mitomycin C in Black and Afro-Latino Patients with Glaucoma: 40% Required Secondary Glaucoma Surgery at 1 Year. *Middle East Afr. J. Ophthalmol.* **2020**, *26*, 229–234. [CrossRef] [PubMed]
57. Smith, M.; Charles, R.; Abdel-Hay, A.; Shah, B.; Byles, D.; Lim, L.A.; Rossiter, J.; Kuo, C.H.; Chapman, P.; Robertson, S. 1-year outcomes of the Xen45 glaucoma implant. *Eye* **2019**, *33*, 761–766. [CrossRef]
58. Teus, M.A.; Moreno-Arrones, J.P.; Castaño, B.; Castejon, M.A.; Bolivar, G. Optical coherence tomography analysis of filtering blebs after long-term, functioning trabeculectomy and XEN®stent implant. *Graefes Arch. Clin. Exp. Ophthalmol.* **2019**, *257*, 1005–1011. [CrossRef]
59. Mansouri, K.; Bravetti, G.E.; Gillmann, K.; Rao, H.L.; Ch'ng, T.W.; Mermoud, A. Two-Year Outcomes of XEN Gel Stent Surgery in Patients with Open-Angle Glaucoma. *Ophthalmol. Glaucoma* **2019**, *2*, 309–318. [CrossRef]

60. Gillmann, K.; Bravetti, G.E.; Rao, H.L.; Mermoud, A.; Mansouri, K. Combined and stand-alone XEN 45 gel stent implantation: 3-year outcomes and success predictors. *Acta Ophthalmol.* **2021**, *99*, e531–e539. [CrossRef]
61. Post, M.; Lubiński, W.; Śliwiak, D.; Podborączyńska-Jodko, K.; Mularczyk, M. XEN Gel Stent in the management of primary open-angle glaucoma. *Doc. Ophthalmol.* **2020**, *141*, 65–76. [CrossRef]
62. Bravetti, G.E.; Mansouri, K.; Gillmann, K.; Rao, H.L.; Mermoud, A. XEN-augmented Baerveldt drainage device implantation in refractory glaucoma: 1-year outcomes. *Graefes Arch. Clin. Exp. Ophthalmol.* **2020**, *258*, 1787–1794. [CrossRef] [PubMed]
63. Scheres, L.M.J.; Kujovic-Aleksov, S.; Ramdas, W.D.; de Crom, R.M.P.C.; Roelofs, L.C.G.; Berendschot, T.T.J.M.; Webers, C.A.B.; Beckers, H.J.M. XEN® Gel Stent compared to PRESERFLO™ MicroShunt implantation for primary open-angle glaucoma: Two-year results. *Acta Ophthalmol.* **2021**, *99*, e433–e440. [CrossRef]
64. Chao, Y.J.; Ko, Y.C.; Chen, M.J.; Lo, K.J.; Chang, Y.F.; Liu, C.J. XEN45 Gel Stent implantation in eyes with primary open angle glaucoma: A study from a single hospital in Taiwan. *J. Chin. Med. Assoc.* **2021**, *84*, 108–113. [CrossRef] [PubMed]
65. Olgun, A.; Aktas, Z.; Ucgul, A.Y. XEN gel implant versus gonioscopy-assisted transluminal trabeculotomy for the treatment of open-angle glaucoma. *Int. Ophthalmol.* **2020**, *40*, 1085–1093. [CrossRef] [PubMed]
66. Schargus, M.; Theilig, T.; Rehak, M.; Busch, C.; Bormann, C.; Unterlauft, J.D. Outcome of a single XEN microstent implant for glaucoma patients with different types of glaucoma. *BMC Ophthalmol.* **2020**, *20*, 490. [CrossRef]
67. Theilig, T.; Rehak, M.; Busch, C.; Bormann, C.; Schargus, M.; Unterlauft, J.D. Comparing the efficacy of trabeculectomy and XEN gel microstent implantation for the treatment of primary open-angle glaucoma: A retrospective monocentric comparative cohort study. *Sci. Rep.* **2020**, *10*, 19317. [CrossRef]
68. Theillac, V.; Blumen-Ohana, E.; Akesbi, J.; Hamard, P.; Sellam, A.; Brasnu, E.; Baudouin, C.; Labbe, A.; Nordmann, J.P. Cataract and glaucoma combined surgery: XEN® gel stent versus nonpenetrating deep sclerectomy, a pilot study. *BMC Ophthalmol.* **2020**, *20*, 231. [CrossRef]
69. Subaşı, S.; Yüksel, N.; Özer, F.; Tugan, B.Y.; Pirhan, D. A Retrospective Analysis of Safety and Efficacy of XEN 45 Microstent Combined Cataract Surgery in Open-Angle Glaucoma over 24 Months. *Turk. J. Ophthalmol.* **2021**, *51*, 139–145. [CrossRef]
70. Fea, A.M.; Bron, A.M.; Economou, M.A.; Laffi, G.; Martini, E.; Figus, M.; Oddone, F. European study of the efficacy of a cross-linked gel stent for the treatment of glaucoma. *J. Cataract. Refract. Surg.* **2020**, *46*, 441–450. [CrossRef]
71. Rauchegger, T.; Angermann, R.; Willeit, P.; Schmid, E.; Teuchner, B. Two-year outcomes of minimally invasive XEN Gel Stent implantation in primary open-angle and pseudoexfoliation glaucoma. *Acta Ophthalmol.* **2021**, *99*, 369–375. [CrossRef] [PubMed]
72. Wagner, F.M.; Schuster, A.K.; Emmerich, J.; Chronopoulos, P.; Hoffmann, E.M. Efficacy and safety of XEN®–Implantation vs. trabeculectomy: Data of a "real-world" setting. *PLoS ONE* **2020**, *15*, e0231614. [CrossRef] [PubMed]
73. Busch, T.; Skiljic, D.; Rudolph, T.; Bergström, A.; Zetterberg, M. Learning Curve and One-Year Outcome of XEN 45 Gel Stent Implantation in a Swedish Population. *Clin. Ophthalmol.* **2020**, *14*, 3719–3733. [CrossRef] [PubMed]
74. Barão, R.C.; José, P.; Teixeira, F.J.; Ferreira, N.P.; Sens, P.; Pinto, L.A. Automated Gonioscopy Assessment of XEN45 Gel Stent Angle Location After Isolated XEN or Combined Phaco-XEN Procedures: Clinical Implications. *J. Glaucoma* **2020**, *29*, 932–940. [CrossRef] [PubMed]
75. Ucar, F.; Cetinkaya, S. Xen implantation in patients with primary open-angle glaucoma: Comparison of two different techniques. *Int. Ophthalmol.* **2020**, *40*, 2487–2494. [CrossRef] [PubMed]
76. Navero-Rodríguez, J.M.; Espinosa-Barberi, G.; Morilla-Grasa, A.; Anton, A. Efficacy of the Ologen collagen matrix in combination with the XEN gel stent implantation in the treatment of open-angle glaucoma: A case-control study. *Clin. Exp. Ophthalmol.* **2020**, *48*, 1003–1005. [CrossRef]
77. Stoner, A.M.; Young, C.E.C.; SooHoo, J.R.; Pantcheva, M.B.; Patnaik, J.L.; Kahook, M.Y.; Seibold, L.K. A Comparison of Clinical Outcomes After XEN Gel Stent and EX-PRESS Glaucoma Drainage Device Implantation. *J. Glaucoma* **2021**, *30*, 481–488. [CrossRef] [PubMed]
78. Düzgün, E.; Olgun, A.; Karapapak, M.; Alkan, A.A.; Ustaoğlu, M. Outcomes of XEN Gel Stent Implantation in the Inferonasal Quadrant after Failed Trabeculectomy. *J. Curr. Glaucoma Pract.* **2021**, *15*, 64–69. [CrossRef] [PubMed]
79. Schargus, M.; Busch, C.; Rehak, M.; Meng, J.; Schmidt, M.; Bormann, C.; Unterlauft, J.D. Functional Monitoring after Trabeculectomy or XEN Microstent Implantation Using Spectral Domain Optical Coherence Tomography and Visual Field Indices-A Retrospective Comparative Cohort Study. *Biology* **2021**, *10*, 273. [CrossRef]
80. Nuzzi, R.; Gremmo, G.; Toja, F.; Marolo, P. A Retrospective Comparison of Trabeculectomy, Baerveldt Glaucoma Implant, and Microinvasive Glaucoma Surgeries in a Three-Year Follow-Up. *Semin. Ophthalmol.* **2021**, *36*, 839–849. [CrossRef]
81. Eraslan, M.; Özcan, A.A.; Dericioğlu, V.; Çiloğlu, E. Multicenter case series of standalone XEN implant vs. combination with phacoemulsification in Turkish patients. *Int. Ophthalmol.* **2021**, *41*, 3371–3379. [CrossRef]
82. Bormann, C.; Schmidt, M.; Busch, C.; Rehak, M.; Scharenberg, C.T.; Unterlauft, J.D. Implantation of XEN After Failed Trabeculectomy: An Efficient Therapy? *Klin. Monbl. Augenheilkd.* **2022**, *239*, 86–93. [CrossRef]
83. Lewczuk, K.; Konopińska, J.; Jabłońska, J.; Rudowicz, J.; Laszewicz, P.; Dmuchowska, D.A.; Mariak, Z.; Rękas, M. XEN Glaucoma Implant for the Management of Glaucoma in Naïve Patients versus Patients with Previous Glaucoma Surgery. *J. Clin. Med.* **2021**, *10*, 4417. [CrossRef] [PubMed]
84. Wanichwecharungruang, B.; Ratprasatporn, N. 24-month outcomes of XEN45 gel implant versus trabeculectomy in primary glaucoma. *PLoS ONE* **2021**, *16*, e0256362. [CrossRef]

85. Lewczuk, K.; Konopińska, J.; Jabłońska, J.; Rudowicz, J.; Laszewicz, P.; Mariak, Z.; Rękas, M. XEN Glaucoma Implant for the Management of Operated Uncontrolled Glaucoma: Results and Complications during a Long-Term Follow-Up. *J. Ophthalmol.* **2021**, *2021*, 2321922. [CrossRef] [PubMed]
86. Reitsamer, H.; Vera, V.; Ruben, S.; Au, L.; Vila-Arteaga, J.; Teus, M.; Lenzhofer, M.; Shirlaw, A.; Bai, Z.; Balaram, M.; et al. Three-year effectiveness and safety of the XEN gel stent as a solo procedure or in combination with phacoemulsification in open-angle glaucoma: A multicentre study. *Acta Ophthalmol.* **2022**, *100*, e233–e245. [CrossRef]
87. Gabbay, I.E.; Goldberg, M.; Allen, F.; Lin, Z.; Morley, C.; Pearsall, T.; Muraleedharan, V.; Ruben, S. Efficacy and safety data for the Ab interno XEN45 gel stent implant at 3 Years: A retrospective analysis. *Eur. J. Ophthalmol.* **2021**, *32*, 11206721211014381. [CrossRef]
88. José, P.; Teixeira, F.J.; Barão, R.C.; Sens, P.; Pinto, L.A. Needling after XEN gel implant: What's the efficacy? A 1-year analysis. *Eur. J. Ophthalmol.* **2021**, *31*, 3087–3092. [CrossRef] [PubMed]
89. Nicolaou, S.; Khatib, T.Z.; Lin, Z.; Sheth, T.; Ogbonna, G.; Hamidovic, L.; Zaheer, A.; Dimitriou, C. A retrospective review of XEN implant surgery: Efficacy, safety and the effect of combined cataract surgery. *Int. Ophthalmol.* **2022**, *42*, 881–889. [CrossRef]
90. Olsen, L.P.; Ruhlmann, P.B.; Vestergaard, A.H. Implantation of the XEN® 45 Gel Stent in patients with glaucoma at a University Hospital—A retrospective quality control study. *Acta Ophthalmol.* **2021**, *99*, e968–e969. [CrossRef]
91. Franco, F.G.S.; Branchetti, M.; Spagnuolo, V.; Piergentili, M.; Serino, F.; De Vitto, M.L.; Bertelli, E.; Virgili, G.; Giasanti, F. Efficacy and safety of Ab interno XEN gel implant after a failed filtering surgery. *Romnian J. Ophthalmol.* **2021**, *65*, 365–370. [CrossRef]
92. Steiner, S.; Resch, H.; Kiss, B.; Buda, D.; Vass, C. Needling and open filtering bleb revision after XEN-45 implantation–A retrospective outcome comparison. *Graefes Arch. Clin. Exp. Ophthalmol.* **2021**, *259*, 2761–2770. [CrossRef] [PubMed]
93. Cappelli, F.; Cutolo, C.A.; Olivari, S.; Testa, V.; Sindaco, D.; Pizzorno, C.; Ciccione, S.; Traaverso, C.E.; Iester, M. Trabeculectomy versus Xen gel implant for the treatment of open-angle glaucoma: A 3-year retrospective analysis. *BMJ Open Ophthalmol.* **2022**, *7*, e000830. [CrossRef] [PubMed]
94. Szigiato, A.A.; Touma, S.; Jabbour, S.; Lord, F.; Agoumi, Y.; Singh, H. Efficacy of ab-interno gelatin microstent implantation in primary and refractory glaucoma. *Can. J. Ophthalmol.* **2022**, *58*, 328–337. [CrossRef] [PubMed]
95. Monja-Alarcón, N.; Perucho-Martínez, S.; Buenasmañanas-Maeso, M.; Toledano-Fernández, N. Does mitomycin-C concentration have any influence on XEN45 gel stent outcomes in a real-world setting? *Graefes Arch. Clin. Exp. Ophthalmol.* **2022**, *260*, 2649–2661. [CrossRef]
96. Buenasmañanas-Maeso, M.; Perucho-Martínez, S.; Monja-Alarcón, N.; Toledano-Fernández, N. Impact of Primary Needling on the XEN Implant Clinical Outcomes: A Real-Life Retrospective Study. *Clin. Ophthalmol.* **2022**, *16*, 935–946. [CrossRef]
97. Hüppi, R.; Wagels, B.; Todorova, M. Two-Year Outcome of Surgery in Glaucoma Patients. *Klin. Monbl. Augenheilkd.* **2022**, *239*, 435–442. [CrossRef]
98. Gillmann, K.; Bravetti, G.E.; Mermoud, A.; Rao, H.L.; Mansouri, K. XEN Gel Stent in Pseudoexfoliative Glaucoma: 2-Year Results of a Prospective Evaluation. *J. Glaucoma* **2019**, *28*, 676–684. [CrossRef]
99. Almendral-Gómez, J.; Perucho-Martínez, S.; Martín-Giral, E.; Fernández-Escámez, C.; Buenasmañanas-Maeso, M.; Monja-Alarcón, N.; Toledano-Fernández, N. XEN Gel Stent Versus Non-penetrating Deep Sclerectomy in Ocular-hypertension and Open-angle Glaucoma Patients. *J. Glaucoma* **2023**, *32*, 511–519. [CrossRef]
100. Marcos-Parra, M.T.; Salinas-López, J.A.; Mateos-Marcos, C.; Moreno-Castro, L.; Mendoza-Moreira, A.L.; Pérez-Santonja, J.J. Long-Term Effectiveness of XEN 45 Gel-Stent in Open-Angle Glaucoma Patients. *Clin. Ophthalmol.* **2023**, *17*, 1223–1232. [CrossRef]
101. Vukmirovic, A.; Ong, J.; Mukhtar, A.; Yu, D.Y.; Morgan, W.H. Outcomes of 45 μm gelatin stent surgery over 24-monthfollow-up. *Clin. Exp. Ophthalmol.* **2023**, *51*, 19–30. [CrossRef]
102. Yang, X.; Zhao, Y.; Zhong, Y.; Duan, X. The efficacy of XEN gel stent implantation in glaucoma: A systematic review and meta-analysis. *BMC Ophthalmol.* **2022**, *22*, 305. [CrossRef]
103. Panarelli, J.F.; Vera, V.; Sheybani, A.; Radcliffe, N.; Fiscella, R.; Francis, B.A.; Smith, O.U.; Noecker, R.J. Intraocular Pressure and Medication Changes Associated with Xen Gel Stent: A Systematic Review of the Literature. *Clin. Ophthalmol.* **2023**, *17*, 25–46. [CrossRef] [PubMed]
104. Huth, A.; Viestenz, A. Hohe Myopie bei vitrektomiertem Auge: Kontraindikation für minimal-invasive glaukomchirurgische Implantate? *Ophthalmologe* **2020**, *117*, 461–466. [CrossRef]
105. Sacchi, M.; Fea, A.M.; Monsellato, G.; Tagliabue, E.; Villani, E.; Ranno, S.; Nucci, P. Safety and Efficacy of Ab Interno XEN 45 Gel Stent in Patients with Glaucoma and High Myopia. *J. Clin. Med.* **2023**, *12*, 2477. [CrossRef]
106. Fea, A.; Sacchi, M.; Franco, F.; Laffi, G.L.; Oddone, F.; Costa, G.; Serino, F.; Giansanti, F. Effectiveness and Safety of XEN45 in Eyes With High Myopia and Open Angle Glaucoma. *J. Glaucoma* **2023**, *32*, 178–185. [CrossRef] [PubMed]
107. Wang, B.; Leng, X.; An, X.; Zhang, X.; Liu, X.; Lu, X. XEN gel implant with or without phacoemulsification for glaucoma: A systematic review and meta-analysis. *Ann. Transl. Med.* **2020**, *8*, 1309. [CrossRef]
108. Sheybani, A.; Vera, V.; Grover, D.S.; Vold, S.D.; Cotter, F.; Bedrood, S.; Sawhney, G.; Piette, S.D.; Simonyi, S.; Gu, X.; et al. Gel Stent vs Trabeculectomy: The Randomized, Multicenter, Gold Standard Pathway Study (GPS) of Effectiveness and Safety at 12 Months: Gel Stent vs Trabeculectomy: A Prospective Randomized Study. *Am. J. Ophthalmol.* **2023**, *252*, 306–325. [CrossRef] [PubMed]
109. Schlenker, M.B.; Gulamhusein, H.; Conrad-Hengerer, I.; Somers, A.; Lenzhofer, M.; Stalmans, I.; Reitsamer, H.; Hengerer, F.H.; Ahmed, I.I.K. Efficacy, Safety, and Risk Factors for Failure of Standalone Ab Interno Gelatin Microstent Implantation versus Standalone Trabeculectomy. *Ophthalmology* **2017**, *124*, 1579–1588. [CrossRef]

110. Sacchi, M.; Agnifili, L.; Brescia, L.; Oddone, F.; Villani, E.; Nucci, P.; Mastropasqua, L. Structural imaging of conjunctival filtering blebs in XEN gel implantation and trabeculectomy: A confocal and anterior segment optical coherence tomography study. *Graefes Arch. Clin. Exp. Ophthalmol.* **2020**, *258*, 1763–1770. [CrossRef]
111. Olgun, A.; Duzgun, E.; Yildiz, A.M.; Atmaca, F.; Yildiz, A.A.; Sendul, S.Y. XEN Gel Stent versus trabeculectomy: Short-term effects on corneal endothelial cells. *Eur. J. Ophthalmol.* **2021**, *31*, 346–353. [CrossRef]
112. Cabourne, E.; Clarke, J.C.; Schlottmann, P.G.; Evans, J.R. Mitomycin C versus 5-Fluorouracil for wound healing in glaucoma surgery. *Cochrane Database Syst. Rev.* **2015**, *2015*, CD006259. [CrossRef] [PubMed]
113. Bell, K.; Bezerra, B.d.P.S.; Mofokeng, M.; Montesano, G.; Nongpiur, M.E.; Marti, M.V.; Lawlor, M. Learning from the past: Mitomycin C use in trabeculectomy and its application in bleb-forming minimally invasive glaucoma surgery. *Surv. Ophthalmol.* **2021**, *66*, 109–123. [CrossRef] [PubMed]
114. Midha, N.; Gillmann, K.; Chaudhary, A.; Mermoud, A.; Mansouri, K. Efficacy of Needling Revision After XEN Gel Stent Implantation: A Prospective Study. *J. Glaucoma* **2020**, *29*, 11–14. [CrossRef] [PubMed]
115. Feldman, R.M.; Tabet, R.R. Needle revision of filtering blebs. *J. Glaucoma* **2008**, *17*, 594–600. [CrossRef]
116. Kerr, N.M.; Lim, S.; Simos, M.; Ward, T. Primary Needling of the Ab Interno Gelatin Microstent Reduces Postoperative Needling and Follow-up Requirements. *Ophthalmol. Glaucoma* **2021**, *4*, 581–588. [CrossRef]
117. Gedde, S.J.; Herndon, L.W.; Brandt, J.D.; Budenz, D.L.; Feuer, W.J.; Schiffman, J.C. Surgical complications in the Tube Versus Trabeculectomy Study during the first year of follow-up. *Am. J. Ophthalmol.* **2007**, *143*, 23–31.e2. [CrossRef] [PubMed]
118. Kim, M.S.; Kim, K.N.; Kim, C.S. Changes in Corneal Endothelial Cell after Ahmed Glaucoma Valve Implantation and Trabeculectomy: 1-Year Follow-up. *Korean J. Ophthalmol.* **2016**, *30*, 416–425. [CrossRef]
119. Shaheer, M.; Amjad, A.; Ahmed, N. Comparison of Mean Corneal Endothelial Cell Loss after Trabeculectomy with and without Mitomycin C. *J. Coll. Physicians Surg. Pak.* **2018**, *28*, 301–303. [CrossRef]
120. Iwasaki, K.; Arimura, S.; Takihara, Y.; Takamura, Y.; Inatani, M. Prospective cohort study of corneal endothelial cell loss after Baerveldt glaucoma implantation. *PLoS ONE* **2018**, *13*, e0201342. [CrossRef]
121. Gillmann, K.; Bravetti, G.E.; Rao, H.L.; Mermoud, A.; Mansouri, K. Impact of Phacoemulsification Combined with XEN Gel Stent Implantation on Corneal Endothelial Cell Density: 2-Year Results. *J. Glaucoma* **2020**, *29*, 155–160. [CrossRef]
122. Oddone, F.; Roberti, G.; Posarelli, C.; Agnifili, L.; Mastropasqua, L.; Carnevale, C.; Micelli Ferrari, T.; Pace, V.; Sacchi, M.; Cremonesi, E.; et al. Endothelial Cell Density After XEN Implant Surgery: Short-term Data from the Italian XEN Glaucoma Treatment Registry (XEN-GTR). *J. Glaucoma* **2021**, *30*, 559–565. [CrossRef] [PubMed]
123. Lenzhofer, M.; Motaabbed, A.; Colvin, H.P.; Hohensinn, M.; Steiner, V.; Hitzl, W.; Runge, C.; Moussa, S.; Reitsamer, H.A. Five-year follow-up of corneal endothelial cell density after transscleral ab interno glaucoma gel stent implantation. *Graefes Arch. Clin. Exp. Ophthalmol.* **2023**, *261*, 1073–1082. [CrossRef] [PubMed]
124. Gedde, S.J.; Herndon, L.W.; Brandt, J.D.; Budenz, D.L.; Feuer, W.J.; Schiffman, J.C.; Tube Versus Trabeculectomy Study Group. Postoperative complications in the Tube Versus Trabeculectomy (TVT) study during five years of follow-up. *Am. J. Ophthalmol.* **2012**, *153*, 804–814.e1. [CrossRef] [PubMed]
125. Kirwan, J.F.; Lockwood, A.J.; Shah, P.; Macleod, A.; Broadway, D.C.; King, A.J.; Trabeculectomy Outcomes Group Audit Study Group. Trabeculectomy in the 21st century: A multicenter analysis. *Ophthalmology* **2013**, *120*, 2532–2539. [CrossRef]
126. Gedde, S.J.; Feuer, W.J.; Lim, K.S.; Barton, K.; Goyal, S.; Ahmed, I.I.K.; Primary Tube Versus Trabeculectomy Study Group. Treatment Outcomes in the Primary Tube Versus Trabeculectomy Study after 3 Years of Follow-up. *Ophthalmology* **2020**, *127*, 333–345. [CrossRef]

Disclaimer/Publisher's Note: The statements, opinions and data contained in all publications are solely those of the individual author(s) and contributor(s) and not of MDPI and/or the editor(s). MDPI and/or the editor(s) disclaim responsibility for any injury to people or property resulting from any ideas, methods, instructions or products referred to in the content.

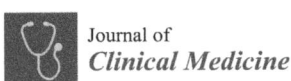

Article

Mid-Term Results of Ab Interno Trabeculectomy among Japanese Glaucoma Patients

Kazuyoshi Kitamura, Yoshiko Fukuda, Yuka Hasebe, Mio Matsubara and Kenji Kashiwagi *

Department of Ophthalmology, Faculty of Medicine, University of Yamanashi, Chuo 409-3898, Japan
* Correspondence: kenjik@yamanashi.ac.jp; Tel.: +81-55-273-1111; Fax: +81-55-273-6757

Abstract: Background: The evaluation of ab interno trabeculectomy, referred to as trabectome®, among Japanese patients is insufficient. Subjects and methods: Japanese patients who underwent trabectome® at the University of Yamanashi Hospital were included. The investigated parameters were intraocular pressure (IOP), best corrected visual acuity, glaucoma medications, visual field, and corneal endothelial cell density. The success rate and its associated factors were investigated. Results: A total of 250 eyes from 197 patients were enrolled. The trabectome® significantly reduced IOP and glaucoma medications up to 48 months. Concomitant cataract extraction enhanced the reduction in IOP and glaucoma medications up to 42 months. At 36 months postoperatively, 40.8% satisfied IOP of the same or less than 18 mmHg or more than a 20% IOP reduction with the same or less use of glaucoma medications as preoperatively. Preoperative IOP and combined cataract extraction were significantly associated with the success rate. The trabectome® alone did not show a significant reduction in corneal endothelial cells. Eyes with postoperative transient IOP elevation and removal of anterior chamber hemorrhage were 11.2% and 1.2%, respectively. Twenty-four eyes (9.6%) underwent additional glaucoma surgeries. Conclusions: The trabectome® could be considered an effective and safe surgery. Compared to trabectome® alone, combined cataract surgery was superior in lowering IOP and reducing glaucoma medications.

Keywords: ab interno trabeculectomy; glaucoma; intraocular pressure

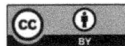

1. Introduction

Glaucoma is a high-ranking cause of blindness with irreversible optic neuropathy. Although glaucoma eye drops are commonly used to lower intraocular pressure (IOP), surgical treatment is often required due to inadequate IOP reduction or side effects. Trabeculectomy is a major glaucoma surgery. Though it is beneficial for lowering IOP, it is a procedure with a high risk of postoperative complications such as bleb infection, complications related to low IOP, and expulsive bleeding [1]. Trabectome® is an ab interno trabeculectomy and is considered a minimally invasive glaucoma surgery (referred to as MIGS) that is performed through a small corneal incision. Trabectome® was approved by the FDA in 2004 and by the Japanese Ministry of Health, Labor, and Welfare in 2010.

The purpose of this study was to evaluate the mid-term efficacy and safety of trabectome®.

2. Materials and Methods

2.1. Study Design

All patients who underwent trabectome® at the University of Yamanashi Hospital between March 2016 and December 2017 and met the following criteria were included in the retrospective study. The study was approved by the Ethics Committee of the University of Yamanashi School of Medicine. It was performed in accordance with the Declaration of Helsinki:

Approval Code: 1974;
Approval Date: 20 March 2019.

2.2. Entry and Exclusion Criteria

Entry criteria included consecutive patients aged 20 years or older who underwent trabectome® at the University of Yamanashi Hospital between March 2016 and December 2017. Accurate intraocular pressure measurement by Goldman Applanation Tonometry (GAT) was possible before and after surgery. Patients who underwent surgery on both eyes were included in the analysis.

2.3. Surgical Technique and Postoperative Management

Surgery was performed by three surgeons (K.K., M.M., and K.K.) using the trabectome® system (Neomedix, Inc., Tustin, CA, USA) at the University of Yamanashi Hospital. In the case of pseudophakic eyes before surgery, Trabectome® alone is indicated. In the case of phakic eyes before surgery, combined cataract surgery with trabectome® is indicated when cataracts are recognized. The presence or absence of cataracts was determined by the surgeon before surgery. A 1.7 mm temporal corneal incision was made, viscoelastic material was inserted intraocularly, the trabectome® was inserted, and a Swan Jacob Gonioprism was used to resect the nasal trabecular meshwork in the 90–120-degree range. In the trabectome® alone group, the surgery was completed after aspiration and removal of reflux hemorrhage and residual viscoelastic material using the trabectome®. In the combined cataract surgery group, conventional lens reconstruction was performed through the same corneal incision. After surgery, steroid eye drops (Betamethasone Sodium Phosphate Ophthalmic Solution 0.1%) and topical antibiotic eye drops (Levofloxacin Ophthalmic Solution 1.5%) were administered four times a day for one month, and 2% pilocarpine hydrochloride ophthalmic solution was started four times a day and gradually decreased. In the combined cataract group, NSAID eye drops (Bromfenac Sodium Hydrate Ophthalmic Solution 0.1%) were used twice a day for 3 months after surgery. All preoperative glaucoma eye drops and oral medications were discontinued, and additional medications were added at the discretion of the surgeon when an increase in IOP was observed.

2.4. Outcome Measures and Safety Evaluation

The primary outcome measures in this study were IOP values measured by GAT and the number of glaucoma medications. Preoperative data were collected based on the last preoperative visit. Patients used glaucoma medications until the day before surgery, with no washout period. The number of glaucoma medications was counted as two for combination eye drops and one for oral carbonic anhydrase inhibitors. Postoperative data were collected from patients at 1 week, 2 weeks, 1 month, and every 3 months thereafter. Secondary endpoints included visual acuity tests, visual field tests, and corneal endothelial cell density before and after surgery. Safety endpoints included surgical complications, adverse events, and additional glaucoma surgeries. Visual field measurements were performed using a Humphrey visual field analyzer (HFA) SITA-standard (Carl Zeiss Meditec, Dublin, CA, USA), and mean deviation (MD) values were included in the analysis.

2.5. Statistical Analyses

Statistical analyses were performed using JMP12.0.1 (SAS Institute, Cary, NC, USA), and changes in IOP and glaucoma medications before and after surgery were analyzed using repeated ANOVA. Corneal endothelial cell density before and after surgery was analyzed using a paired t-test. Changes in visual field defects before and after the surgery were compared using a paired t-test or repeated ANOVA. Factors related to survival were analyzed using logistic regression analysis. A p value < 0.05 was considered statistically significant.

3. Results

3.1. Demographics and Preoperative Ocular Parameters

Table 1 shows the preoperative data of the patients studied. The study population consisted of 107 male and 90 female patients with a mean age of 70.7 ± 12.6 years (16–93 years). The postoperative observation period ranged from 1 to 60 months. There were 201 phakic eyes and 48 pseudophakic eyes. There were 154 eyes that underwent combined cataract surgery with trabectome® and 96 eyes that underwent trabectome® alone. The preoperative IOP was 20.6 ± 6.8 mmHg.

Table 1. Demographics and Preoperative Ocular Parameters.

Eye (Subjects)	250 (197)	Male/Female: 107/90
Age (range)		70.7 ± 12.6(16–93)
Right eye:Left eye		126:124
Glaucoma subtype % (n)	POAG	63% (158)
	PXG	16% (41)
	SOAG	12% (31)
	NVG	1% (2)
	Mixed	3% (8)
	Others	4% (10)
Pre-operative lens status		Phakia (201):IOL (48)
Phaco combi:Single		154:96
IOP (mmHg) (range)		20.6 ± 6.8 (11–58)
BCVA (logMAR)		0.20 ± 0.36
Visual field test (HFA24-2) MD (dB) (range)		−10.5 ± 7.0 (1.31–−31.48)
Number of medications		4.1 ± 1.3

POAG: primary open angle glaucoma, PXG: pseudoexfoliation glaucoma, SOAG: secondary open angle glaucoma, NVG: neovascular glaucoma, IOP: intraocular pressure, BCVA: best corrected visual acuity, LogMAR: logarithm of the minimum angle of resolution, HFA: Humphrey Field Analyzer, MD: mean deviation, numbers after ±: standard deviation.

Glaucoma types were primary open-angle glaucoma (POAG) in 158 eyes (63%), pseudoexfoliative glaucoma (PXG) in 41 eyes (16%), neovascular glaucoma (NVG) in 2 eyes (1%), mixed glaucoma in 8 eyes (3%), secondary glaucoma (SG) in 31 eyes (12%), and glaucoma of undetermined type in 10 eyes (4%). We performed trabectome® for open-angle glaucoma without extensive peripheral anterior synechia (PAS). In the case of NVG, Trabectome is performed if there is no active angle neovascularization. Patients with NVG showed burn-out status of their NGV, and we confirmed that their angle was open without severe PAS formation. We used topical oxybuprocaine hydrochloride eyedrops for anaesthetizing. The mean preoperative best corrected visual acuity (BCVA) (logMAR) was 0.20 ± 0.36, and the mean preoperative HFA24-2MD value was −10.5 ± 7.0 dB (1.31 to –31.48). The mean number of glaucoma medications administered preoperatively was 4.1 ± 1.3.

3.2. Changes in IOP and Medications

Figure 1 shows the mean IOP before and after surgery (Figure 1a) and the rate of IOP reduction (Figure 1b). The mean IOP decreased from 20.6 ± 6.8 mmHg preoperatively to 15.0 ± 4.1 mmHg at 6 months, 15.6 ± 4.0 mmHg at 12 months, 15.6 ± 3.2 mmHg at 24 months, 16.5 ± 5.3 mmHg at 36 months, and 17.5 ± 6.2 mmHg at 48 months after surgery, and the differences in decreases were statistically significant from 6 to 51 months postoperatively ($p < 0.05$). The IOP reduction rate averaged 23.4% for the entire postoperative period, ranging from 20 to 25%.

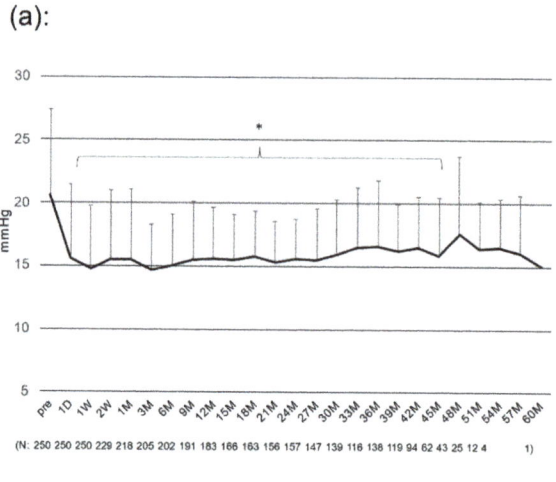

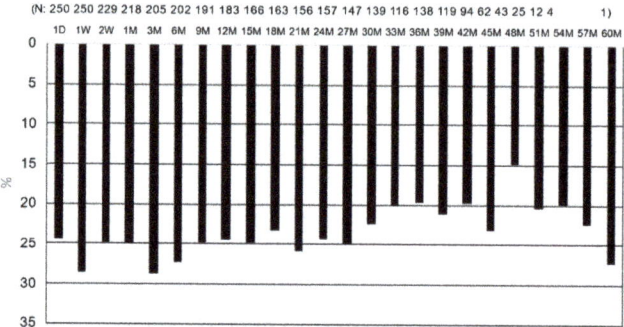

Figure 1. Postoperative changes in IOP and IOP reduction rate: (**a**) postoperative changes in IOP, * $p < 0.05$ vs. preoperative value (repeated ANOVA), (**b**) postoperative IOP reduction rate. Bar = SD.

Figure 2 shows the number of glaucoma medications (Figure 2a) and the percentage of patients who were medication free (Figure 2b) before and after surgery. The number of glaucoma medications decreased from 4.1 ± 1.3 preoperatively to 1.5 ± 1.4 at 6 months, 1.5 ± 1.6 at 12 months, 1.9 ± 1.6 at 24 months, 2.4 ± 1.8 at 36 months, and 2.7 ± 1.9 at 48 months after surgery. The mean of all postoperative periods was significantly lower ($p < 0.001$). The average decrease in the number of glaucoma medications during the entire postoperative period was 48.0% (−1.96). The number of postoperative glaucoma medications tended to gradually increase over time (Figure 2a). The percentage of postoperative glaucoma medication-free patients was up to 38.3% at 9 months and 38.2% at 12 months, followed by a gradual decrease (Figure 2b).

(a):

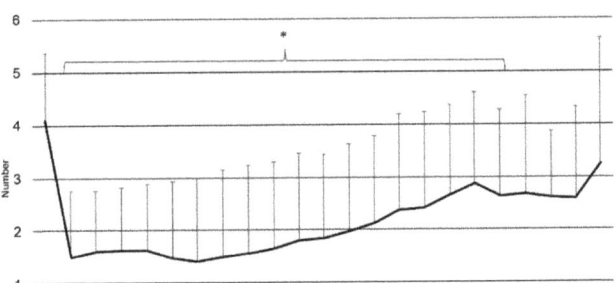

pre 1W 2W 1M 3M 6M 9M 12M 15M 18M 21M 24M 27M 30M 33M 36M 39M 42M 45M 48M 51M 54M 57M
(N: 250 250 229 218 205 202 191 183 166 163 156 157 147 139 116 138 119 94 62 43 25 12 4)

(b):

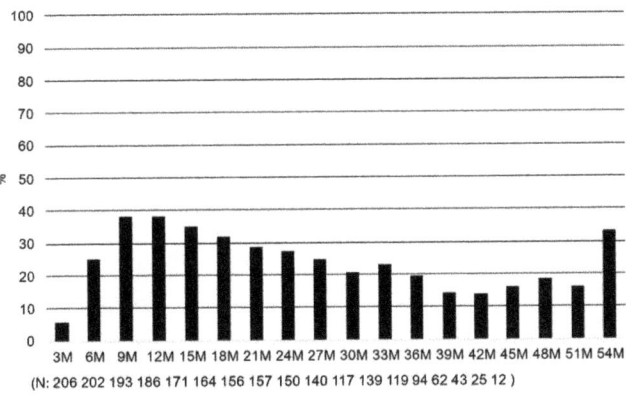

3M 6M 9M 12M 15M 18M 21M 24M 27M 30M 33M 36M 39M 42M 45M 48M 51M 54M
(N: 206 202 193 186 171 164 156 157 150 140 117 139 119 94 62 43 25 12)

Figure 2. Postoperative changes in the number of antiglaucoma medications and the rate of medication-free eyes: (**a**) postoperative reduction in the number of antiglaucoma medications, * $p < 0.001$ vs. preoperative value (repeated ANOVA), (**b**) postoperative rates of medication-free eyes. Bar = SD.

3.3. Preoperative IOP and IOP Reduction

Figure 3 shows the results of the postoperative IOP changes after dividing the preoperative IOP into three groups: Group A: less than 15 mmHg, Group B: 15–20 mmHg, and Group C: 21 mmHg or higher. Pre-IOP value means last preoperative visit IOP. Postoperative IOP in Groups B and C significantly decreased for most of the time periods (Group B: 1D-54 M ($p < 0.05$), Group C: 1D-57 M ($p < 0.05$)), whereas Group A showed no significant decrease in all measured time periods. The number of postoperative medications decreased significantly in all three groups for most of the time periods compared to the preoperative period (Group A: 1D-39 M, 48 M ($p < 0.05$); Group B: 1D-45 M ($p < 0.05$); Group C: 1D-54 M ($p < 0.05$)).

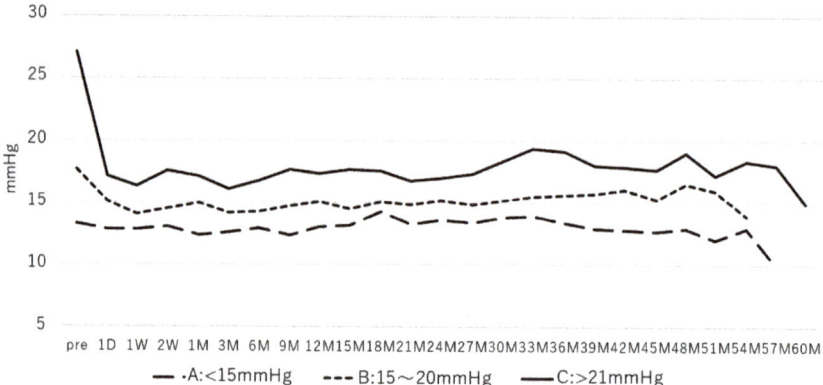

Figure 3. Postoperative changes: comparison by pre-IOP values: Group B: 15–20 mmHg and Group C: 21 mmHg or higher showed a significant decrease in postoperative IOP for the majority of the time periods (Group B: 1D-54 M ($p < 0.05$), Group C: 1D-57 M ($p < 0.05$)), whereas Group A: <15 mmHg showed no significant descent in all measurement periods (repeated ANOVA).

3.4. Success Rate

Figure 4 shows the results of the success rate study as defined below.

Complete Success was defined as no glaucoma medications, IOP less than 15 mmHg, and at least a 20% reduction from preoperative IOP.

Qualified success 1 was defined as IOP less than or equal to 15 mmHg and at least a 20% reduction from preoperative IOP. Postoperative glaucoma medications were equal to or less than preoperative.

Qualified success 2 was defined as IOP less than or equal to 18 mmHg and at least a 20% reduction from preoperative IOP. Postoperative glaucoma medications were equal to or less than preoperative.

The percentage of patients who achieved complete success was 25.4% at 12 months, 13.1% at 24 months, 6.9% at 36 months, 4.6% at 48 months, and 4.6% at 60 months.

The percentage of patients who achieved qualified success 1 was 39.2% at 12 months, 27.6% at 24 months, 24.6% at 36 months, 16.1% at 48 months, and 10.6% at 60 months.

The percentage of patients who achieved qualified success 2 was 60.6% at 12 months, 49.6% at 24 months, 42.5% at 36 months, 36.0% at 48 months, and 32.2% at 60 months.

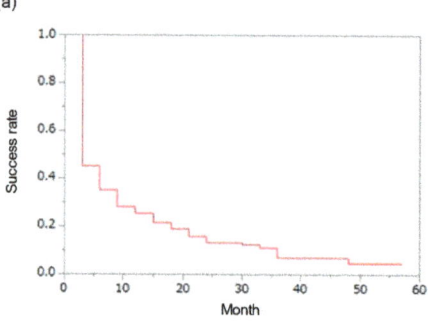

Figure 4. *Cont.*

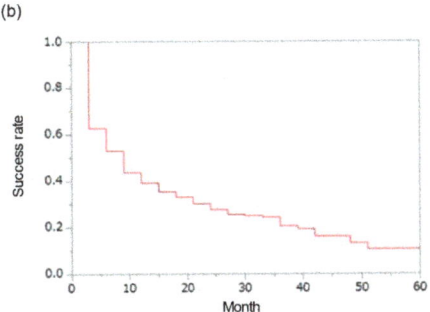

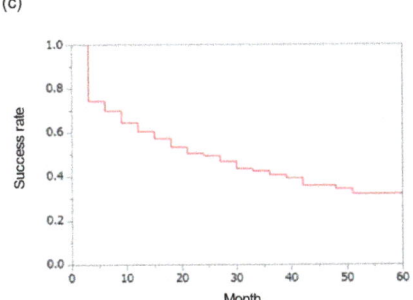

Figure 4. Comparison of survival curves by success definitions. (**a**) Complete success; (**b**) qualified success 1; (**c**) qualified success 2; Kaplan—Meier analysis.

The percentage of patients who achieved qualified success 2 in the POAG and PXG groups and for other types of glaucoma was evaluated (Figure 5a).

In the POAG and PXG groups, 74.9% of patients achieved qualified success 2: 61.1% at 12 months, 49.6% at 24 months, 40.3% at 36 months, 32.9% at 48 months, and 29.3% at 57 months.

In the other glaucoma groups, the rates of qualified success 2 were 58.2% at 12 months, 49.5% at 24 months, 43.1% at 36 months, 39.8% at 48 months, and 39.8% at 57 months.

Comparison using the log-rank test between the POAG and PE groups and the other glaucoma groups showed no significant difference in survival rates. There were also no significant differences in survival rates between the POAG and PXG groups ($p = 0.35$).

Next, the percentage of patients who achieved qualified success 2 in the combined cataract group and the Trabectome® alone group was examined (Figure 5b).

In the combined cataract group, the percentage of patients who achieved qualified success 2 was 69.0% at 12 months, 61.0% at 24 months, 51.1% at 36 months, 47.2% at 48 months, and 43.3% at 60 months.

In the Trabectome® alone group, the percentage of patients who achieved qualified success 2 was 46.9% at 12 months, 31.8% at 24 months, 24.7% at 36 months, 15.2% at 48 months, and 39.8% at 54 months.

When compared using the log-rank test for the combined cataract and trabectome® alone groups, the combined cataract group had a significantly higher survival rate ($p < 0.0001$).

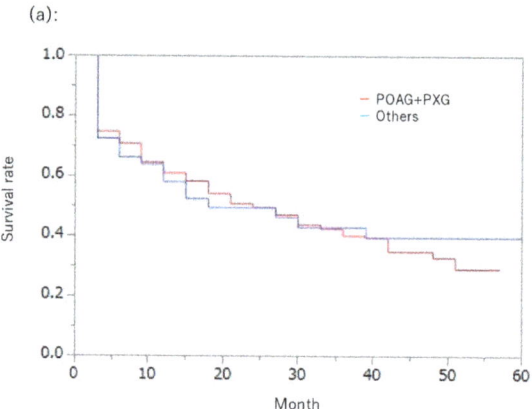

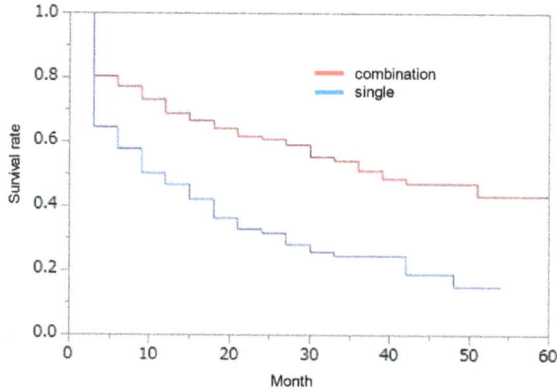

Figure 5. Comparison of survival curves between (**a**) type of glaucoma and (**b**) single vs. combination with cataract surgery in the qualified success 2 definition; Kaplan—Meier method.

3.5. Examination of Factors Related to Success

Factors associated with success in the above definition were examined. Logistic regression analysis was used to examine factors associated with success at 3 years postoperatively, including age, sex, glaucoma type, trabectome® alone/combined cataract, preoperative IOP, number of preoperative medications, and postoperative complications.

There were no significant factors associated with complete success, including age ($p = 0.19$), sex ($p = 0.09$), glaucoma type ($p = 0.93$), trabectome® alone/combined cataract ($p = 0.41$), preoperative IOP ($p = 0.36$), preoperative medications ($p = 0.45$), or postoperative complications ($p = 0.96$).

Preoperative IOP was significantly associated with qualified success 1 ($p = 0.02$). No significant associations were found for other factors, including age ($p = 0.65$), sex ($p = 0.47$), glaucoma type ($p = 0.64$), trabectome® alone/combined cataract ($p = 0.41$), number of preoperative medications ($p = 0.72$), or postoperative complications ($p = 0.62$).

The presence of combined cataract surgery was significantly associated with qualified success 2 ($p < 0.01$). No significant associations were found for other factors, including age ($p = 0.80$), sex ($p = 0.98$), glaucoma type ($p = 0.90$), preoperative IOP ($p = 0.40$), number of preoperative medications ($p = 0.70$), or postoperative complications ($p = 0.44$).

3.6. Comparison between Combined Cataract Surgery and Trabectome® Alone Surgery

Figure 6 shows the changes in IOP (Figure 6a) and the number of glaucoma medications (Figure 6b) in the combined cataract group and the trabectome® alone group. In the combined cataract group, IOP significantly decreased from the day after surgery to 48 months postoperatively, and in the trabectome® alone group, IOP significantly decreased from the day after surgery to 45 months postoperatively ($p < 0.05$). The mean postoperative IOP reduction rate was 22.2% in the combined cataract group and 24.0% in the trabectome® alone group, with both groups showing greater IOP reductions, significantly more so in the combined cataract group ($p < 0.001$).

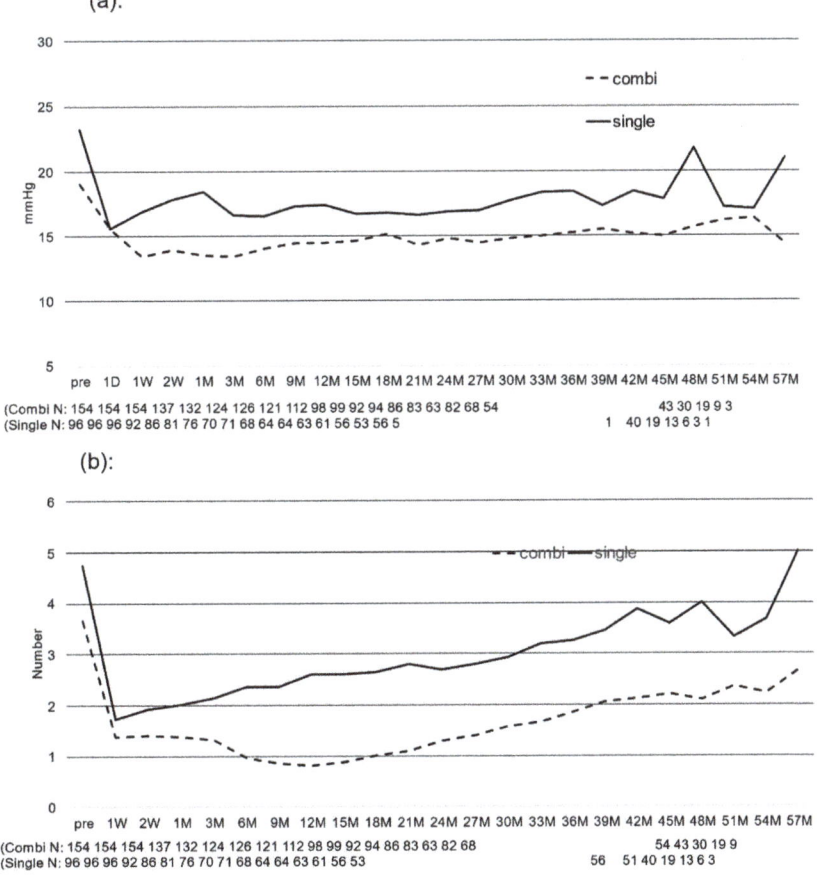

Figure 6. Postoperative changes in (**a**) IOP and (**b**) the number of medications between single vs. combination with cataract surgery. (**a**) IOP significantly decreased from the day after surgery to 48 months postoperatively in the combined cataract group and significantly decreased from the day after surgery to 45 months postoperatively in the trabectome® alone group ($p < 0.05$). (**b**) The number of glaucoma drugs also significantly decreased from 1 week to 51 months postoperatively in the combined cataract surgery group and from 1 week to 39 months postoperatively in the trabectome® alone group ($p < 0.05$).

The number of glaucoma medications also significantly decreased from 1 week to 51 months postoperatively in the combined cataract group and significantly decreased from 1 week to 39 months postoperatively in the trabectome® alone group ($p < 0.05$). The mean postoperative reduction in the number of drugs was 55.4% (−2.0) in the combined cataract group and 37.9% (−1.8) in the trabectome® alone group, which was significantly higher in the combined cataract group (Figure 6b).

The mean postoperative reduction in IOP was similar in both groups, but the decrease in the number of glaucoma medications was greater in the combined cataract group. A comparison of the two groups at each measurement period showed that IOP was significantly lower in the combined cataract group than in the trabectome® alone group for most periods from preoperative to 42 months postoperative ($p < 0.05$). In addition, the number of glaucoma medications was significantly lower in the combined cataract group at all time points from preoperative to 42 months ($p < 0.01$).

3.7. Changes in BCVA and Visual Field

Figure 7 shows the changes in BCVA in the combined cataract surgery group and the trabectome® alone group. BCVA significantly improved in the combined cataract group from 1 to 30 months postoperatively ($p < 0.05$). The BCVA significantly decreased in the trabectome® alone group ($p < 0.001$) during the first postoperative week, but the significant difference from the preoperative period disappeared from 2 weeks to 57 months postoperatively (Figure 7).

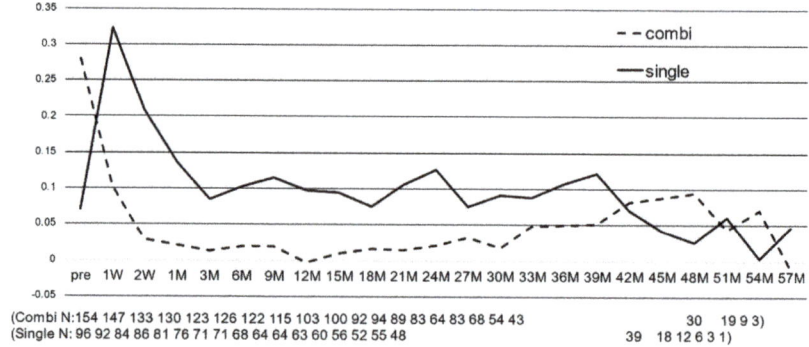

Figure 7. Postoperative changes in BCVA (logMAR) between single vs. combined cataract surgery. Repeated ANOVA; BCVA significantly improved from 1 to 30 months postoperatively in the combined cataract group ($p < 0.05$). In the trabectome® alone group, BCVA significantly decreased during the first postoperative week ($p < 0.001$), but the significant difference from the preoperative period disappeared from 2 weeks to 57 months postoperatively.

Overall, HFA24-2MD values were −10.5 ± 7.0 dB (1.31–31.48) preoperatively and −10.3 ± 7.0 dB (1.69–28.46) at 12 months postoperatively, with no significant deterioration in visual field defects ($p = 0.81$, paired t-test). In the long-term follow-up, HFA24-2MD values were 10.2 ± 7.1 dB (0.96–27.61) at 24 months postoperatively, 11.4 ± 7.4 dB (0.08–29.93) at 36 months postoperatively, and 11.4 ± 7.8 dB (−0.67–30.77) at 48 months postoperatively, with no significant deterioration of any visual field defect (repeated ANOVA).

The HFA24-2MD value was −11.7 ± 6.5 dB (−0.02–31.48) preoperatively and −11.4 ± 6.9 dB (−1.12–28.46) at 12 months postoperatively in the combined cataract group, with no significant deterioration of visual field defects ($p = 0.72$).

In the trabectome® alone group, the preoperative HFA24-2MD value was −8.77 ± 7.2 dB (1.31–29.79), and the 12-month postoperative value was −8.84 ± 7.0 dB (1.69–27.33), showing no significant deterioration of visual field defects ($p = 0.95$).

3.8. Safety Profile

Surgical complications are shown in Table 2. Postoperative transient elevation of IOP ($\geq$30 mmHg) was observed in 28 eyes (11.2%). The transient elevation of IOP occurred from the day after surgery to 1 month after surgery. Transient elevation of IOP occurred in 4 (2.6%) eyes in the combined cataract group and 24 (25%) eyes in the trabectome® alone group, with a significantly higher incidence in the trabectome® alone group ($p < 0.01$). Severe anterior chamber hemorrhage requiring anterior chamber wash out was observed in three eyes, all in the trabectome® alone group. No serious complications, such as endophthalmitis, expulsive bleeding, or choroidal detachment, were observed.

Table 2. Surgical complications and postoperative procedures.

	Number	%
Endophthalmitis	0	0
Choroidal hemorrhage	0	0
IOP elevation (IOP ≧ 30 mmHg)	28	11
Hypotomy (<5 mmHg)	0	0
Anterior chamber irrigation due to severe hyphema	3	1
Additional surgery	24 (trabeculectomy 19, trabectome 3, trabectome + GSL 1, trabeculotomy 1)	10

GSL: goniosynechialysis.

Of the 24 eyes that underwent additional glaucoma surgery due to poor postoperative IOP control, most (19) underwent trabeculectomy, 3 underwent additional trabectome®, 1 underwent trabectome® + goniosynechialysis (GSL), and 1 underwent trabeculotomy. The average time of additional surgery was 27.8 months postoperatively (2 weeks to 42 months postoperatively). We excluded the following information from analysis at the time of additional surgery. Five eyes (2%) underwent additional procedures: yttrium aluminum garnet (YAG) in one eye, cyclo photo coagulation (CPC) in two eyes, and selective laser trabeculoplasty (SLT) in two eyes, ranging from 1 month to 21 months postoperatively.

Changes in corneal endothelial cell density are shown in Table 3. In all patients, corneal endothelial cell density significantly decreased from $2465.6 \pm 376.3/mm^2$ preoperatively to $2378.6 \pm 378.2/mm^2$ postoperatively (-3.52%) ($p < 0.001$). The combined cataract group significantly decreased from $2518.4 \pm 333.6/mm^2$ preoperatively to $2381.0 \pm 359.9/mm^2$ postoperatively (-5.45%) ($p < 0.001$), whereas the trabectome® alone group showed no significant difference, from $2353.4 \pm 435.5/mm^2$ preoperatively to $2374.6 \pm 408.2/mm^2$ postoperatively. Therefore, the decrease in corneal endothelial cell density was considered to be an effect of cataract surgery.

Table 3. Changes of Corneal endothelial cell density.

	Pre-Operation	Post-Operation	Reduction Rate (%)	p Value
Total	2465.6 ± 376.3	2378.6 ± 378.2	−3.52	<0.001
Combi.	2518.4 ± 333.6	2381.0 ± 359.9	−5.45	<0.001
Single.	2353.4 ± 435.5	2374.6 ± 408.2	0.9	0.69

4. Discussion

4.1. Summary of Results: Intraocular Pressure and Number of Medications

This study examined the postoperative results of trabectome® surgery in Japanese glaucoma patients treated at our hospital up to 60 months postoperatively. IOP and the number of glaucoma medications were significantly decreased during most of the follow-up period compared to the preoperative period. It is thought that the reason for which the significant difference disappeared after 50 months was due to the decrease in the number of subjects for analysis. The average IOP reduction was 23.4% for the entire period, ranging from 20 to 25%, and the reduction in the number of glaucoma medications during the entire postoperative period was 48.0%. The percentage of patients who were free of glaucoma medication after surgery was 38.2% at 12 months, which continued to gradually decrease. IOP reduction was greater in the combined cataract surgery group, and the number of glaucoma drugs decreased substantially.

In previous reports by Avar M, Minckler D et al., a baseline IOP of approximately 23.0 mmHg was reduced to 16.5–17.2 mmHg (−26 to −28%) [2,3]. Esfandiari et al. and Bendel et al. reported a decrease in baseline IOP from 18.0~20.0 mmHg to 13.9~15.6 mmHg (−19~22%) [4,5]. In a study of Japanese subjects, Kono et al. reported a reduction from a baseline IOP of 29.2 mmHg to 16.4 mmHg (−43.8%) after 72 months [6]. Tojo et al. also reported a decrease from a baseline IOP of 23.0 mmHg to 13.6 mmHg after 24 months [7]. In our results, the rate of IOP reduction was somewhat less than that previously reported, but this may be because the preoperative IOP in our study was somewhat lower than that in other reports. The postoperative IOP was almost the same as that in a previous report. In both our study and previous reports, the rate of IOP reduction was lower than that of trabeculectomy [8]. Trabectome® is a surgical technique that promotes aqueous humor outflow in the main aqueous humor pathway by resecting the trabecular meshwork, and the outflow resistance of the outflow tracts (collecting channel and superior scleral vein) after the trabecular meshwork is constant, which may explain why the lower limit of IOP reduction was higher than that in trabeculectomy.

In the present study, preoperative IOP was divided into three groups: Group A: <15 mmHg, Group B: 15–20 mmHg, and Group C: >20 mmHg, and postoperative IOP changes were examined. The number of glaucoma medications in all three groups decreased significantly, and IOP also decreased significantly in groups A and B. However, in group C, there was no significant decrease in all postoperative periods. These results are similar to those of Tojo et al. and suggest that trabectome® should be indicated in patients with a preoperative IOP of 16 mmHg or higher [7].

Previous reports have reported higher postoperative success rates in the combined cataract surgery group than in the trabectome® alone group, similar to our results [6,9,10]. This may be because cataract surgery itself has an IOP-lowering effect, and the increase in IOP during cataract surgery after trabectome® surgery reduces postoperative anterior chamber hemorrhage and transient IOP elevation [11].

4.2. Factors Involved in Trabectome® Outcome

In this study, IOP control was considered to be successful at 3 years postoperatively in 6.9% of patients in the complete success group, 20.6% in qualified success group 1, and 40.8% in qualified success group 2. An analysis of the factors associated with success showed no significant association in the complete success group, but preoperative IOP was significantly associated with success in qualified success group 1 ($p = 0.02$), and the presence or absence of combined cataract surgery in qualified success group 2 was significantly associated ($p < 0.01$). Preoperative IOP may affect the success rate of the trabectome®, and therefore, patients with high preoperative IOPs should be treated with the possibility of poor success rates in trabectome® procedures. In addition, the presence or absence of combined cataract surgery is significantly related to the success rate of trabectome® and should be actively considered in patients who are eligible for combined cataract surgery.

Kono et al. reported that 26% of their patients had an IOP of 16 mmHg and achieved an IOP reduction of 20% or greater at 3 years postoperatively, and 46% had an IOP of 18 mmHg and achieved an IOP reduction of 20% or greater, with our results showing a slightly lower success rate [6][6]. In addition, our results showed no significant differences by glaucoma type, and the survival rate was significantly higher in the combined cataract group than in the trabectome® alone group, all of which are similar to previously reported results.

4.3. Advantages of the Trabectome®

Among the subjects in the current study, up to 38.3% of the patients did not require postoperative glaucoma medications. Although glaucoma medication has made significant progress in recent years, problems associated with multiple-medication therapy, such as poor adherence, dropout from medication therapy, and side effects of eye drops and oral medications, have become apparent. Therefore, very few medications should be used. In the present study, a maximum of 38.3% of patients achieved medication-free treatment, and the number of glaucoma medications was reduced from the preoperative level in most patients. This is very useful for glaucoma treatment in terms of improving adherence, preventing dropouts, and reducing the side effects of eye drops and oral medications.

4.4. Summary of Complications and Comparison with Previous Reports

In the present study, transient postoperative IOP elevation ($\geq$30 mmHg) was observed in 28 eyes (11.2%), and severe anterior chamber hemorrhage requiring anterior chamber wash out was observed in 3 eyes, but there were no cases of serious complications, such as endophthalmitis or expulsive bleeding, which were similar to those in previous reports [12,13]. Compared to the combined cataract group, the rate of transient postoperative IOP elevation and severe anterior chamber hemorrhage was higher in the trabectome® alone group, but this may be because, as mentioned above, the increase in IOP during cataract surgery can reduce transient IOP elevation by reducing postoperative anterior chamber hemorrhage. Trabectome® is a safe, low-patient-load technique with low surgical invasiveness and an infrequent need for postoperative surgical procedures (9.6% of patients required such procedures).

In addition, corneal endothelial cell density was significantly decreased in all patients and in the combined cataract group but not in the trabectome® alone group, suggesting that the effects of cataract surgery were not significant, and that trabectome® caused little damage to corneal endothelial cells.

4.5. Limitations of the Present Study

Limitations of the current study include the following: the lack of a control group in a retrospective study. There were three surgeons, and there may be differences in surgical techniques among the surgeons. Although the results were obtained during a period of up to 60 months, the follow-up period varied from patient to patient. Multiple types of disease were entered. There are no criteria for the resumption of glaucoma medication after surgery, and resumption is at the discretion of the surgeon. The corneal endothelial cell density was not compared to that in the cataract surgery group.

However, trabectome® is a safe procedure with a short operative time and few intraoperative and postoperative complications.

Trabectome® is suitable for patients who are unable to continue long-term medication therapy, who are concerned about side effects or poor adherence to multiple medications, or who are expected to drop out of treatment. However, since this is a surgical procedure to promote aqueous humor outflow in the main aqueous humor pathway, and since the outflow resistance of the outflow tracts (collecting channels and superior scleral vein) after the trabecular meshwork is constant, there is a lower limit to IOP reduction and a limit to IOP reduction value, so care should be taken in selecting cases. Trabeculectomy should be carefully considered for patients whose IOP before surgery is stable at 15 mmHg or lower but whose visual field is progressing or whose glaucoma is at the end stage and whose target IOP of approximately 10 mmHg is desired.

In addition, our results showed that trabectome® was performed in patients who were using more than four medications before surgery and in patients who were using multiple types of medications. As the number of glaucoma medications increases, patient adherence declines, and the side effects of eye drops worsen. In addition, the results of the present study showed that the combined cataract group had greater IOP reductions and fewer drugs than the trabectome® alone group. Therefore, the use of trabectome® in patients who require cataract surgery may be actively considered regardless of glaucoma type. In the future, we may consider performing trabectome® surgery for a wide range of indications, from patients with early-stage glaucoma who are receiving single-drug therapy to patients with end-stage glaucoma who cannot undergo trabeculectomy due to advanced age or poor general condition. Kashiwagi et al. reported that trabectome® surgery, both in combined cataract surgery and as a stand-alone procedure, not only lowers IOP but also improves practical vision by improving ocular surface conditions such as corneal epithelial damage due to a decrease in the number of medications [14]. We believe that this may further contribute to the improvement of patient QOV after surgery.

In Japan, following trabectome®, various MIGS, such as iStent®, iStent inject W®, Kahook dual blade®, and μ-hook®, are now available.

According to Iwasaki et al., IOP significantly decreased from 19.8 ± 7.3 mm Hg to 13.0 ± 3.1 mm Hg, and the mean number of medications significantly decreased from 2.5 ± 1.4 to 1.6 ± 1.6 in the Kahook Dual Blade® procedure. IOP significantly decreased from 17.8 ± 2.9 mmHg to 14.3 ± 2.3 mmHg, and the mean number of medications significantly decreased from 2.2 ± 1.1 to 0.9 ± 1.4. The IOP reduction rate was 26.2% with Kahook Dual Blade® and 19.0% with iStent® surgery [15], which were comparable to our results.

Nitta et al. reported that the iStent procedure with cataracts reduced IOP by 18% from 16.5 ± 3.4 mmHg preoperatively to 13.6 ± 3.0 mmHg and reduced the number of glaucoma drugs by 81% from 1.96 ± 0.98 preoperatively to 0.37 ± 0.74, with 77% of the patients being glaucoma medication free [16]. Although our results showed a greater IOP reduction, the percentage of patients who became glaucoma medication free was lower. The reason for this may be that the number of preoperative glaucoma medications in our study was higher, and although the number of medications could be significantly reduced, the patients did not become glaucoma medication free.

iStent inject W® has been available in Japan since 2020. Overseas reports have shown that iStent inject W® is superior to iStent® in lowering IOP and significantly reducing the number of glaucoma medications [17,18]. There are also reports that iStent inject W® and trabectome® are equivalent and others that iStent inject W® is superior to trabectome® [19,20]. In Japan, there are still few reports on iStent injection W®, so further studies are needed, including comparisons with trabectome®.

Tanito et al. reported that IOP decreased from 25.9 mmHg preoperatively to 14.5 mmHg at 6 months postoperatively for μ-hook surgery alone and from 16.4 ± 2.9 mmHg preoperatively to 11.8 ± 4.5 mmHg at 9.5 months postoperatively for combined cataract surgery [21,22]. In addition, Tojo et al. compared surgical outcomes between μ-hook and trabectome® and reported that trabectome® had significantly better surgical outcomes, although no significant difference was found for postoperative IOP [23].

Although there are differences in the results of IOP reduction and reduction in the number of glaucoma medications among the various techniques, we believe that the various MIGS techniques are minimally invasive and useful, resulting in good reductions in IOP and the number of glaucoma medications and fewer surgical complications.

5. Conclusions

Trabectome® is a minimally invasive and useful procedure that leads to a reduction in the number of glaucoma medications without serious complications, a significantly lower IOP, and improved visual acuity compared to preoperative visual acuity. Compared to trabectome® surgery alone, combined cataract surgery was superior in lowering IOP and reducing the number of glaucoma medications. However, there is a limit to the amount of IOP reduction, so the indication for trabectome® surgery should be carefully evaluated in patients with low target IOP.

Author Contributions: Conception of the study, K.K. (Kenji Kashiwagi); Data collection, K.K. (Kazuyoshi Kitamura), Y.F., Y.H. and M.M.; Statistical analysis, K.K. (Kazuyoshi Kitamura); Writing—original draft, K.K. (Kazuyoshi Kitamura); Writing—review and editing of manuscript, Y.F., Y.H., M.M. and K.K. (Kenji Kashiwagi). All authors have read and agreed to the published version of the manuscript.

Funding: This research received no external funding.

Institutional Review Board Statement: The study was conducted according to the guidelines of the Declaration of Helsinki and approved by the Ethics Committee of University of Yamanashi (protocol code 1974 and date of approval 20 March 2019).

Informed Consent Statement: Patient consent was waived due to this study being performed anonymously.

Data Availability Statement: Not applicable.

Conflicts of Interest: The authors declare no conflict of interest.

References

1. Yamamoto, T.; Sawada, A.; Mayama, C.; Araie, M.; Ohkubo, S.; Sugiyama, K.; Kuwayama, Y.; Collaborative Bleb-Related Infection Incidence; Treatment Study Group. The 5-year incidence of bleb-related infection and its risk factors after filtering surgeries with adjunctive mitomycin C: Collaborative bleb-related infection incidence and treatment study 2. *Ophthalmology* **2014**, *121*, 1001–1006. [CrossRef]
2. Minckler, D.; Mosaed, S.; Francis, B.; Loewen, N.; Weinreb, R.N. Clinical results of ab interno trabeculotomy using the Trabectome for open-angle glaucoma: The mayo clinic series in Rochester, Minnesota. *Am. J. Ophthalmol.* **2014**, *157*, 1325–1326. [CrossRef]
3. Avar, M.; Jordan, J.F.; Neuburger, M.; Engesser, D.; Lubke, J.; Anton, A.; Wecker, T. Long-term follow-up of intraocular pressure and pressure-lowering medication in patients after ab-interno trabeculectomy with the Trabectome. *Graefes Arch. Clin. Exp. Ophthalmol.* **2019**, *257*, 997–1003. [CrossRef]
4. Bendel, R.E.; Patterson, M.T. Long-term Effectiveness of Trabectome (Ab-interno Trabeculectomy) Surgery. *J. Curr. Glaucoma Pract.* **2018**, *12*, 119–124. [CrossRef]
5. Esfandiari, H.; Shah, P.; Torkian, P.; Conner, I.P.; Schuman, J.S.; Hassanpour, K.; Loewen, N.A. Five-year clinical outcomes of combined phacoemulsification and trabectome surgery at a single glaucoma center. *Graefes Arch. Clin. Exp. Ophthalmol.* **2019**, *257*, 357–362. [CrossRef]
6. Kono, Y.; Kasahara, M.; Hirasawa, K.; Tsujisawa, T.; Kanayama, S.; Matsumura, K.; Morita, T.; Shoji, N. Long-term clinical results of trabectome surgery in patients with open-angle glaucoma. *Graefes Arch. Clin. Exp. Ophthalmol.* **2020**, *258*, 2467–2476. [CrossRef]
7. Tojo, N.; Hayashi, A. The Outcomes of Trabectome Surgery in Patients with Low, Middle, and High Preoperative Intraocular Pressure. *Clin. Ophthalmol.* **2020**, *14*, 4099–4108. [CrossRef]
8. Sugimoto, Y.; Mochizuki, H.; Ohkubo, S.; Higashide, T.; Sugiyama, K.; Kiuchi, Y. Intraocular Pressure Outcomes and Risk Factors for Failure in the Collaborative Bleb-Related Infection Incidence and Treatment Study. *Ophthalmology* **2015**, *122*, 2223–2233. [CrossRef]
9. Minckler, D.; Mosaed, S.; Dustin, L.; Ms, B.F.; Trabectome Study, G. Trabectome (trabeculectomy-internal approach): Additional experience and extended follow-up. *Trans. Am. Ophthalmol. Soc.* **2008**, *106*, 149–159.
10. Ahuja, Y.; Ma Khin Pyi, S.; Malihi, M.; Hodge, D.O.; Sit, A.J. Clinical results of ab interno trabeculotomy using the trabectome for open-angle glaucoma: The Mayo Clinic series in Rochester, Minnesota. *Am. J. Ophthalmol.* **2013**, *156*, 927–935.e2. [CrossRef]
11. Yang, H.S.; Lee, J.; Choi, S. Ocular biometric parameters associated with intraocular pressure reduction after cataract surgery in normal eyes. *Am. J. Ophthalmol.* **2013**, *156*, 89–94.e1. [CrossRef]
12. Kaplowitz, K.; Bussel, I.I.; Honkanen, R.; Schuman, J.S.; Loewen, N.A. Review and meta-analysis of ab-interno trabeculectomy outcomes. *Br. J. Ophthalmol.* **2016**, *100*, 594–600. [CrossRef]
13. Lavia, C.; Dallorto, L.; Maule, M.; Ceccarelli, M.; Fea, A.M. Minimally-invasive glaucoma surgeries (MIGS) for open angle glaucoma: A systematic review and meta-analysis. *PLoS ONE* **2017**, *12*, e0183142. [CrossRef]
14. Kashiwagi, K.; Matsubara, M. Reduction in Ocular Hypotensive Eyedrops by Ab Interno Trabeculotomy Improves Not Only Ocular Surface Condition But Also Quality of Vision. *J. Ophthalmol.* **2018**, *2018*, 8165476. [CrossRef]
15. Iwasaki, K.; Takamura, Y.; Orii, Y.; Arimura, S.; Inatani, M. Performances of glaucoma operations with Kahook Dual Blade or iStent combined with phacoemulsification in Japanese open angle glaucoma patients. *Int. J. Ophthalmol.* **2020**, *13*, 941–945. [CrossRef]
16. Nitta, K.; Yamada, Y.; Morokado, S.; Sugiyama, K. iStent Trabecular Micro-Bypass Stent Implantation with Cataract Surgery in a Japanese Glaucoma Population. *Clin. Ophthalmol.* **2020**, *14*, 3381–3391. [CrossRef]
17. Guedes, R.A.P.; Gravina, D.M.; Lake, J.C.; Guedes, V.M.P.; Chaoubah, A. One-Year Comparative Evaluation of iStent or iStent inject Implantation Combined with Cataract Surgery in a Single Center. *Adv. Ther.* **2019**, *36*, 2797–2810. [CrossRef]

18. Manning, D. Real-world Case Series of iStent or iStent inject Trabecular Micro-Bypass Stents Combined with Cataract Surgery. *Ophthalmol. Ther.* **2019**, *8*, 549–561. [CrossRef]
19. Khan, M.; Saheb, H.; Neelakantan, A.; Fellman, R.; Vest, Z.; Harasymowycz, P.; Ahmed, I.I.K. Efficacy and safety of combined cataract surgery with 2 trabecular microbypass stents versus ab interno trabeculotomy. *J. Cataract. Refract. Surg.* **2015**, *41*, 1716–1724. [CrossRef]
20. Gonnermann, J.; Bertelmann, E.; Pahlitzsch, M.; Maier-Wenzel, A.B.; Torun, N.; Klamann, M.K. Contralateral eye comparison study in MICS & MIGS: Trabectome(R) vs. iStent inject(R). *Graefes Arch. Clin. Exp. Ophthalmol.* **2017**, *255*, 359–365.
21. Tanito, M.; Ikeda, Y.; Fujihara, E. Effectiveness and safety of combined cataract surgery and microhook ab interno trabeculotomy in Japanese eyes with glaucoma: Report of an initial case series. *Jpn. J. Ophthalmol.* **2017**, *61*, 457–464. [CrossRef]
22. Tanito, M.; Sano, I.; Ikeda, Y.; Fujihara, E. Short-term results of microhook ab interno trabeculotomy, a novel minimally invasive glaucoma surgery in Japanese eyes: Initial case series. *Acta Ophthalmol.* **2017**, *95*, e354–e360. [CrossRef]
23. Tojo, N.; Otsuka, M.; Hayashi, A. Comparison of trabectome and microhook surgical outcomes. *Int. Ophthalmol.* **2021**, *41*, 21–26. [CrossRef]

Disclaimer/Publisher's Note: The statements, opinions and data contained in all publications are solely those of the individual author(s) and contributor(s) and not of MDPI and/or the editor(s). MDPI and/or the editor(s) disclaim responsibility for any injury to people or property resulting from any ideas, methods, instructions or products referred to in the content.

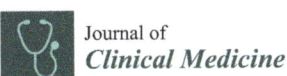

Article

Long-Term Outcomes of the PRESERFLO MicroShunt Implant in a Heterogeneous Glaucoma Cohort

Jens Julian Storp [1,*], Friederike Elisabeth Vietmeier [1], Ralph-Laurent Merté [1], Raphael Koch [2], Julian Alexander Zimmermann [1], Nicole Eter [1] and Viktoria Constanze Brücher [1]

[1] Department of Ophthalmology, University of Muenster Medical Center, 48149 Muenster, Germany; friederikeelisabeth.vietmeier@ukmuenster.de (F.E.V.); ralph-laurent.merte@ukmuenster.de (R.-L.M.); julian.zimmermann@ukmuenster.de (J.A.Z.); nicole.eter@ukmuenster.de (N.E.); viktoria.bruecher@ukmuenster.de (V.C.B.)

[2] Institute of Biostatistics and Clinical Research, University of Muenster, 48149 Muenster, Germany; raphael.koch@ukmuenster.de

* Correspondence: jens.storp@ukmuenster.de; Tel.: +49-251-83-56001

Abstract: The Preserflo MicroShunt represents a novel glaucoma treatment device, necessitating long-term follow-up data to accurately assess its efficacy. The aim of this study is to report real-world data of a heterogenous glaucoma cohort who received Preserflo implantation at a specialized glaucoma clinic. A total of 160 eyes of 160 patients who underwent Preserflo MicroShunt implantation were retrospectively enrolled in this study. Patient characteristics, as well as success and failure rates, were assessed. The numbers of adverse events and revision procedures were recorded, along with any reduction in supplementary medication. The progression of intraocular pressure (IOP) was assessed over the course of 12 months, and fluctuations were analyzed. The overall success rate was 61.9% (complete success: 51.3%, qualified success: 10.6%). Revision surgery was performed in 25% of cases. Excessive hypotony occurred postoperatively in 54.4% of patients and regressed after 7 days in 88.8% of all cases. Median IOP decreased from 22 (interquartile range (IQR): 17–27) mmHg preoperatively to 14 (IQR 12–16) mmHg at 12 months postoperatively ($p < 0.01$). The median number of antiglaucomatous agents decreased from three to zero at latest follow-up. The Preserflo MicroShunt achieved a noticeable reduction in IOP over the course of 12 months in glaucoma patients, irrespective of disease severity or disease subtype. The frequency of postoperative adverse events and number for revision surgeries over the course of the follow-up period were low.

Keywords: success; failure; MIGS; microinvasive glaucoma surgery; intraocular pressure; IOP; real-world; PEX; POAG; secondary

Citation: Storp, J.J.; Vietmeier, F.E.; Merté, R.-L.; Koch, R.; Zimmermann, J.A.; Eter, N.; Brücher, V.C. Long-Term Outcomes of the PRESERFLO MicroShunt Implant in a Heterogeneous Glaucoma Cohort. J. Clin. Med. 2023, 12, 4474. https://doi.org/10.3390/jcm12134474

Academic Editor: Eun Ji Lee

Received: 28 May 2023
Revised: 14 June 2023
Accepted: 1 July 2023
Published: 4 July 2023

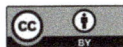

Copyright: © 2023 by the authors. Licensee MDPI, Basel, Switzerland. This article is an open access article distributed under the terms and conditions of the Creative Commons Attribution (CC BY) license (https://creativecommons.org/licenses/by/4.0/).

1. Introduction

Glaucoma is a worldwide leading cause of blindness [1]. An increased intraocular pressure (IOP) is regarded as one of the main risk factors associated with the disease [2], which is why the majority of treatment options focus on IOP reduction. The latter can be achieved via the administration of IOP lowering drugs, nonpenetrating approaches, such as laser procedures, or penetrating surgical intervention. To date, trabeculectomy remains the gold standard for penetrating glaucoma surgery [3–5], despite requiring intensive post-surgical follow-up [4,5]. Microinvasive glaucoma surgery (MIGS) treatment options are intended to provide an acceptable IOP reduction for patients, while reducing intra- and postoperative care burden [5].

Recent years have seen a number of these MIGS devices being developed. One novel innovation is the Preserflo MicroShunt (Santen, Miami, FL, USA), an 8.5 mm long tubular structure with a 350 µm outer diameter and 70 µm lumen made from biocompatible (poly)styrene-block-isobutylene-block-styrene [5,6]. The Preserflo system is placed into the subconjunctival space and acts as a drainage device, transporting aqueous humor from the anterior chamber to the subconjunctival space. The system has been reported to lower IOP during long-term observation in different types of glaucoma [7–10]. Due to its size, the Preserflo MicroShunt is expected to be associated with a faster recovery time and fewer postoperative adverse events in comparison to larger penetrating interventions, such as trabeculectomy [10].

Although a number of studies have already demonstrated the effectiveness of the Preserflo system [9–11], further studies are needed to assess long-term efficacy in clinical settings. This is especially true, as most of the studies available today investigated the efficacy of the Preserflo system in open-angle glaucoma patients only [8,12,13]. Yet, in clinical routine, practitioners might want to be able to offer any patient surgical therapy using the Preserflo system, regardless of the type of glaucoma. Therefore, studies reporting real-world data for heterogeneous glaucoma populations are required. In this study, we report real-world outcomes of the Preserflo MicroShunt in a large patient cohort consisting of patients with various types of glaucoma and disease severity levels.

This study investigates success rates, failure rates, the decrease in intraocular pressure (IOP), and the clinical development observed in a glaucoma patient group who underwent Preserflo implantation at a specialized glaucoma clinic in Germany over a 1 year period.

2. Materials and Methods

2.1. Design and Setting

All procedures were performed in accordance with the ethical standards issued by the ethics committee of the Medical Association of Westfalen-Lippe and the University of Münster, as well as the 1964 Helsinki declaration and its later amendments. Informed consent was waived due to the retrospective nature of this study. Data in this retrospective, monocentric trial were collected from glaucoma patients visiting the Department of Ophthalmology at the University Hospital Münster, Germany from July 2020 to December 2022. Data were obtained from electronic patient records in the digital documentation system FIDUS (Arztservice Wente GmbH, Darmstadt, Germany).

All patients older than 18 years of age, who received implantation of the Preserflo MicroShunt during this time span, were eligible for study inclusion. In accordance with the guidelines of the World Glaucoma Association, all fellow eye surgeries were excluded from the database of this study [14].

2.2. Surgical Procedure

In the preoperative phase, patients at our clinic stop taking any antiglaucomatous eye drops 4 weeks before Preserflo implantation to ensure the absence of any conjunctival hyperemia on the day of surgery. Instead, they are given oral azetacolamide for four weeks and corticoid eye drops 3 days prior to surgery. Then, 2–3 h before the operation, they receive intravenous acetazolamide and mannitol, in order to lower the pre- to postoperative pressure gradient. The subsequent surgical procedure of the implantation of the Preserflo Microshunt has been explained in detail elsewhere [9,10,15]. In short, after dissection of the conjunctiva and Tenon's capsule, mitomycin-C (MMC) 0.2 mg/mL is applied to the bare sclera for 3 min by placing sponges into the conjunctival flap. After subsequent rinsing with a balanced salt solution, a 2 mm deep scleral tunnel is created using a 1 mm lance. A 25 gauge needle is then guided through this tract to enter the anterior chamber, thus forming a tunnel between the anterior chamber and the subconjunctival pocket 3.5–4 mm from the limbus. The microshunt is inserted ab externo into the tunnel with its tip reaching approximately 2 mm into the anterior chamber, while its wings are kept inside the scleral pocket. After confirmation of flow through the device, seen by the formation of drops at the external end of the tube, Tenon's capsule and conjunctiva are closed. Figure 1 shows the correct postoperative placement of the Preserflo MicroShunt.

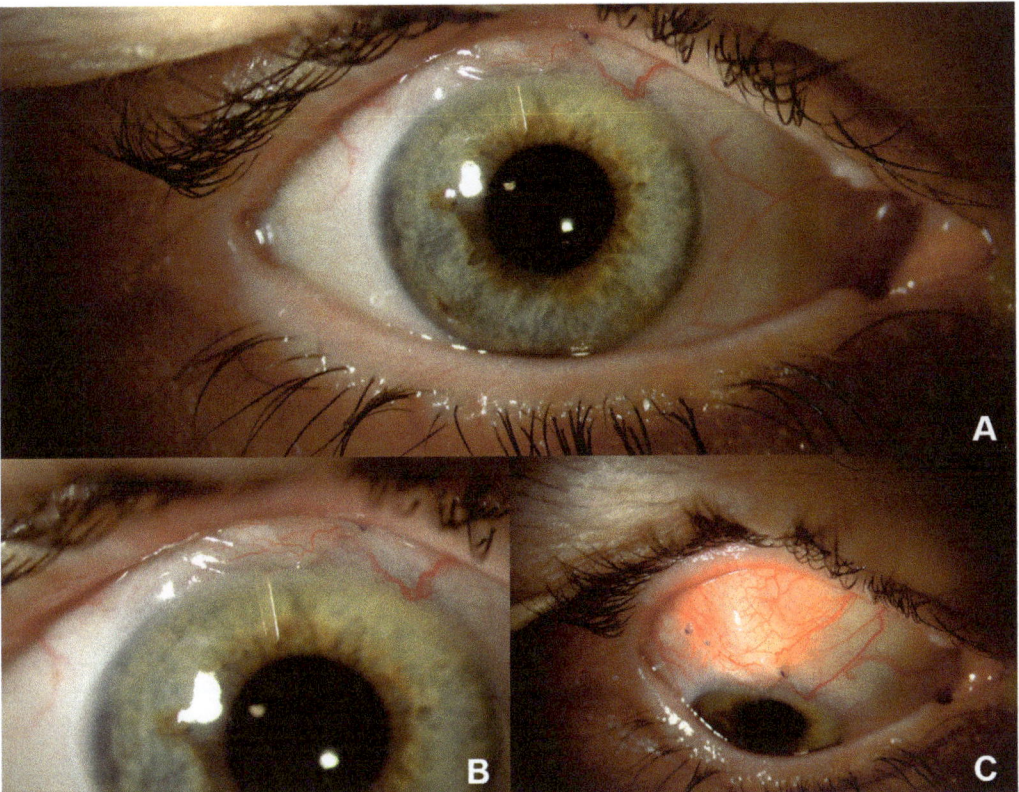

Figure 1. Situs after Preserflo Microshunt implantation in a right eye 1 day after surgery. (**A**) Macroscopic view: the scleral pocket is partly covered by the upper eyelid. (**B**) Close-up view: the shunt reaches into the anterior chamber without touching the iris or cornea. The scleral pocket is partly covered by the upper eyelid. (**C**) View of the prominent scleral pocket during downward gaze.

In our clinic, we regularly give 5-fluoruracil injections into the subtenonal space postoperatively if corkscrew vessels are present, or if the scleral pocket appears encapsulated.

2.3. Data Collection

Data on age, gender, ethnicity, type of glaucoma, and previous ocular surgeries including laser treatments were compiled from the electronic patient files. Surgeries were defined as all interventions used to treat conditions of the eyes, including laser treatment, such as selective laser-trabeculoplasty and other MIGS procedures, as well as cataract surgery and other penetrating procedures. Clinical information included results of slit-lamp examination, best corrected visual acuity, applanatory IOP, perimetric testing results including mean deviation, lens status, number of postoperative 5-fluoruracil injections, and number of antiglaucoma medications (topical and oral). Information was assessed preoperatively and at each of five postoperative timepoints: day 1, month 1, month 3, month 8, and month 12. After discharge, patients were scheduled to revisit 1, 3, 8, and 12 months after surgery. If patients reconsulted with our clinic more often than they were scheduled to, the IOP values closest to the whole month mark were drawn into the statistical analysis of IOP development. However, unscheduled visits were considered in the calculation of success rates. The occurrence of postoperative adverse events, as well as the necessity for revision surgeries, were noted. Adverse events were defined as hypotony ≤5 mmHg at any of the given timepoints, postoperative hyphemia, choroidal detachments, vitreous hemorrhage, or opening of Tenon's capsule. Revision surgeries were defined as surgical procedures that succeeded Preserflo implantation and that were conducted in order to achieve therapeutic success. Trabeculectomy, bleb revision, pars-plana vitrectomy, cyclophotocoagulation, implantation of another microshunt, and rinsing of the anterior chamber were regarded as revision procedures. The number of subconjunctival 5-fluoruracil injections was noted, but not counted as a revision procedure.

Visual field testing was conducted using the automated Humphrey Visual Field Analyzer II (HFA II, model 750; Carl Zeiss Meditec AG, Jena, Germany) with the standard program of the 30–2 Swedish interactive threshold algorithm (SITA fast).

2.4. Outcome Measures

The main outcome after 12 months was the overall success rate. Clinical outcome was classified as complete success (CS), qualified success (QS), or failure in accordance with the Primary Tube versus Trabeculectomy Study [16]. CS was achieved if, from month 1 onward, a patient's IOP reached values of 6–21 mmHg on two consecutive follow-up visits with a reduction of $\geq 20\%$ in comparison to mean preoperative IOP in both visits. If patients fulfilled the abovementioned criteria, but required further supplemental medical therapy, they were considered as having achieved QS. Overall success rate was defined as all cases of CS and QS. Failure was defined as IOP >21 mmHg in any of two consecutive postoperative visits after 1 month postoperatively, an IOP reduction of less than 20% on any of two consecutive postoperative visits in comparison to baseline 1 month postoperatively, a necessity for revision surgery, or loss of light perception following microshunt implantation from day 1 postoperatively.

Additionally, overall IOP reduction (mmHg) at 12 months after surgery was investigated in comparison to preoperative values in the entire patient cohort and in the disease severity subgroups. The median IOP of the date closest to the predefined intervals was calculated and drawn into the study. Eyes were allocated to disease severity groups (early, moderate, or severe) on the basis of the results of perimetric testing (Hodapp–Parrish–Anderson classification) [17]. We further report the number of postoperative supplemental antiglaucoma medications, number of postoperative adverse events, number of postoperative 5-FU injections, and number of revision procedures within 1 year of follow-up.

2.5. Statistical Analysis

Statistical analyses were performed using IBM SPSS Statistics for Windows, Version 28.0 (IBM Corp.: Armonk, NY, USA). All p-values and confidence limits were two-sided and intended to be exploratory rather than confirmatory. Therefore, no adjustment for multiplicity was made. Exploratory two-sided p-values ≤ 0.05 were considered statistically noticeable.

In descriptive analysis, continuous variables are reported as the median (25% quantile–75% quantile, interquartile range (IQR)). Categorical variables are presented as absolute and relative frequencies. Subgroup comparisons for continuous variables were performed using the Kruskal–Wallis test and Fisher's exact test for categorical variables. A comparison of pairwise IOP changes between two timepoints was performed using Wilcoxon signed-rank tests. Boxplots were used for graphical representation. Missing values were regarded as missing completely at random.

3. Results

3.1. Baseline Characteristics

A total of 160 eyes of 160 patients from the Department of Ophthalmology, University of Münster Medical Center, Germany, were included in this study. Patient characteristics are summarized in Table 1. The median follow-up time was 9 (IQR 5–12) months.

Table 1. General patient characteristics. Data are presented as the median (25% quartile–75% quartile) or as absolute and relative values.

Characteristics	Total Cohort
Eyes (n)	160
Patients (n)	160
Age (years)—median (IQR)	69 (62–77)
Gender (M:F) (n,%)	80 (50%):80 (50%)
Study eye (R:L) (n; %)	83 (52%):77 (48%)
Disease severity groups (n; %)	
Early	50 (31%)
Moderate	26 (16%)
Severe	84 (53%)
Type of glaucoma (n, %)	
POAG	111 (69%)
PEX glaucoma	28 (18%)
Secondary glaucoma	9 (6%)
Pigment-dispersion glaucoma	8 (5%)
Primary angle-closure glaucoma	4 (2%)
Previous surgery (n, %)	
None	38 (24%)
Total	122 (76%)
1–2 operations	85 (53%)
>2 operations	37 (23%)

n = number, % = percentage, M = male; F = female, R = right, L = left, POAG = primary open-angle glaucoma, PEX = pseudo-exfoliation.

3.2. Outcome: Success Rates

The overall success rate for the entire study population was 61.9% (CS: 51.3%, QS: 10.6%). Overall success was highest in patients with early glaucoma, followed by moderate and severe glaucoma. Overall success rate was lowest for secondary glaucoma patients (Table 2). The overall success rate differed noticeably among disease severity groups ($p = 0.04$) and among glaucoma subtypes ($p = 0.02$); however, it did not differ noticeably among eyes grouped according to the number of prior surgical interventions ($p = 0.35$).

Table 2. Success and failure rates for the entire study population and according to disease severity groups, type of glaucoma, and number of previous surgeries. Data are presented as absolute and relative values.

	Complete Success	Qualified Success	Failure
Total study population, (n, %)	82 (51%)	17 (11%)	61 (38%)
Disease severity groups			
early (n, %)	29 (58%)	4 (8%)	17 (34%)
moderate (n, %)	14 (54%)	1 (4%)	11 (42%)
severe (n, %)	39 (46%)	12 (14%)	33 (39%)
Type of glaucoma			
POAG (n, %)	65 (59%)	9 (8%)	37 (33%)
PEX glaucoma (n, %)	9 (31%)	5 (18%)	14 (50%)
Secondary glaucoma (n, %)	2 (22%)	0 (0%)	7 (78%)
Pigment-dispersion glaucoma (n, %)	3 (38%)	3 (38%)	2 (25%)
Primary angle-closure glaucoma (n, %)	3 (75%)	0 (0%)	1 (25%)

Table 2. Cont.

	Complete Success	Qualified Success	Failure
Previous surgical interventions			
None	21 (53%)	5 (13%)	14 (35%)
1–2	24 (49%)	7 (14%)	18 (37%)
>2	37 (52%)	5 (7%)	29 (41%)

n = number, % = percentage, POAG = primary open-angle glaucoma, PEX = pseudo-exfoliation.

3.3. Outcome: IOP Reduction

The median IOP reduction for the entire patient cohort over 1 year was 6 (IQR 2–13) mmHg with median IOP values of 22 (IQR 17–27) mmHg preoperatively and values of 14 (IQR 12–16) mmHg at 12 months postoperatively ($p < 0.001$; Figure 2, Table 3).

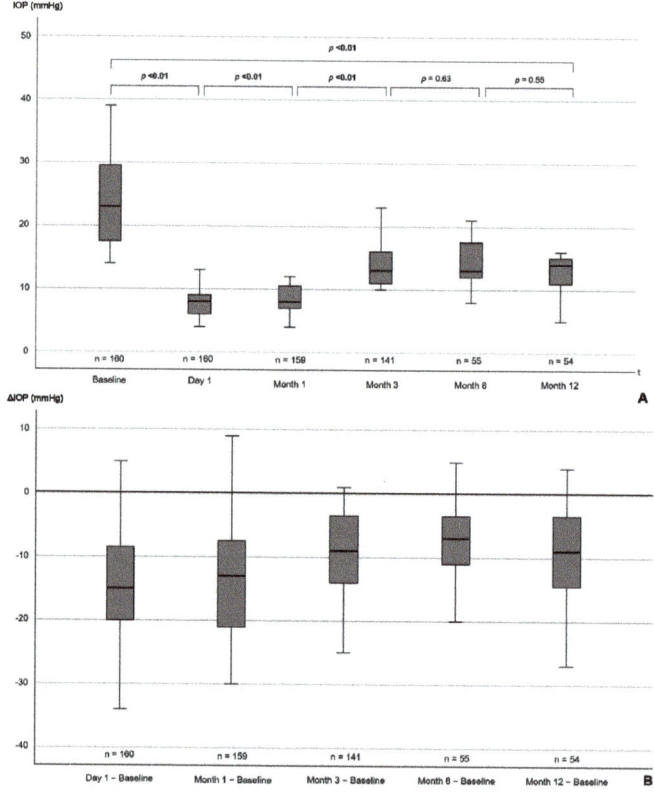

Figure 2. (**A**) Boxplots showing IOP from baseline to 12 months postoperatively. p-values for the difference between individual follow-up timepoints, as well as for the baseline comparison to 12 months, are presented. (**B**) Boxplots showing the reduction in IOP from baseline at the distinct follow-up timepoints. p-values are from Wilcoxon signed-rank tests. p-values ≤ 0.05 are highlighted in bold. Note that distances between the time intervals are not to scale. IOP = intraocular pressure, mmHg = millimeters of mercury, t = time, Δ = difference.

Table 3. IOP reduction at 12 months postoperatively in comparison to baseline for the entire patient population and according to disease severity groups, type of glaucoma, and number of previous surgeries. Data are presented as numbers and medians (25–75% quantile). p-values are reported from the Wilcoxon signed-rank test. p-values < 0.05 are highlighted in bold.

	IOP Baseline	IOP 12 Months	IOP Reduction	p-Value
Total study population (mmHg)	n = 160 22 (17–27)	n = 54 14 (12–16)	n = 54 6 (2–13)	**<0.01**
Disease severity groups				
Early (mmHg)	n = 50 21 (17–26)	n = 17 14 (12–15)	n = 17 4 (1–10)	**0.01**
Moderate (mmHg)	n = 26 19 (16–27)	n = 10 14 (14–19)	n = 10 4 (2–5)	**0.02**
Severe (mmHg)	n = 84 23 (18–28)	n = 27 14 (11–15)	n = 27 10 (2–14)	**0.01**
Type of glaucoma				
POAG (mmHg)	n = 111 21 (17–27)	n = 37 14 (12–16)	n = 37 6 (1–11.3)	**<0.01**
PEX (mmHg)	n = 28 24 (22–28)	n = 9 13 (13–14)	n = 9 9 (4–13.5)	**<0.01**
Secondary (mmHg) *	n = 9 26 (24–29)	n = 4 20 (15–24)	n = 4 11 (7.3–14.3)	
Pigment dispersion (mmHg) *	n = 8 18 (17–22)	n = 2 14 (14–14)	n = 2 3 (3–5)	
Primary angle closure (mmHg) *	n = 4 22 (18–28)	n = 2 8 (8–8)	n = 2 8 (3–15.8)	
Previous surgical interventions				
None	n = 40 23 (20–26)	n = 10 14 (10–16)	n = 10 10 (7–11)	**<0.01**
1–2	n = 49 23 (17–28)	n = 13 15 (13–17)	n = 13 13 (6–15)	**<0.01**
>2	n = 71 21 (17–28)	n = 21 14 (12–15)	n = 21 3 (1–6)	**0.01**

mmHg = millimeter mercury, POAG = primary open-angle glaucoma, PEX = pseudo-exfoliation. * p value not calculated, due to the small sample size.

IOP was noticeably reduced at 12 months postoperatively irrespective of disease severity group or type of glaucoma (Table 3, Figure 3). The median IOP reduction differed noticeably among disease severity groups ($p < 0.01$) and glaucoma subtypes ($p = 0.01$).

3.4. Postoperative Development

3.4.1. Supplemental Medications

Changes in supplemental medications were analyzed for the 54 patients who were present at the 12 month follow-up visit. The number of supplemental medications decreased noticeably from three (IQR 2.8–4) medications at baseline to zero (IQR 0–2) medications at 12 months postoperatively ($p < 0.01$).

3.4.2. Postoperative Complications

Postoperatively, 87 eyes (54%) were affected with hypotony (IOP $\leq$ 5 mmHg), with 30 eyes (19%) showing a choroidal detachment. Central choroidal detachment was observed in three eyes (2%). In the majority of cases, hypotony and choroidal detachment resolved spontaneously or with support of intensified locally applied steroidal therapy in the first weeks postoperatively. Hypotony persisted after 1 week in 18 eyes (11%) and after 90 days in four eyes (2%). Hyphemia was observed in 38 eyes (24%) (Table 4).

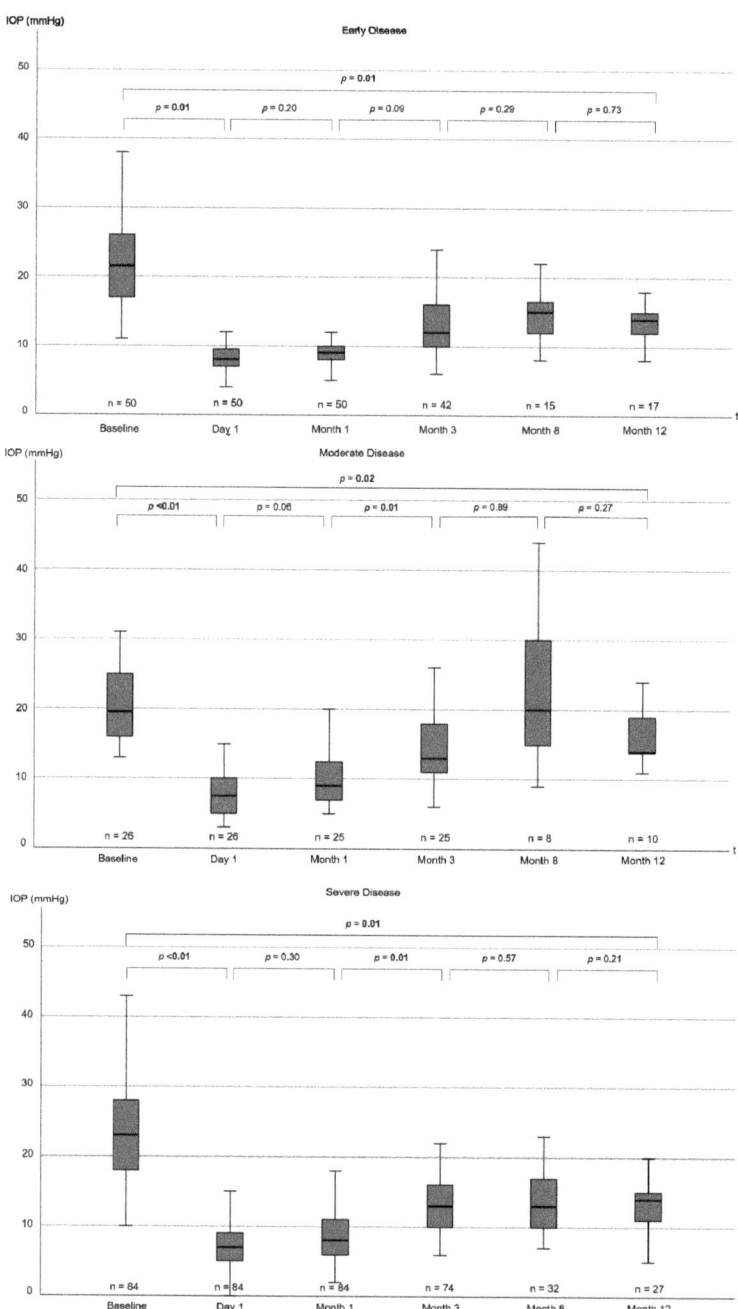

Figure 3. Boxplots showing IOP from baseline to 12 months postoperatively for disease severity cohorts (early, moderate, and severe). Note that distances between the time intervals are not to scale. p-values for the difference between individual follow-up timepoints, as well as for the comparison of baseline to the 12 month follow-up date, are displayed. p-values are from Wilcoxon signed-rank tests. p-values ≤ 0.05 are highlighted in bold. IOP = intraocular pressure, mmHg = millimeters of mercury, t = time.

Table 4. Number of eye-related postoperative adverse events in the entire study population and according to disease severity groups, type of glaucoma, and number of previous surgeries within 1 year. Data are presented as absolute and relative values.

Eye-Related Postoperative Adverse Events	n (%)
Total	106 (66%)
Hypotony (IOP $\leq$ 5 mmHg)	87 (54%)
Hypotony (IOP $\leq$ 5 mmHg) persistent after 1 week	18 (11%)
Hypotony (IOP $\leq$ 5 mmHg) persistent after 3 months	4 (3%)
Choroidal detachment	30 (19%)
Central choroidal detachment	3 (2%)
Peripheral choroidal detachment	27 (17%)
Hyphemia	38 (24%)
Disease severity groups	
Early (n = 50)	34 (68%)
Moderate (n = 26)	15 (58%)
Severe (n = 84)	57 (68%)
Type of glaucoma	
POAG (n = 111)	71 (64%)
PEX (n = 28)	20 (71%)
Secondary (n = 9)	7 (78%)
Pigment dispersion (n = 8)	6 (75%)
Primary angle closure (n = 4)	2 (50%)
Previous surgical interventions	
None (n = 40)	26 (65%)
1–2 (n = 49)	32 (65%)
>2 (n = 71)	48 (68%)

n = number, % = percentage, POAG = primary open-angle glaucoma, PEX = pseudo-exfoliation.

The number of eye-related adverse events differed noticeably among disease severity groups (p = 0.05) and glaucoma subtypes (p = 0.01), but did not differ noticeably among eyes grouped according to the number of prior surgical interventions (p = 0.72) (Table 4).

We would like to highlight two cases with unusual problems following Preserflo implantation that happened in our tertiary referral center.

One patient suffered from bleb infection with conjunctival necrosis followed by Preserflo explantation and scleral patch. The patient's history contained herpetic keratouveitis, and XEN Implant in the same eye. The conjunctiva was avascular prior to the Preserflo implantation, which likely predisposed to infection and necrosis.

Another patient with secondary glaucoma after perforating eye injury, aphakia, and pretreatment with two cyclophotocoagulations developed hypotony and phthisis bulbi in the further course after Preserflo implantation. The patient required numerous further procedures, including perforating keratoplasty, Eckhardt prosthesis, and vitrectomy. As a result, in our opinion, phthisis bulbi should be regarded as a result of the perforating damage rather than a complication of Preserflo implantation.

3.4.3. 5-FU Injections and Postoperative Interventions

A total of 123 eyes (77%) received at least one subconjunctival injection of 5-FU (range: 0–21; median: 2) (Table 5). We did not count subconjunctival injections of 5-FU as revision surgery. Furthermore, 73% of all 5-FU injections were given within 1 week after surgery, 88% were given within 14 days after surgery, 97% were given within the first month after surgery, and 100% were given within the first 3 months after surgery.

Table 5. Number of postoperative 5-FU injections and revisory operations in the entire study population within 1 year. Results are reported as numbers and percentages.

Postoperative Interventions within 1 Year	n (%)
Subconjunctival injection of 5-FU, total	123 (77%)
None	37 (23%)
1–3	83 (52%)
≥4	40 (25%)
Revision surgeries within 1 year	**n (%)**
Total	40 (25%)
Anterior chamber surgery	12 (8%) *
Bleb revision surgery	28 (18%) *
Trabeculectomy	5 (3%) *
Cyclophotocoagulation	6 (4%) *
Vitrectomy	3 (2%) *
Percentage of revision surgeries by disease severity group	
Early ($n = 50$)	9 (18%)
Moderate ($n = 26$)	8 (31%)
Severe ($n = 84$)	23 (27%)
Percentage of revision surgeries by type of glaucoma	
POAG ($n = 111$)	25 (23%)
PEX glaucoma ($n = 28$)	11 (39%)
Secondary glaucoma ($n = 9$)	4 (44%)
Pigment-dispersion glaucoma ($n = 8$)	0
Primary angle-closure glaucoma ($n = 4$)	0
Percentage of revision surgeries by number of previous surgical interventions	
None ($n = 40$)	8 (20%)
1–2 ($n = 49$)	16 (33%)
>2 ($n = 71$)	16 (23%)

n = number, % = percentage, POAG = primary open-angle glaucoma, PEX = pseudo-exfoliation. * Percentage values reported as the proportion of the entire study population ($n = 160$).

Overall, 40 patients (25%) needed ophthalmological revision surgery. Bleb revision surgery was required in 28 eyes (18%). A total of 12 eyes (8%) underwent anterior chamber surgery, due to hyphemia or hyperfiltration with shallow anterior chamber. Subsequent trabeculectomy was performed in five eyes (3%), and cyclophotocoagulation was performed in six eyes (4%). Postoperative vitrectomy was performed in three eyes, due to vitreous body prolapse (2%) (Table 5). The percentage of revision surgeries differed noticeably among disease severity groups ($p = 0.01$), glaucoma groups ($p < 0.01$), and eyes with differences in the number of previous surgical interventions ($p = 0.01$) (Table 5).

4. Discussion

In this retrospective study, the Preserflo MicroShunt achieved an overall success rate of 61.9% (CS: 51.3%, QS: 10.6%) in a heterogenous glaucoma cohort. Median IOP reduction was 6 (IQR 2–13) mmHg after 12 months, and revision surgery was required in 25% of all cases. Postoperative adverse events were noted in almost two-thirds of patients. Compared to baseline, the number of supplemental glaucoma medications taken 12 months postoperatively was noticeably lower in the 54 patients who were present at 12 months follow-up.

Among the first trials to report success rates for this novel concept, Battle et al. achieved an overall success rate of 100% after 1 year of follow-up, which has since not been replicable [18]. Consisting of only 23 patients, the overall success rate of their Preserflo trial remains among the highest in the literature, with consistent overall success rates ≥ 91% throughout a 3 year follow-up period [8]. Meanwhile, the CS rate was high with 91% after 1 year.

Success rates of later trials with bigger study cohorts ranged 53.9% to 92.3% for CS and 68.3% to 92.6% for overall success rates [7,9–13]. These numbers are similar to success rates in this trial. Some of these authors further distinguished among different types of glaucoma. Nobl et al. reported success rates for both PEX glaucoma patients and POAG glaucoma patients. Interestingly, both CS and QS were comparable between PEX patients and POAG patients, which contrasts earlier studies reporting on success rates in penetrating glaucoma surgery, such as trabeculectomy [19]. The authors attribute this observation to the fact that the minimally invasive approach does not aggravate the already compromised blood–aqueous barrier in PEX glaucoma as much as penetrating glaucoma surgery, resulting in lower inflammatory cytokine levels in the anterior chamber and, as a result, lower rates of fibrosis and scarring [7,20].

Conversely, in this trial, patients with POAG had higher overall success rates than PEX glaucoma patients. PEX patients had a noticeably higher proportion of QS and failure cases than the POAG cohort. It should, however, be noted that comparability among subpopulations in this trial is limited, as patient characteristics across subgroups were not matched; thus, parameters, such as age, gender, or disease severity might explain the differences seen here. Nevertheless, this explorative analysis allows an estimate of real-world performance of the Preserflo Microshunt system in different glaucoma group constellations. We observed secondary glaucoma patients to have the lowest overall success rate, despite featuring the highest median IOP decrease. This is because the rate of revision surgery in secondary glaucoma eyes was the highest of all with 44%. We assume that, as glaucoma in these patients developed secondary to another underlying cause, the surgical procedure oftentimes is more complicated, and the postoperative development is influenced by factors not present in other types of glaucoma. Success rates for pigment-dispersion and primary angle-closure glaucoma eyes were high, yet the small population in these cohorts limits the generalizability of this observation.

The level of IOP reduction after 1 year in this trial is comparable to other trials [10,11,21,22]. When differentiating among disease severity groups, IOP reduction at 12 months follow-up was greatest in patients with severe glaucoma. This might in part be explained by the behavior of ophthalmologists during postoperative follow-up visits, as most experts might tend to prescribe supplemental, IOP-lowering medication in patients with advanced optical nerve damage rather than in patients with an early form of glaucoma.

Schlenker et al. reported secondary OAG and a lower dose of intraoperative MMC to be associated with a higher failure rate [9]. This association might in part explain the comparatively low success rate reported by Baker et al., who used a low dosage of MMC in their trial (0.2 mg/mL) [12]. Durr et al. investigated the influence of different concentrations of MMC and found that a lower dosage of MMC was associated with higher rates for needling [11]. They also found that the association between disease severity and failure rate was high in mild to moderate disease [11]. This is in line with reports by Tanner et al., who described an association between higher mean deviation and failure [10]. However, in this trial, this association was not as present, as described by previous studies. Although CS rates were higher in less advanced glaucoma stages, failure rates were comparable among all severity groups. This deviation from previous reports might be attributable to the composition of the population in this study, as it was more heterogeneous than in other trials, which oftentimes only included one type of glaucoma.

The rate of postoperative hypotony in this trial (54%) was high in comparison to other studies, with highest rates not exceeding 40% [7–9,11,12,18,23]. Likewise, choroidal detachment also occurred noticeably more often in this trial (19%), compared to most reports in the literature [8,9,11,18,23], with only Nobl et al. reporting higher choroidal detachment rates of 30% for PEX glaucoma patients [7]. Central choroidal detachment occurred in three cases (2%) in this trial, which is comparable to rates reported in other studies [7,13]. We report real-world data of patients treated at a tertiary care referral center. Therefore, the number of complicated glaucoma cases, e.g., involving eyes with secondary glaucoma or with history of previous glaucoma surgery, was naturally high and might at least in part explain the large number of cases with postoperative hypotony. The frequent usage of 5-FU in this study might also have contributed to this observation. Likewise, the pre-operative administration of acetazolamide and mannitol might have had an influence on postoperative IOP development. With a half-life of 6–8 h [24], intravenous acetazolamide might have affected the IOP in our study population within the first days after surgery. Nonetheless, over the course of 1 week, hypotony resolved in 89% of cases and in 95% of affected cases after 3 months without any sequelae.

The rates for revision surgery were higher in our study than reported by Nobl et al. [7] and Durr et al. [11], albeit lower than that described by Baker et al., who reported a rate of 40.8% of patients requiring postoperative interventions [12]. Comparison of postoperative revision procedures is difficult across studies, as there is a wide variety of what authors consider a postoperative intervention. Tanner et al. separately reported the rate of bleb revisions to be 11.5% in their study [10], which is lower than in our study (17.5%). We included a proportionally large number of patients who had undergone previous ocular surgery (76%), in comparison to the 66.3% of patients in the trial by Tanner et al. [10]. The difference in baseline study characteristics might explain the differences in postoperative bleb revisions seen in this particular case and in other postoperative procedures. Eventually, the decision to perform surgical revision is not standardizable and is left to the discretion of the treating surgeon, making comparison with other trials, even with those that apply the same definitions, difficult.

Limitations

This study had some limitations. Firstly, due to its retrospective design, we are limited in the possibility to comment on future IOP development. Although we do not expect IOP and, therefore, success rates to fluctuate strongly in the period after 12 months of follow-up, recent trials have seen a decrease in success rates over a follow-up period of 5 years [8]. Further longitudinal studies with larger follow-up periods are required for adequate prognoses.

Secondly, even though we accounted for most of the factors known to exert an influence on glaucoma surgery results, such as age, sex, severity of glaucoma, type of glaucoma, and previous surgery, individual factors and individual postoperative behaviour might have had an influence on IOP development. Future studies are needed to replicate the findings reported in this trial.

Thirdly, we saw a relatively large dropout rate after the third postoperative month. In our experience, this very well represents the clinical reality in postoperative care. Patients with insufficient IOP regulation after surgery will usually attend most, if not all, prescheduled follow-up visits. However, those patients with an unproblematic postoperative development tend to not keep further appointments from a certain point onward if they do not see the necessity to revisit. The overall patient compliance should, therefore, be kept in mind when interpreting the results depicted in this study.

5. Conclusions

To summarize, the Preserflo MicroShunt achieved an overall success rate of 61.9% in a study cohort consisting of patients with various types and severity stages of glaucoma. It showed noticeable reductions in both IOP and number of medications. The Preserflo device is still new to many professionals; therefore, comparison to other established invasive glaucoma treatments is limited. As surgeons become more experienced in the implantation of the system, long-term outcomes might change.

Author Contributions: Conceptualization, J.J.S., F.E.V. and V.C.B.; data curation, J.J.S. and F.E.V.; formal analysis, J.J.S. and F.E.V.; investigation, J.J.S., F.E.V. and J.A.Z.; methodology, J.J.S., F.E.V. and V.C.B.; project administration, R.-L.M., N.E. and V.C.B.; resources, N.E.; software, R.K.; validation, R.K.; writing—original draft, J.J.S. and F.E.V.; writing—review and editing R.-L.M., R.K., J.A.Z., N.E. and V.C.B. All authors have read and agreed to the published version of the manuscript.

Funding: We acknowledge support from the Open Access Publication Fund of the University of Muenster.

Institutional Review Board Statement: Ethical review and approval were waived for this study due to the retrospective design of the trial.

Informed Consent Statement: Patient consent was waived due to local regulations of the Ethics Committee of the University of Muenster, Germany, as this study met the criteria of the §6 health data protection law, North-Rhine Westphalia.

Data Availability Statement: Not applicable.

Acknowledgments: The authors thank Monika Vuko for her technical support in this study.

Conflicts of Interest: The authors declare no conflict of interest.

References

1. Weinreb, R.N.; Aung, T.; Medeiros, F.A. The pathophysiology and treatment of glaucoma: A review. *JAMA* **2014**, *311*, 1901–1911. [CrossRef] [PubMed]
2. Fechtner, R.D.; Weinreb, R.N. Mechanisms of optic nerve damage in primary open angle glaucoma. *Surv. Ophthalmol.* **1994**, *39*, 23–42. [CrossRef]
3. Lusthaus, J.; Goldberg, I. Current management of glaucoma. *Med. J. Aust.* **2019**, *210*, 180–187. [CrossRef] [PubMed]
4. Rao, A.; Cruz, R.D. Trabeculectomy: Does It Have a Future? *Cureus* **2022**, *14*, 27834. [CrossRef] [PubMed]
5. Gambini, G.; Carlà, M.M.; Giannuzzi, F.; Caporossi, T.; De Vico, U.; Savastano, A.; Baldascino, A.; Rizzo, C.; Kilian, R.; Caporossi, A.; et al. PreserFlo® MicroShunt: An Overview of This Minimally Invasive Device for Open-Angle Glaucoma. *Vision* **2022**, *6*, 12. [CrossRef] [PubMed]
6. Green, W.; Lind, J.T.; Sheybani, A. Review of the Xen Gel Stent and InnFocus MicroShunt. *Curr. Opin. Ophthalmol.* **2018**, *29*, 162–170. [CrossRef]
7. Nobl, M.; Freissinger, S.; Kassumeh, S.; Priglinger, S.; Mackert, M.J. One-year outcomes of microshunt implantation in pseudoexfoliation glaucoma. *PLoS ONE* **2021**, *16*, 0256670. [CrossRef]
8. Batlle, J.F.; Corona, A.; Albuquerque, R. Long-term results of the PRESERFLO MicroShunt in patients with primary open-angle glaucoma from a single-center nonrandomized Study. *J. Glaucoma* **2021**, *30*, 281–286. [CrossRef]
9. Schlenker, M.B.; Durr, G.M.; Michaelov, E.; Ahmed, I.I.K. Intermediate Outcomes of a Novel Standalone Ab Externo SIBS Microshunt With Mitomycin C. *Am. J. Ophthalmol.* **2020**, *215*, 141–153. [CrossRef]
10. Tanner, A.; Haddad, F.; Fajardo-Sanchez, J.; Nguyen, E.; Thong, K.X.; Ah-Moye, S.; Perl, N.; Abu-Bakra, M.; Kulkarni, A.; Trikha, S.; et al. One-year surgical outcomes of the PreserFlo MicroShunt in glaucoma: A multicentre analysis. *Br. J. Ophthalmol.* **2022**, *2021*, 320631. [CrossRef]
11. Durr, G.M.; Schlenker, M.B.; Samet, S.; Ahmed, I.I.K. One-year outcomes of stand-alone ab externo SIBS microshunt implantation in refractory glaucoma. *Br. J. Ophthalmol.* **2022**, *106*, 71–79. [CrossRef]
12. Baker, N.D.; Barnebey, H.S.; Moster, M.R.; Stiles, M.C.; Vold, S.D.; Khatana, A.K.; Flowers, B.E.; Grover, D.S.; Strouthidis, N.G.; Panarelli, J.F.; et al. Ab-Externo MicroShunt versus Trabeculectomy in Primary Open-Angle Glaucoma: One-Year Results from a 2-Year Randomized, Multicenter Study. *Ophthalmology* **2021**, *128*, 1710–1721. [CrossRef]
13. Pillunat, K.R.; Herber, R.; Haase, M.A.; Jamke, M.; Jasper, C.S.; Pillunat, L.E. PRESERFLO™ MicroShunt versus trabeculectomy: First results on efficacy and safety. *Acta Ophthalmol.* **2022**, *100*, 779–790. [CrossRef]
14. Shaarawy, T.M.; Sherwood, M.B.; Grehn, F. *World Glaucoma Association Guidelines on Design & Reporting Glaucoma Trials*; Kugler Publications: Amsterdam, The Netherlands, 2009.
15. Kerr, N.M.; Ahmed, I.I.K.; Pinchuk, L. PRESERFLO MicroShunt. In *Minimally Invasive Glaucoma Surgery*; Springer: Singapore, 2021; pp. 91–103.
16. Gedde, S.J.; Feuer, W.J.; Shi, W.; Lim, K.S.; Barton, K.; Goyal, S.; Ahmed, I.I.K.; Brandt, J.; Primary Tube Versus Trabeculectomy Study Group. Treatment Outcomes in the Primary Tube Versus Trabeculectomy Study after 1 Year of Follow-up. *Ophthalmology* **2018**, *125*, 650–663. [CrossRef]
17. Hodapp, E.; Parrish, R.K.; Anderson, D.R. *Clinical Decisions in Glaucoma*; Mosby Incorporated: Maryland Heights, MO, USA, 1993.
18. Batlle, J.F.; Fantes, F.; Riss, I.; Pinchuk, L.; Alburquerque, R.; Kato, Y.P.; Arrieta, E.; Peralta, A.C.; Palmberg, P.; Parrish, R.K., 2nd; et al. Three-Year Follow-up of a Novel Aqueous Humor MicroShunt. *J. Glaucoma* **2016**, *25*, 58–65. [CrossRef]
19. Li, F.; Tang, G.; Zhang, H.; Yan, X.; Ma, L.; Geng, Y. The Effects of Trabeculectomy on Pseudoexfoliation Glaucoma and Primary Open-Angle Glaucoma. *J. Ophthalmol.* **2020**, *2020*, 1723691. [CrossRef]
20. Gillmann, K.; Meduri, E.; Niegowski, L.J.; Mermoud, A. Surgical Management of Pseudoexfoliative Glaucoma: A Review of Current Clinical Considerations and Surgical Outcomes. *J. Glaucoma* **2021**, *30*, 32–39. [CrossRef]
21. Beckers, H.J.M.; Aptel, F.; Webers, C.A.B.; Bluwol, E.; Martínez-de-la-Casa, J.M.; García-Feijoó, J.; Lachkar, Y.; Méndez-Hernández, C.D.; Riss, I.; Shao, H.; et al. Safety and Effectiveness of the PRESERFLO® MicroShunt in Primary Open-Angle Glaucoma: Results from a 2-Year Multicenter Study. *Ophthalmol. Glaucoma* **2022**, *5*, 195–209. [CrossRef]

22. Martínez-de-la-Casa, J.M.; Saenz-Francés, F.; Morales-Fernandez, L.; Perucho, L.; Mendez, C.; Fernandez-Vidal, A.; Garcia-Saenz, S.; Sanchez-Jean, R.; García-Feijoo, J. Clinical outcomes of combined Preserflo Microshunt implantation and cataract surgery in open-angle glaucoma patients. *Sci. Rep.* **2021**, *11*, 15600. [CrossRef]
23. Scheres, L.M.J.; Kujovic-Aleksov, S.; Ramdas, W.D.; de Crom, R.; Roelofs, L.C.G.; Berendschot, T.; Webers, C.A.B.; Beckers, H.J.M. XEN® Gel Stent compared to PRESERFLO™ MicroShunt implantation for primary open-angle glaucoma: Two-year results. *Acta Ophthalmol.* **2021**, *99*, 433–440. [CrossRef]
24. Shukralla, A.A.; Dolan, E.; Delanty, N. Acetazolamide: Old drug, new evidence? *Epilepsia Open* **2022**, *7*, 378–392. [CrossRef] [PubMed]

Disclaimer/Publisher's Note: The statements, opinions and data contained in all publications are solely those of the individual author(s) and contributor(s) and not of MDPI and/or the editor(s). MDPI and/or the editor(s) disclaim responsibility for any injury to people or property resulting from any ideas, methods, instructions or products referred to in the content.

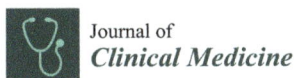

Journal of
Clinical Medicine

Article

MicroShunt versus Trabeculectomy for Surgical Management of Glaucoma: A Retrospective Analysis

Michael X. Fu [1,2,*], Eduardo M. Normando [1,3], Sheila M. H. Luk [4], Mira Deshmukh [4], Faisal Ahmed [1,3], Laura Crawley [1,3], Sally Ameen [1,3], Niten Vig [1,3], Maria Francesca Cordeiro [1,3] and Philip A. Bloom [1,3,4]

1. Department of Surgery and Cancer, Imperial College London, London SW7 2AZ, UK
2. Nuffield Department of Medicine, University of Oxford, Oxford OX1 3SY, UK
3. Imperial College Ophthalmology Research Group, Western Eye Hospital, London NW1 5QH, UK
4. The Hillingdon Hospitals NHS Foundation Trust, Uxbridge UB8 3NN, UK
* Correspondence: michael.fu18@imperial.ac.uk or michael.fu@sjc.ox.ac.uk

Abstract: This case-control study aims to compare the efficacy, safety, and postoperative burden of MicroShunt versus trabeculectomy. The first consecutive cohort of MicroShunt procedures (n = 101) was matched to recent historical trabeculectomy procedures (n = 101) at two London hospital trusts. Primary endpoints included changes in intraocular pressure (IOP) and glaucoma medications. Secondary outcome measures included changes in retinal nerve fibre layer (RNFL) thickness, rates of complications, further theatre interventions, and the number of postoperative visits. From the baseline to Month-18, the median [interquartile range] IOP decreased from 22 [17–29] mmHg (on 4 [3–4] medications) to 15 [10–17] mmHg (on 0 [0–2] medications) and from 20 [16–28] mmHg (on 4 [3–4] medications) to 11 [10–13] mmHg (on 0 [0–0] medications) in the MicroShunt and trabeculectomy groups, respectively. IOP from Month-3 was significantly higher in the MicroShunt group (p = 0.006), with an increased number of medications from Month-12 (p = 0.024). There were greater RNFL thicknesses from Month-6 in the MicroShunt group (p = 0.005). The rates of complications were similar (p = 0.060) but with fewer interventions (p = 0.031) and postoperative visits (p = 0.001) in the MicroShunt group. Therefore, MicroShunt has inferior efficacy to trabeculectomy in lowering IOP and medications but provides a better safety profile and postoperative burden and may delay RNFL loss.

Keywords: glaucoma; surgical glaucoma treatment; filtration surgery; minimally penetrating glaucoma surgery

Citation: Fu, M.X.; Normando, E.M.; Luk, S.M.H.; Deshmukh, M.; Ahmed, F.; Crawley, L.; Ameen, S.; Vig, N.; Cordeiro, M.F.; Bloom, P.A. MicroShunt versus Trabeculectomy for Surgical Management of Glaucoma: A Retrospective Analysis. *J. Clin. Med.* **2022**, *11*, 5481. https://doi.org/10.3390/jcm11185481

Academic Editors: Michele Figus and Karl Mercieca

Received: 31 August 2022
Accepted: 15 September 2022
Published: 18 September 2022

Publisher's Note: MDPI stays neutral with regard to jurisdictional claims in published maps and institutional affiliations.

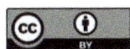

Copyright: © 2022 by the authors. Licensee MDPI, Basel, Switzerland. This article is an open access article distributed under the terms and conditions of the Creative Commons Attribution (CC BY) license (https://creativecommons.org/licenses/by/4.0/).

1. Introduction

Glaucoma is a leading cause of blindness worldwide [1]. Lowering the intraocular pressure (IOP) has long been held to be the only effective strategy to reduce glaucomatous progression [2]. In patients showing advancing visual field (VF) loss, inadequate IOP control, or experiencing side effects or non-adherence to medication, surgical intervention is often advocated to halt the disease progression [3]. Trabeculectomy with intraoperative mitomycin-C (MMC) has long been regarded as the gold standard surgical modality [4]. Despite well-documented IOP-lowering effectiveness and cost efficiency [5], trabeculectomy may be associated with lengthy postoperative care [4]. There is an increasingly perceived need for safer alternative surgical techniques, but also the recognition that any new procedure must be rigorously assessed for efficacy.

Several alternatives have been proposed, such as minimally invasive glaucoma surgeries (MIGSs). However, the IOP reductions achieved with MIGSs are modest and largely targeted at patients with mild-to-moderate glaucoma [6], often in combination with lens surgery. For more advanced glaucoma, minimally penetrating glaucoma surgeries (MPGSs) have demonstrated initial efficacy and safety [7], tending to reduce postoperative visits [8].

Compared to trabeculectomy, MPGSs used in the UK have increased significantly, particularly during the coronavirus pandemic [8]. The *ab interno* XEN® Gel Stent (Allergan Inc., Irvine, CA, USA), although initially popular, is less commonly used due to early failure, necessitating numerous postoperative manoeuvres [9]. The *ab externo* PRESERFLO™ MicroShunt ("MicroShunt," Santen Pharmaceutical) is an alternative MPGS that has shown early promise [10].

Despite similarities between MicroShunt and trabeculectomy, such as subconjunctival dissection and MMC usage, MicroShunt implantation does not require scleral flap formation, sclerostomy, or iridectomy [7]. The posterior placement of the MPGS device may also influence the bleb position and morphology, which may affect issues such as the risk of bleb leaks, bleb-related infections, and bleb dysaesthesia; MicroShunts tend to drain more posteriorly, which may be associated with an improved safety profile. Controlling the aqueous outflow through flow resistance without relying on the precise suture-tensioning techniques used in trabeculectomy [11] may mitigate postoperative care and variations in surgical skill.

However, a paucity of literature compares MicroShunt to trabeculectomy, the gold standard [3,12,13]. A favourable safety profile was found with the MicroShunt, with conflicting evidence on its efficacy [3,12,13]. However, these studies had short follow-up periods of 6 months [3,13] and 12 months [12], with only one study investigating the VF mean deviation (VF/MD), and this was with 6-month data [3], which is insufficient to detect meaningful changes [14]. No previous studies have analysed the retinal nerve fibre layer (RNFL) thickness.

The purpose of this study was to compare MicroShunt to trabeculectomy as the primary glaucoma surgery in terms of efficacy, safety, and postoperative burden. To the best of our knowledge, this is the first study to compare a comprehensive set of outcome measures between both procedures in all glaucoma diagnoses, including RNFL thickness and number of postoperative visits, with an 18-month follow-up.

2. Materials and Methods

2.1. Study Design

This study adhered to the tenets of the Declaration of Helsinki and was given local regulatory approval. Consecutive MicroShunt procedures from August 2020 at the Imperial College Healthcare NHS Trust (ICH) and July 2021 at the Hillingdon Hospitals NHS Foundation Trust (THH) were identified from Medisoft electronic records and theatre records, corresponding to the initial procedure performed at each trust. Recent historical consecutive trabeculectomy procedures were also identified. Lists were then cross-checked against search-generated data obtained from Medisoft. If both eyes were eligible, the first operated eye was included [3,13]. Only patients undergoing primary incisional glaucoma surgery with a minimum 3-month follow-up until May 2022 were included. Patients were listed for both procedures based on surgeons' discretion.

Using the case-control matching function in SPSS (IBM, Armonk, NY, USA, version 28.0.0), matching was performed using the variables' age (with a ten-year match tolerance), sex, ethnic group, glaucoma diagnosis, and the first or second eye undergoing an IOP-lowering operation (where the first eye was operated before the observed timeframe). According to the available MicroShunt follow-up, identical follow-up durations were analysed for the corresponding trabeculectomy match. Patients who underwent post-procedural secondary IOP-lowering surgeries were analysed up until the point at which the intervening decision was made since the outcomes after secondary surgery no longer reflected the initial procedure. Manual data collection from clinic letters was cross-checked with search-generated data.

2.2. Surgery

All cases were performed by glaucoma consultants or fellows under direct supervision in both surgical centres. Similar standardised methods were used by all surgeons.

For trabeculectomy, access was obtained by the creation of a fornix-based conjunctival flap. Using a soaked sponge, 0.4 mg/mL MMC was applied for 3 min below Tenon's capsule, followed by irrigation with 40 mL of sterile saline. After cautery, a rectangular partial-thickness scleral flap was created. A paracentesis was performed to allow anterior chamber (AC) refilling as required. The AC was entered with a sharp blade under the scleral flap, followed by sclerostomy and peripheral iridectomy. The scleral flap was closed with 2 releasable and 1 fixed 10-0 nylon sutures, and Tenon's capsule and the conjunctiva were closed together using 10-0 nylon sutures.

For MicroShunt, following the creation of a fornix-based conjunctival flap, a soaked sponge with 0.4 mg/mL MMC was applied below Tenon's capsule for 3 min, followed by irrigation with 40 mL of sterile saline. After cautery, the sclera was marked 3 mm from the limbus. A shallow scleral pocket was prepared with a 1 mm-width knife at the distally marked point. A needle was then used to create a transscleral tunnel from the apex of the scleral pocket into the AC to insert the MicroShunt, with the MicroShunt fin tucked tightly into the scleral pocket. Tenon's and conjunctiva were then closed with 10-0 nylon sutures after verifying for continuous aqueous flow at the distal MicroShunt end.

The postoperative visits schedule for both procedures was guided by the department protocol, with modifications by the surgeons according to individuals' needs. Visits closest to established time points were chosen to amalgamate heterogeneous data from both trusts [15]: Day-1, Week-1, Month-1, Month-3, Month-6, Month-12, and Month-18. Due to the paucity of data for other time points, the time points of 6, 12, and 18 months were chosen for VF measurements. Postoperative glaucoma medications (medications) were discontinued post-surgery immediately and reintroduced at surgeons' discretion for inadequately controlled IOP.

2.3. Outcome Measures

Baseline demographics were recorded for the visit where patients were listed. Primary outcome measures included changes in IOP and medications. Secondary outcomes included: VF/MD, average RNFL thickness, success rates, complications and theatre interventions, duration of surgery, and the number of postoperative glaucoma visits.

In keeping with current standards [4,12,15], 'complete success' criteria were: [1] IOP $\leq$ 21 mmHg; [2] no further surgical reintervention for glaucoma; [3] no loss of light perception vision; [4] no chronic hypotony (IOP $\leq$ 5 mmHg at two consecutive follow-ups from Month-3); and [5] no usage of medications to maintain adequate IOP. Surgical interventions were those performed in an operating room setting, including needling. Qualified success followed the same 'complete success' criteria but allowed for the use of medications.

Since this study did not use washout IOPs and the baseline IOP was not significantly high for many patients with medications, defining success with an additional IOP percentage reduction was deemed unsuitable [3]. However, to enable comparability with other studies with differing definitions, 'strict success' was defined as the 'complete success' criterion but with a $\geq$20% IOP reduction compared to the baseline [3]. The three success criteria were also assessed using 18 mmHg and 14 mmHg as the upper limit of the criteria.

2.4. Statistical Methods

Data were entered into Excel (Microsoft Corp.,Washington, DC, USA, version 16.60) and analysed using GraphPad Prism (LLC, Manhattan, KS, USA, version 9.3.1). Histograms and Shapiro–Wilk tests confirmed non-normal distributions for every outcome except VF/MD. Continuous data were reported as median [interquartile range (IQR)] or mean $\pm$ standard deviation and categorical variables as proportions. Mann–Whitney U/unpaired t-tests (group comparisons) and Wilcoxon/paired t-tests (longitudinal samples) were performed for continuous variables. Fisher's exact and Chi-squared tests compared categorical data. Probabilities of success were analysed using Kaplan–Meier survival curves. As matched patients had identical follow-up duration, loss to follow-up was not a censoring criterion, but failure at one visit was a censoring criterion. Two-sided $p \leq 0.050$ was considered statistically significant.

3. Results

3.1. Baseline Characteristics

Included were 202 eyes from 202 patients, with 101 eyes in each group. Table 1 shows the baseline comparisons between the groups. The MicroShunt group had higher American Society of Anaesthesiology (ASA) grades than the trabeculectomy group. At months 6, 12, and 18, respectively, 142, 92, and 36 eyes were available for analysis.

Table 1. Baseline demographics and characteristics. Data are expressed as proportions, means ± standard deviation, or medians [interquartile range] where appropriate. For the type of medications, ethnic groups, type of glaucoma, previous procedures, co-morbidities, and lens status, data represent the number of patients; '-' denotes matched variables.

Patient Characteristics	MicroShunt	Trabeculectomy	p-Value
Age (years)	69 [57–78]	66 [57–76]	0.250 *
IOP (mmHg)	22 [17–29]	20 [16–28]	0.182 *
Number of medications	4 [3–4]	4 [3–4]	0.273 *
- Prostaglandins	94 (93.1%)	96 (95.0%)	0.767 #
- Beta-blockers	76 (75.2%)	85 (84.2%)	0.161 #
- Alpha-2-agonists	53 (52.5%)	63 (62.4%)	0.200 #
- Carbonic anhydrase inhibitors	91 (90.1%)	92 (91.1%)	>0.999 #
- Parasympathomimetics	0 (0.0%)	1 (1.0%)	>0.999 #
Ethnic group			
- White	41 (40.6%)	41 (40.6%)	
- Black	17 (16.8%)	17 (16.8%)	
- Asian	14 (13.9%)	14 (13.9%)	-
- Other	15 (14.9%)	15 (14.9%)	
- Not stated	14 (13.9%)	14 (13.9%)	
Identify as female	37 (36.6%)	37 (36.6%)	-
Identify as male	64 (63.4%)	64 (63.4%)	-
Best-corrected visual acuity (logMAR)	0.2 [0.0–0.5]	0.2 [0.0–0.5]	0.814 *
Visual field mean deviation (dB)	−13.35 ± 8.10	−14.38 ± 8.13	0.546 **
Average RNFL thickness (microns)	57 [47–71]	55 [47–68]	0.670 *
Type of glaucoma			
- Primary open-angle glaucoma	74 (73.3%)	74 (73.3%)	
- Angle-closure glaucoma	12 (11.9%)	12 (11.9%)	-
- Secondary open-angle glaucoma	14 (13.9%)	14 (13.9%)	
- Normal tension glaucoma	1 (1.0%)	1 (1.0%)	

Table 1. Cont.

Patient Characteristics	MicroShunt	Trabeculectomy	p-Value
Previous laser treatment	37 (36.6%)	29 (28.7%)	0.294 #
- Selective laser trabeculoplasty	13 (12.9%)	7 (6.9%)	0.238 #
- Cyclodiode laser	7 (6.9%)	8 (7.9%)	>0.999 #
- Micropulse diode laser	14 (13.9%)	10 (9.9%)	0.515 #
- Laser peripheral iridotomy	8 (7.9%)	6 (5.9%)	0.783 #
- Endoscopic Cyclophotocoagulation	1 (1.0%)	0 (0.0%)	>0.999 #
Previous MIGS	12 (11.9%)	10 (9.9%)	0.822 #
- iStent	8 (7.9%)	5 (5.0%)	0.568 #
- Cypass	4 (4.0%)	6 (5.0%)	0.748 #
First or second eye undergoing glaucoma surgery			
- First eye	77 (76.2%)	77 (76.2%)	-
- Second eye	24 (23.8%)	24 (23.8%)	
Co-morbidities			
- Diabetes	20 (19.8%)	22 (21.8%)	0.863 #
- Hypertension	48 (47.5%)	42 (41.6%)	0.479 #
- Anti-coagulant use	3 (3.0%)	2 (2.0%)	>0.999 #
ASA grade			
- Grade 1	18 (17.8%)	34 (33.7%)	
- Grade 2	69 (68.3%)	53 (52.5%)	0.030 +
- Grade 3	13 (12.9%)	13 (12.9%)	
Pseudophakic lens status	51 (50.5%)	41 (40.6%)	0.220 #

* Mann–Whitney U test; ** unpaired t-test; # Fisher's exact test; + Chi-squared test.

3.2. Primary Outcomes

3.2.1. IOP

IOP was significantly lower than the baseline at all time points ($p \leq 0.001$) for both groups. In the MicroShunt group, IOP decreased from 22 [17–29] mmHg at the baseline to 15 [10–17] mmHg at Month-18 (Figure 1). In the trabeculectomy group, IOP decreased from 20 [16–28] at the baseline to 11 [10–13] mmHg. On Day-1, the MicroShunt group had lower IOPs than the trabeculectomy group (6 [4–8] mmHg vs. 8 [5–12] mmHg, respectively, $p < 0.001$). At Month-3 (11 [9–15] mmHg vs. 10 [7–13] mmHg, $p = 0.006$) and Month-6 (12 [10–16] mmHg vs. 11 [8–14] mmHg, $p = 0.048$), the IOP in the MicroShunt group was higher, although the Month-12 IOP was still higher but not statistically significant (13 [10–16] mmHg vs. 11 [8–14] mmHg, $p = 0.183$). Month-18 IOP was also higher in the MicroShunt group but not statistically significant ($p = 0.060$). Figure 1 shows a trend toward a higher median IOP with time in the MicroShunt compared to the trabeculectomy group. When comparing the cumulative number of eyes undergoing bleb revision as a proportion of the total number of available eyes for analysis between the groups, this was only significantly more in the trabeculectomy at Month-6 ($p = 0.004$).

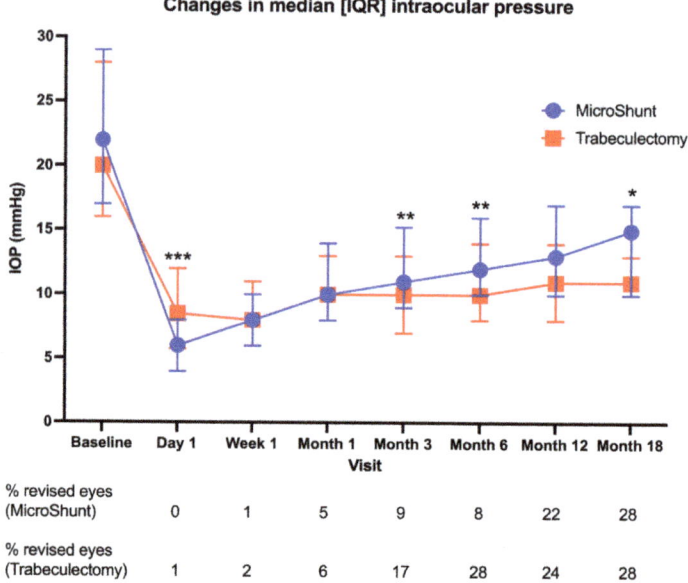

Figure 1. Changes in median IOP during follow-up after MicroShunt and trabeculectomy (* denotes $p \leq 0.050$ between groups; ** denotes $p \leq 0.010$ between groups, *** denotes $p \leq 0.001$ between groups, assessed using Mann–Whitney U tests). Error bars represent interquartile ranges. The cumulative percentage of eyes undergoing bleb revision for each group as the proportion of the total number of available eyes for analysis is displayed under each time point.

3.2.2. Medications

Both procedures were associated with a significantly lower need for medications than at the baseline for all time points ($p < 0.001$). Medications were reduced from four [3–4] at the baseline to zero [0–0] in both groups immediately post-surgery (Figure 2), with no significant differences between the groups until Month-12, when the trabeculectomy group used fewer medications than the MicroShunt group (0 [0–0] vs. 0 [0–1], respectively, $p = 0.024$), continued at Month-18 (0 [0–0] vs. 0 [0–2], $p = 0.019$).

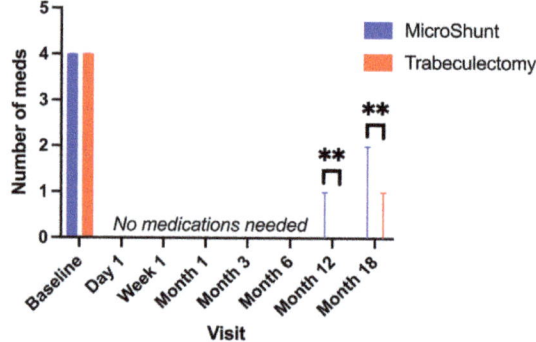

Figure 2. Changes in the median number of glaucoma medications during follow-up after MicroShunt and trabeculectomy (** denotes $p \leq 0.010$ between groups, assessed using Mann–Whitney U tests). Error bars represent interquartile ranges.

3.3. Secondary Outcomes

3.3.1. VF/MD

The VF/MD was similar to the baseline at Month-6 and Month-12 in both groups but worsened at Month-18 compared to the baseline, with no differences between the groups at any time point (Table 2). A sub-analysis of pseudophakic and non-pseudophakic eyes showed similar results; however, the VF/MD was similar to the baseline at Month-18 in the non-pseudophakic MicroShunt eyes.

Table 2. Changes in mean ± standard deviation VF/MD and median [IQR] RNFL thicknesses during follow-up after MicroShunt and trabeculectomy (* Mann–Whitney U test; ** unpaired *t*-test; # Wilcoxon test, ## paired *t*-test).

	MicroShunt	*p*-Value (Comparison with Baseline)	Trabeculectomy	*p*-Value (Comparison with Baseline)	*p*-Value (Comparison between Groups)
Baseline					
VF MD (dB)	−13.35 ± 8.10	-	−14.38 ± 8.13	-	0.546 **
RNFL (μm)	57 [47–71]	-	55 [47–68]	-	0.670 *
Day-1					
RNFL (μm)	59 [46–78]	<0.001 #	59 [49–75]	0.002 #	0.795 *
Week-1					
RNFL (μm)	64 [52–75]	<0.001 #	56 [46–78]	0.011 #	0.151 *
Month-1					
RNFL (μm)	56 [49–71]	0.732 #	56 [48–68]	0.181 #	0.947 *
Month-3					
RNFL (μm)	56 [46–66]	0.012 #	54 [47–65]	<0.001 #	0.663 *
Month-6					
VF MD (dB)	−13.80 ± 7.53	0.668 ##	−14.47 ± 8.56	0.147 ##	0.735 **
RNFL (μm)	57 [48–66]	0.072 #	50 [44–55]	<0.001 #	0.005 *
Month-12					
VF MD (dB)	−14.52 ± 8.18	0.348 ##	−15.73 ± 7.39	0.192 ##	0.638 **
RNFL (μm)	55 [47–69]	0.114 #	50 [43–55]	0.003 #	0.046 *
Month-18					
VF MD (dB)	−15.97 ± 8.26	0.009 ##	−16.45 ± 8.08	0.026 ##	0.882 **
RNFL (μm)	52 [46–63]	0.101 #	51 [46–61]	0.016 #	0.674 *

3.3.2. RNFL Thickness

The average RNFL thicknesses transiently increased postoperatively in both groups (Table 2) and returned to baseline levels per Month-1. At Month-3, the average thicknesses were lower than the baseline in both groups. However, thicknesses in the MicroShunt group were comparable to the baseline from Month-6, whereas thicknesses continued to be lower than the baseline in the trabeculectomy group. Month-6 and Month-12 thicknesses were lower in the trabeculectomy group compared to the MicroShunt group.

3.3.3. Success

Using the 21 mmHg upper limit, the probabilities of complete success were 65.3%, 55.1%, and 42.8% for MicroShunt and 63.9%, 58.1%, and 53.9% for trabeculectomy at Month-6, Month-12, and Month-18, respectively. Figure 3 shows a divergence between the groups with time, with lower complete success in the MicroShunt group. The probabilities of qualified success were 72.0%, 68.2%, and 68.2% for MicroShunt and 68.1%, 62.1%, and 62.1% for trabeculectomy at Month-6, Month-12, and Month-18, respectively. The probabilities of strict success were 52.9%, 44.5%, and 35.6% for MicroShunt and 46.4%,

40.1%, and 35.6% for trabeculectomy at Month-6, Month-12, and Month-18, respectively. No significant differences were found between the groups for all the success criteria. With 18 mmHg and 14 mmHg upper limits, similar results were obtained.

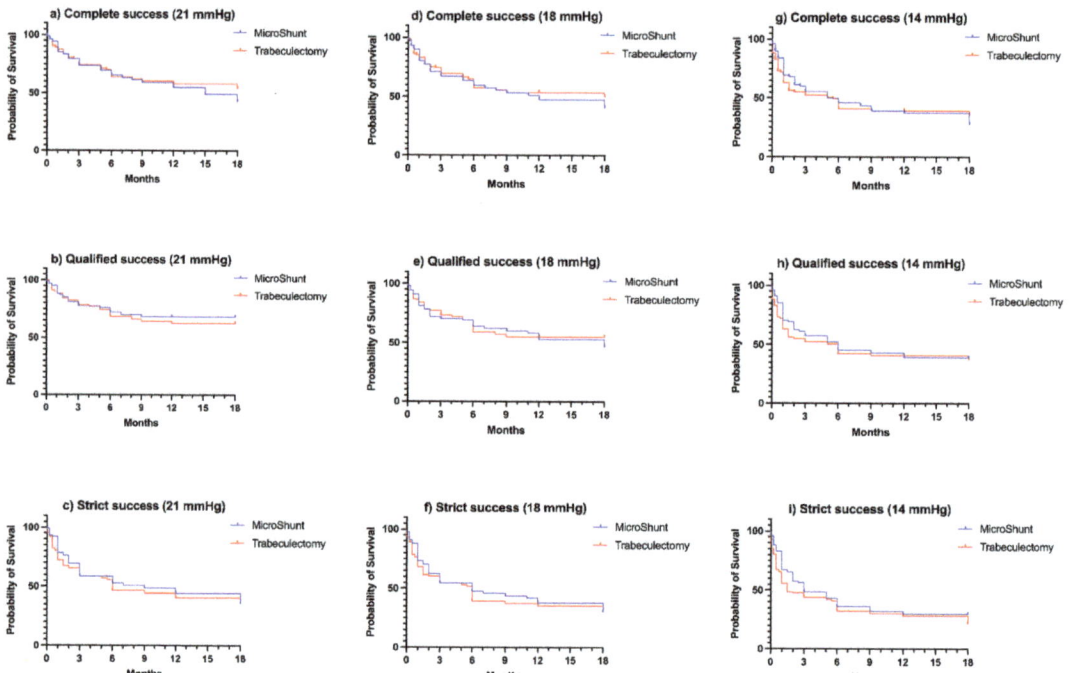

Figure 3. Kaplan–Meier survival curve of both groups during follow-up after MicroShunt and trabeculectomy: (**a**) complete success (IOP $\leq$ 21 mmHg; no theatre reoperation for glaucoma; no loss of light perception vision; no chronic hypotony (defined as IOP $\leq$ 5 mmHg on 2 consecutive follow-up visits from 3 months); and no use of postoperative adjunct medications to maintain adequate IOP), (**b**) qualified success (the aforementioned criteria, but with use of postoperative medications), (**c**) strict success ('complete success' criteria with at least 20% IOP reduction from baseline), (**d**) same as '(**a**)' but with IOP $\leq$ 18 mmHg, (**e**) same as '(**b**)' but with IOP $\leq$ 18 mmHg, (**f**) same as '(**c**)' but with IOP $\leq$ 18 mmHg, (**g**) same as '(**a**)' but with IOP $\leq$ 14 mmHg, (**h**) same as '(**b**)' but with IOP $\leq$ 14 mmHg, and (**i**) same as '(**c**)' but with IOP $\leq$ 14 mmHg. Log-rank (Mantel–Cox) test p-values were (**a**) $p = 0.715$, (**b**) $p = 0.595$, (**c**) $p = 0.489$, (**d**) $p = 0.645$, (**e**) $p = 0.828$, (**f**) $p = 0.494$, (**g**) $p = 0.616$, (**h**) $p = 0.464$, and (**i**) $p = 0.464$.

3.3.4. Complications and Interventions

Although more trabeculectomy than MicroShunt eyes had complications, this was not statistically significant between the groups (Table 3). The hypotony rates were similar, but there were more incidences of hypotony in the trabeculectomy group from Month-3 of the follow-up. Rates of chronic hypotony and maculopathy were higher in the trabeculectomy group. Ten trabeculectomy eyes required laser suture lysis.

Table 3. Numbers and proportions of patients with complications and interventions in both groups (* includes a patient with two occurrences, ** includes one patient with three occurrences, *** includes two patients with two occurrences, **** includes one patient with 5 occurrences).

Complication/Intervention	MicroShunt n (%)	Trabeculectomy n (%)	p-Value
Hypotony	46 (45.5%)	51 (50.5%)	0.573
- <3-months	44 (43.6%)	50 (49.5%)	0.890
- ≥3-months	4 (4.0%)	16 (15.8%)	0.008
Chronic hypotony	0 (0.0%)	10 (9.9%)	0.002
Choroidal effusion	13 (12.9%)	15 (14.9%)	0.839
Choroidal detachment	0 (0.0%)	2 (2.0%)	0.498
Hypotony maculopathy	1 (1.0%)	9 (8.9%)	0.019
Hyphaema	17 (16.8%)	11 (10.9%)	0.309
Malignant glaucoma	1 (1.0%)	0 (0.0%)	>0.999
Laser suture lysis	0 (0.0%)	10 (9.9%) *	0.002
Flat AC	4 (4.0%)	6 (5.9%)	0.748
AC reformation in theatre	0 (0.0%)	4 (4.0%) *	0.121
AC washout in clinic	1 (1.0%)	0 (0.0%)	>0.999
AC washout in theatre	2 (2.0%)	0 (0.0%)	0.498
AC Avastin injection in theatre	0 (0.0%)	2 (2.0%)	0.498
Bleb revision in clinic	3 (3.0%) * **	1 (1.0%)	0.621
Bleb revision in theatre	11 (10.9%) * ***	25 (24.8%) * ** *** ****	0.016
Secondary Cyclodiode treatment	2 (2.0%) *	0 (0.0%)	0.498
Secondary IOP-lowering surgery	2 (2.0%)	0 (0.0%)	0.498
Laser suture lysis	0 (0.0%)	4 (4.0%) *	0.121
Suture removal in theatre	0 (0.0%)	3 (3.0%)	0.246
Total n with complications (excluding hypotony)	32 (31.7%)	46 (45.5%)	0.060
- Including hypotony	59 (48.5%)	66 (65.3%)	0.385
Total n with theatre interventions	17 (16.8%)	31 (30.7%)	0.031

Significantly more trabeculectomy eyes had theatre interventions. Bleb revision was the most common intervention in both groups, with more trabeculectomy eyes requiring this procedure. Two MicroShunt eyes required further IOP-lowering surgery.

3.3.5. Operation Time and Number of Visits

The MicroShunt group had significantly shorter operation times (50 [44–62] vs. 71 [59–87] minutes, respectively, $p < 0.001$) and statistically significant fewer postoperative visits (8 [6–10] vs. 10 [7–13] visits, $p = 0.001$) than the trabeculectomy group.

4. Discussion

This study has found that trabeculectomy reduced the IOP and the need for medications more than MicroShunt. Changes in the VF and success rates were similar, but RNFL's thickness loss slowed after MicroShunt. While complication rates were comparable, there were fewer theatre interventions and postoperative visits post-MicroShunt. These findings have a significant clinical impact, demonstrating that MicroShunt may not be the worthy successor to trabeculectomy in the treatment paradigm of moderate-to-advanced glaucoma.

4.1. IOP

Although IOP reaches low values in both groups, this study found that trabeculectomy had better IOP-lowering efficacy. The greater immediate IOP-lowering efficacy of the MicroShunt on Day-1, also reported in prior studies [16,17], may be attributable to the device's predictable nature against trabeculectomy's complex suture-tensioning techniques. There is clinical significance to the noticeable trend towards higher IOPs in the MicroShunt group over time. The non-significance between groups from Month-12 may be explained by the smaller sample sizes at each subsequent follow-up visit after Month-3, although this study's sample size at Month-18 is comparable to previous retrospective studies with 6-month follow-up [3,13].

Baker et al.'s [12] study with 0.2 mg/mL MMC observed IOP reductions from 21.1 mmHg to 14.3 mmHg in the MicroShunt group at Month-12. We found a greater reduction at Month-12 from 22 [17–29] mmHg to 13 [10–16] mmHg. This suggests that 0.2 mg/mL MMC may be less efficacious for IOP-lowering than the 0.4 mg/mL in this study. Wagner et al.'s [13] study used 0.2 mg/mL MMC but found a similar IOP reduction as this study, suggesting that MMC concentration may have a minimal effect on efficacy. These discrepancies necessitate further investigations into the optimal MMC dose during glaucoma surgery. However, differences in the cohorts' demographics, such as fewer ethnic heterogeneity [12] and medication use [12,13] than in this study, decrease scarring risk and subsequent IOP control [12] and thus may confound MMC comparisons. Nonetheless, the clinical significance of the greater IOPs from Month-3 and the trend toward greater IOP increases in the MicroShunt group found in this study constitutes a significant finding, suggesting that trabeculectomy should still be utilised as the preferred surgery when a lower target pressure is sought, such as those patients with normal-tension glaucoma. Although this study is the first to present Month-18 results comparing both procedures, longer-term investigations are required to investigate whether IOP continues to increase after Month-18 following MicroShunt when compared to trabeculectomy since trabeculectomy is known to lower IOP effectively over up to 20 years [18].

4.2. Medications

Although both groups significantly reduced medication use, greater medication-lowering efficacy was observed with trabeculectomy at Month-3, Month-12, and Month-18. The reductions are higher than in previous studies; for example, Baker et al. [12] reported reductions from 3.1 to 0.6 medications at Month-12 in their MicroShunt groups, compared to 4 [3–4] to 0 [0–1] medications in this study. The higher reductions found in this study may be due to higher baseline medications, enabling the medication-lowering efficacy of both procedures to be more pronounced. Our findings differ from previous comparative studies [3,12,13] that showed similar medication-lowering efficacy of MicroShunt and trabeculectomy. Whether this is due to conflicts of interest in previous studies on the MicroShunt [3,12] or small sample sizes [3,13], future prospective studies are necessitated to investigate whether the increase in medications following the MicroShunt procedure is a longer-term effect.

4.3. VF/MD

The VF/MD was not different between the groups at any time point, suggesting similar effects on the functional preservation effect by both surgeries. In the only previous study comparing VF between MicroShunt and trabeculectomy, Pillunat et al. [3] also reported no significant change in either group at Month-6. However, their small sample size of 26 eyes in each group limits the reliability of the conclusions. Furthermore, the inclusion of solely Caucasian patients invalidates the comparison with the present study, which included ≥45.5% non-Caucasians, who have a higher likelihood of subsequent failure after bleb-forming surgery than Caucasians [12]. Studies evaluating VF post-trabeculectomy have come to inconsistent conclusions [19,20], necessitating more studies comparing VF progressions after MicroShunt and trabeculectomy. Furthermore, the VF progression seen at Month-18 in both groups was likely due to natural glaucomatous progression despite

IOP-lowering surgery or due to the decreases in the sample size with time. This may also explain the similarity of the VF/MD at Month-18 compared to the baseline in non-pseudophakic eyes in the MicroShunt group, suggesting that potential cataract progression may not have modulated VF/MD progression.

4.4. RNFL Thickness

The RNFL thickness after MicroShunt implantation has not been studied before. This study shows that MicroShunt may delay RNFL thickness loss compared to trabeculectomy. Similar to our findings, a previous study showed that RNFL thicknesses increased in the first postoperative week following trabeculectomy but decreased to baseline levels in subsequent visits [21]. Potential explanations include the reversal or rebound of the bowing of the laminar cribrosa by the elevated pre-intervention IOP, which manifests as a decreased cup area postoperatively [21]. It may also be due to the transient rebound to the normal shape and size of the retinal ganglion cell axons following dramatic IOP reductions post-surgery [22]. Additionally, Ch'ng et al. [23] attributed transient RNFL thickness increases post-trabeculectomy to postoperative inflammation.

The thinner RNFL values in this study's trabeculectomy cohort from Month-6 may be explained by the higher hypotony levels from the Month-3 follow-up observed with significantly more cases of chronic hypotony and maculopathy, where the formation of retinal folds may have decreased the RNFL thicknesses in the trabeculectomy cohort compared to the MicroShunt. Furthermore, it may have been difficult to measure RNFL thinning with a baseline median RNFL thickness of 57 µm and 55 µm in the MicroShunt and trabeculectomy groups, respectively, since there may be a 'floor effect' at approximately 50 µm with Spectralis OCT [24].

4.5. Success Rates

The trend toward lower 'complete success' in the MicroShunt group is clinically important, supporting that MicroShunt is clinically less efficacious than trabeculectomy. With similar definitions, Wagner et al. [13] also found no differences in 'complete' and 'qualified' successes. However, 'strict success' was significantly higher in their trabeculectomy group, and they observed higher success rates in both groups compared to the present study. This may be because of their small sample size and better baseline VF/MD, affecting comparability. Baker et al. [12] also observed lower 'strict success' in their MicroShunt than trabeculectomy groups (53.9 vs. 72.7%; $p < 0.01$) at Month-12. The prevention of medication reintroduction until a predetermined IOP threshold should have resulted in lower success rates than in the present study, where medications were reintroduced at the surgeons' discretion. However, this study observed similar 'strict success' at Month-12 between the groups. This may be due to Baker et al.'s [12] baseline IOP inclusion threshold of ≥15 mmHg. Therefore, attaining a prespecified 20% IOP reduction may be easier compared to this study, which included all baseline IOP values. Their failure definition of inadequate IOP reduction at two consecutive visits compared to one in this study may also favour higher success. Additionally, their inclusion of solely primary open-angle glaucoma [12] may not reflect real-world results with differing glaucoma subtypes.

This study's trabeculectomy 'strict success' rate at Month-18 (35.6%) was low compared to Kirwan et al.'s [25] 65% at Year-2. Many factors contribute to this difference: Patients had no previous MIGS or diodes, suggesting milder glaucoma, whilst a large proportion of our cohort had these procedures. Additionally, the inclusion of both eyes from each patient, where applicable, may have skewed their results in favour of higher success [26] and violated statistical assumptions [27]; the inclusion of more Caucasians (79% vs. 40.6% in this study) who have a lower risk of scarring after bleb-forming surgery than black patients [12]; and the inclusion of solely open-angle glaucoma.

4.6. Complications and Theatre Interventions

Although the lower complication rate in the MicroShunt group is statistically insignificant, this is still clinically important, and the lower theatre intervention rate for MicroShunt confirms the hypothesis of a better safety profile. Additionally, higher ASA grades in the MicroShunt group, which may have been intentional due to a better-hypothesised speed and safety, may have skewed safety profiles in favour of trabeculectomy.

The posterior MicroShunt bleb has a broad, diffuse, and low elevation with low vascularity, whereas the typical trabeculectomy bleb is anterior with a medium-high diffuse elevation and variable vascularity. Thus, the trabeculectomy bleb is more prone to overdraining and leakage (increasing the risk of infection and bleb dysaesthesia), resulting in more observed cases of chronic hypotony compared to the MicroShunt, which has a controlled lumen size that drains fluid more controllably. This theory makes it plausible that there were fewer postoperative theatre interventions in the MicroShunt group, as found by prior studies [3,12]. Indeed, due to the more problematic bleb, more cases of surgical bleb revision occurred in the trabeculectomy group. Differing definitions of what constituted a 'theatre intervention' and heterogeneity in the reporting hindered comparability with previous studies. Similar to Baker et al.'s [12] findings, laser suture lysis was necessary following trabeculectomy to allow for flow titration. The controlled flow titration of the MicroShunt eliminated the requirement for flow-restricting sutures and subsequent suture lysis.

4.7. Postoperative Visits and Operation Times

As the first study to compare postoperative visits, the findings confirm the hypothesis that MicroShunt results in less postoperative burden. Additionally, despite the potential learning curve with the new MicroShunt technique [12], a shorter MicroShunt operation time was found, contrary to Pillunat et al.'s [3] findings. The larger heterogeneous sample size supports the increased validity of the present study's result. In the context of a significant backlog of glaucoma surgery after the coronavirus pandemic, the reduced operation time, visits, and reinterventions for the MicroShunt cohort mean that this device does constitute a favourable option for managing certain glaucoma patients. Furthermore, these factors may also mitigate the initial MicroShunt acquisition cost compared to the traditional trabeculectomy approach with minimal material costs and could be more cost-effective for lower-risk patients to manage glaucoma more safely. However, a recent cost analysis of Baker et al.'s [12] findings in American healthcare suggests that trabeculectomy is more cost-effective than MicroShunt [28], necessitating the validation of this finding in the UK NHS.

5. Conclusions

For the surgical treatment of refractory glaucoma in a clinically heterogeneous population, MicroShunt has inferior efficacy to trabeculectomy regarding IOP and medications, but MicroShunt has a superior safety profile and reduced postoperative burden. This contributes cautious findings to the paucity of evidence surrounding the MicroShunt's potential to replace trabeculectomy as the gold standard operation in the glaucoma treatment paradigm, suggesting that trabeculectomy should still be reserved for higher-risk or more advanced patients. However, this study has also shown that the MicroShunt can reduce IOP safely with a potentially lesser burden on already stretched glaucoma services. Further longer-term studies are needed to corroborate this study's findings and ascertain MicroShunt's position in the surgical treatment of glaucoma.

Author Contributions: Conceptualisation, P.A.B. and E.M.N.; Methodology and Surgical Protocol, P.A.B., E.M.N., F.A., L.C., N.V., S.A., S.M.H.L., M.F.C. and M.X.F.; Data Acquisition, M.X.F. and M.D.; Data Analysis, M.X.F.; Writing—Original Draft Preparation, M.X.F.; Writing—Critical Revision, P.A.B. and E.M.N. All authors have read and agreed to the published version of the manuscript.

Funding: This research received no external funding.

Institutional Review Board Statement: This study was conducted in accordance with the Declaration of Helsinki and approved by local clinical governance teams at the Imperial College Healthcare NHS Trust and Hillingdon Hospitals NHS Trust, who confirmed that this analysis did not require formal ethics approval as it was conducted as part of a service evaluation.

Informed Consent Statement: Patient consent was waived due to its retrospective nature.

Data Availability Statement: The datasets used and/or analysed during the current study are available from the corresponding author upon reasonable request.

Acknowledgments: Locum consultants Dimitrios Besinis, Alastair Porteous, Joanna Tryfinopoulou, Ahmed Al-Nahrawy, and Nada Mohamed; the fellows and trainees are also acknowledged for their care for the study patients.

Conflicts of Interest: The authors declare no conflict of interest.

References

1. Quigley, H.; Broman, A.T. The Number of People with Glaucoma Worldwide in 2010 and 2020. *Br. J. Ophthalmol.* **2006**, *90*, 262–267. [CrossRef]
2. Gaasterland, D.E.; Ederer, F.; Beck, A.; Costarides, A.; Leef, D.; Closek, J.; Banks, J.; Jackson, S.; Moore, K.; Vela, A.; et al. The Advanced Glaucoma Intervention Study (AGIS): 7. The Relationship between Control of Intraocular Pressure and Visual Field Deterioration.The AGIS Investigators. *Am. J. Ophthalmol.* **2000**, *130*, 429–440. [CrossRef]
3. Pillunat, K.R.; Herber, R.; Haase, M.A.; Jamke, M.; Jasper, C.S.; Pillunat, L.E. PRESERFLO™ MicroShunt versus Trabeculectomy: First Results on Efficacy and Safety. *Acta Ophthalmol.* **2021**, *100*, e779–e790. [CrossRef]
4. Gedde, S.J.; Schiffman, J.C.; Feuer, W.J.; Herndon, L.W.; Brandt, J.D.; Budenz, D.L. Treatment Outcomes in the Tube Versus Trabeculectomy (TVT) Study after Five Years of Follow-Up. *Am. J. Ophthalmol.* **2012**, *153*, 789–803.e2. [CrossRef] [PubMed]
5. Landers, J.; Martin, K.; Sarkies, N.; Bourne, R.; Watson, P. A Twenty-Year Follow-up Study of Trabeculectomy: Risk Factors and Outcomes. *Ophthalmology* **2012**, *119*, 694–702. [CrossRef] [PubMed]
6. Richter, G.M.; Coleman, A.L. Minimally Invasive Glaucoma Surgery: Current Status and Future Prospects. *Clin. Ophthalmol.* **2016**, *10*, 189–206. [CrossRef] [PubMed]
7. Batlle, J.F.; Fantes, F.; Riss, I.; Pinchuk, L.; Alburquerque, R.; Kato, Y.P.; Arrieta, E.; Peralta, A.C.; Palmberg, P.; Parrish, R.K.; et al. Three-Year Follow-up of a Novel Aqueous Humor MicroShunt. *J. Glaucoma* **2016**, *25*, e58–e65. [CrossRef]
8. Holland, L.J.; Mercieca, K.J.; Kirwan, J.F. Effect of COVID-19 Pandemic on Glaucoma Surgical Practices in the UK. *Br. J. Ophthalmol.* **2021**. [CrossRef] [PubMed]
9. Buffault, J.; Graber, M.; Bensmail, D.; Bluwol, É.; Jeanteur, M.N.; Abitbol, O.; Benhatchi, N.; Sauvan, L.; Lachkar, Y. Efficacy and Safety at 6 Months of the XEN Implant for the Management of Open Angle Glaucoma. *Sci. Rep.* **2020**, *10*, 4527. [CrossRef]
10. Schlenker, M.B.; Durr, G.M.; Michaelov, E.; Ahmed, I.I.K. Intermediate Outcomes of a Novel Standalone Ab Externo SIBS Microshunt with Mitomycin C. *Am. J. Ophthalmol.* **2020**, *215*, 141–153. [CrossRef] [PubMed]
11. Fujimoto, T.; Nakashima, K.I.; Watanabe-Kitamura, F.; Watanabe, T.; Nakamura, K.; Maki, K.; Shimazaki, A.; Kato, M.; Tanihara, H.; Inoue, T. Intraocular Pressure-Lowering Effects of Trabeculectomy Versus MicroShunt Insertion in Rabbit Eyes. *Transl. Vis. Sci. Technol.* **2021**, *10*, 9. [CrossRef] [PubMed]
12. Baker, N.D.; Barnebey, H.S.; Moster, M.R.; Stiles, M.C.; Vold, S.D.; Khatana, A.K.; Flowers, B.E.; Grover, D.S.; Strouthidis, N.G.; Panarelli, J.F. Ab-Externo MicroShunt versus Trabeculectomy in Primary Open-Angle Glaucoma: One-Year Results from a 2-Year Randomized, Multicenter Study. *Ophthalmology* **2021**, *128*, 1710–1721. [CrossRef] [PubMed]
13. Wagner, F.M.; Schuster, A.K.; Munder, A.; Muehl, M.; Pfeiffer, N.; Hoffmann, E.M. Comparison of Subconjunctival Microinvasive Glaucoma Surgery and Trabeculectomy. *Acta Ophthalmol.* **2021**, *100*, e1120–e1126. [CrossRef] [PubMed]
14. Lichter, P.R.; Musch, D.C.; Gillespie, B.W.; Guire, K.E.; Janz, N.K.; Wren, P.A.; Mills, M.P.H.R.P. Interim Clinical Outcomes in the Collaborative Initial Glaucoma Treatment Study Comparing Initial Treatment Randomized to Medications or Surgery. *Ophthalmology* **2001**, *108*, 1943–1953. [CrossRef]
15. Shaarawy, T.M.; Sherwood, M.B.; Grehn, F. *Guidelines on Design and Reporting of Glaucoma Surgical Trials*; Kugler Publications: Amsterdam, The Netherlands, 2008.
16. Batlle, J.F.; Corona, A.; Albuquerque, R. Long-Term Results of the PRESERFLO MicroShunt in Patients with Primary Open-Angle Glaucoma from a Single-Center Nonrandomized Study. *J. Glaucoma* **2021**, *30*, 281–286. [CrossRef]
17. Tanner, A.; Haddad, F.; Fajardo-Sanchez, J.; Nguyen, E.; Xin Thong, K.; Ah-Moye, S.; Perl, N.; Abu-Bakra, M.; Kulkarni, A.; Trikha, S.; et al. One-Year Surgical Outcomes of the PreserFlo MicroShunt in Glaucoma: A Multicentre Analysis. *Br. J. Ophthalmol.* **2022**, 1–8. [CrossRef]
18. Gedde, S.J.; Feuer, W.J.; Lim, K.S.; Barton, K.; Goyal, S.; Ahmed, I.I.K.; Brandt, J.D. Treatment Outcomes in the Primary Tube Versus Trabeculectomy Study after 3 Years of Follow-Up. *Ophthalmology* **2020**, *127*, 333–345. [CrossRef]
19. Wanichwecharungruang, B.; Ratprasatporn, N. 24-Month Outcomes of XEN45 Gel Implant versus Trabeculectomy in Primary Glaucoma. *PLoS ONE* **2021**, *16*, e0256362. [CrossRef]

20. Schargus, M.; Busch, C.; Rehak, M.; Meng, J.; Schmidt, M.; Bormann, C.; Unterlauft, J.D. Functional Monitoring after Trabeculectomy or XEN Microstent Implantation Using Spectral Domain Optical Coherence Tomography and Visual Field Indices—A Retrospective Comparative Cohort Study. *Biology* **2021**, *10*, 273. [CrossRef]
21. Raghu, N.; Pandav, S.S.; Kaushik, S.; Ichhpujani, P.; Gupta, A. Effect of Trabeculectomy on RNFL Thickness and Optic Disc Parameters Using Optical Coherence Tomography. *Eye* **2012**, *26*, 1131. [CrossRef]
22. Quigley, H.A.; Addicks, E.M.; Green, W.R.; Maumenee, A.E. Optic Nerve Damage in Human Glaucoma. II. The Site of Injury and Susceptibility to Damage. *Arch. Ophthalmol.* **1981**, *99*, 635–649. [CrossRef] [PubMed]
23. Ch'ng, T.W.; Gillmann, K.; Hoskens, K.; Rao, H.L.; Mermoud, A.; Mansouri, K. Effect of Surgical Intraocular Pressure Lowering on Retinal Structures—Nerve Fibre Layer, Foveal Avascular Zone, Peripapillary and Macular Vessel Density: 1 Year Results. *Eye* **2020**, *34*, 562. [CrossRef] [PubMed]
24. Mwanza, J.C.; Budenz, D.L.; Warren, J.L.; Webel, A.D.; Reynolds, C.E.; Barbosa, D.T.; Lin, S. Retinal Nerve Fibre Layer Thickness Floor and Corresponding Functional Loss in Glaucoma. *Br. J. Ophthalmol.* **2015**, *99*, 732–737. [CrossRef] [PubMed]
25. Kirwan, J.F.; Lockwood, A.J.; Shah, P.; Macleod, A.; Broadway, D.C.; King, A.J.; McNaught, A.I.; Agrawal, P. Trabeculectomy in the 21st Century: A Multicenter Analysis. *Ophthalmology* **2013**, *120*, 2532–2539. [CrossRef]
26. Iwasaki, K.; Takamura, Y.; Nishida, T.; Sawada, A.; Iwao, K.; Shinmura, A.; Kunimatsu-Sanuki, S.; Yamamoto, T.; Tanihara, H.; Sugiyama, K.; et al. Comparing Trabeculectomy Outcomes between First and Second Operated Eyes: A Multicenter Study. *PLoS ONE* **2016**, *11*, e0162569. [CrossRef]
27. Karakosta, A.; Vassilaki, M.; Plainis, S.; Elfadl, N.H.; Tsilimbaris, M.; Moschandreas, J. Choice of Analytic Approach for Eye-Specific Outcomes: One Eye or Two? *Am. J. Ophthalmol* **2012**, *153*, 571–579.e1. [CrossRef]
28. Atik, A.; Fahy, E.; Rhodes, L.A.; Samuels, B.C.; Mennemeyer, S.T.; Girkin, C.A. Comparative Cost-Effectiveness of Trabeculectomy versus MicroShunt in the United States Medicare System. *Ophthalmology* 2022, *in press*. [CrossRef]

Article

Efficacy of the PRESERFLO MicroShunt and a Meta-Analysis of the Literature

Shigeo S. M. Pawiroredjo [1], Wichor M. Bramer [2], Noemi D. Pawiroredjo [3], Jan Pals [1], Huub J. Poelman [1], Victor A. de Vries [1], Roger C. W. Wolfs [1] and Wishal D. Ramdas [1,*]

1. Department of Ophthalmology, Erasmus Medical Center, University Medical Center, 3000 CA Rotterdam, The Netherlands
2. Medical Library, Erasmus Medical Center, University Medical Center, 3000 CA Rotterdam, The Netherlands
3. Faculty of Science, Vrije Universiteit Amsterdam, 1081 HV Amsterdam, The Netherlands
* Correspondence: w.ramdas@erasmusmc.nl; Tel.: +31-10-7033691; Fax: +31-10-7035105

Abstract: Background: Recent studies on the PRESERFLO MicroShunt suggest that it may be effective in lowering intraocular pressure (IOP); however, the number of studies on this device remains limited. Therefore, we assessed the efficacy of the PRESERFLO MicroShunt in patients with glaucoma and performed a meta-analysis of published results. Methods: Prospective study including all patients that underwent PRESERFLO MicroShunt surgery from 2018 onwards. Sub-analyses were performed for cataract-combined procedures. To compare our results, we performed a systematic review and meta-analysis. IOP, IOP-lowering medication and surgical complications reported in the retrieved studies were assessed. Results: A total of 72 eyes underwent PRESERFLO-implant surgery (59 as standalone procedure and 13 as cataract-combined procedure). No significant differences were found in IOP and IOP-lowering medication between both groups. The mean ± standard deviation IOP and IOP-lowering medications of both groups taken together declined from 21.72 ± 8.35 to 15.92 ± 8.54 mmHg ($p < 0.001$, 26.7% reduction) and 3.40 to 0.93 ($p < 0.001$, 72.6% reduction) at 1 year follow-up, respectively. Secondary surgeries were required in 19.4% of eyes, the majority (71.4%) within 6 months. The meta-analysis including 14 studies (totaling 1213 PRESERFLO MicroShunt surgeries) from the systematic review showed a mean preoperative IOP and IOP-lowering medication of 22.28 ± 5.38 and 2.97 ± 1.07, respectively. The three-years postoperative pooled mean was (weighted mean difference, 95% CI) 11.07 (10.27 [8.23–12.32], $p < 0.001$) mmHg and 0.91 (1.77 [1.26–2.28], $p < 0.001$) for IOP and IOP-lowering medication, respectively. The most common reported complication was hypotony (2–39%). Conclusion: The PRESERFLO MicroShunt is effective and safe in lowering IOP and the number of IOP-lowering medications.

Keywords: PRESERFLO; MicroShunt SIBS polymer; ab externo surgery; MIGS; glaucoma; intraocular pressure (IOP)

1. Introduction

Glaucoma is an optic neuropathy which is often caused by a rapid increase and/or prolonged periods of elevated intraocular pressure (IOP) [1]. Treatment of glaucoma is mainly focused on lowering of the IOP [2]. The first-line treatment of glaucoma usually consists of IOP-lowering medication [3]. If the target IOP is not achieved using IOP-lowering medication, laser treatment or incisional surgery is introduced [1]. Trabeculectomy is generally regarded as the gold standard among surgical glaucoma treatments for many years and has shown to drastically reduce IOP; however, postoperative interventions are frequently required because of the high risk of complications [4,5]. Therefore, there has been an increased demand for safer and less invasive surgical treatment options. These are the so-called minimally invasive glaucoma surgeries (MIGS) and aim to reduce the IOP whilst lowering the risk of complications [6,7]. One of these new implants is the PRESERFLO MicroShunt

(Santen Inc., Miami, FL; formerly known as the InnFocus MicroShunt). The PRESERFLO MicroShunt is an 8.5 mm long tube with a 70 µm lumen composed of poly(styrene-block-isobutylene-block-styrene), or SIBS. This device is implanted via an ab externo approach in the anterior chamber-angle, allowing outflow of aqueous humor from the anterior chamber to a posterior subconjunctival bleb [8]. Implantation of the PRESERFLO MicroShunt could be performed standalone or in combination with cataract surgery and is augmented with mitomycin-C to prevent postoperative scarring [9,10]. Recent studies on the PRESERFLO MicroShunt suggest that it is effective in lowering IOP and the number of IOP-lowering medications; however, the number of studies on this device remains limited. The aim of this study is to assess the efficacy and safety of the PRESERFLO MicroShunt as a standalone and a cataract-combined procedure in patients with glaucoma. Furthermore, a systematic review with meta-analysis was conducted to see whether the results of the current study are in line with the available literature and to give an overall view of its performance across multiple studies.

2. Materials and Methods

2.1. Study Design

The current study was conducted in a subset of the Erasmus Glaucoma Cohort [11]. For the current analyses, a prospective single-center study was conducted. All patients who underwent PRESERFLO MicroShunt implantation at the department of ophthalmology of the Erasmus Medical Center, Rotterdam, The Netherlands, from July 2019 till June 2021 were included in the current study.

All patients underwent extensive ophthalmologic examination including best corrected visual acuity, autorefraction, gonioscopy, and applanation tonometry. Data (IOP and number of IOP-lowering medications) on 1 day, 1 week, 1 month, 3 months, 6 months, 1 year, and the last postoperative visit were collected. The Medical Ethics Committee of the Erasmus University had approved the study. Formal consent was not required, because patients did not undergo non-clinically related interventions.

2.2. Surgical Procedure

All surgeries were either performed by one of the two surgeons (RCWW and WDR). First, local or general anesthesia was administered. A 6 to 8 mm incision was made through the conjunctiva at the limbus and the Tenon's capsule was dissected from the sclera using blunt tipped scissors. Three LASIK sponges with 0.2 mg/mL mitomycin-C were then placed beneath the conjunctiva flap for 3 min. The flap was then washed with a sterile saline solution. Bipolar diathermy was used to avoid bleeding (if required). An inked marker was then used to mark a point on the sclera 3 mm posterior from the limbus. Next, a shallow 2 mm scleral pocket was formed using a 1 mm slit knife. A needle tract was made into the anterior chamber using a 25-gauge needle through the scleral pocket, bisecting the iridocorneal angle. The MicroShunt was then inserted through the needle tract using forceps with the bevel up, until the wedge fins of the MicroShunt locked into the scleral pocket to avoid migration. Flow of aqueous humor was confirmed by priming and observing drop formation at the distal end of the MicroShunt. Once the flow was confirmed, the distal end of the MicroShunt was tucked under the Tenon's capsule and the Tenon's capsule was then pulled up and over the MicroShunt. Lastly, the conjunctiva was closed using Vicryl 8-0 sutures.

The main indication for cataract surgery was a narrow anterior chamber or significant cataract. In case of a combined procedure, cataract surgery was performed directly after administrating mitomycin-C and before the needle tract was created.

A secondary surgery was indicated if the MicroShunt failed to achieve the desired reduction in IOP. Secondary surgery was performed as follows: the conjunctiva of the bleb area was opened, and all the tissue adhesions were removed. Mitomycin-C was not used. Next, the PRESERFLO MicroShunt was primed. Lastly, the conjunctiva was closed with Vicryl 8-0 sutures.

2.3. Assessment of Main Outcomes

IOP was assessed using Goldman applanation tonometry (Haag-Streit, Köniz, Switzerland), which had been calibrated according to manufacturer's recommendations. IOP-lowering medications were divided into several categories which included: prostaglandins, beta-blockers, carbonic anhydrase inhibitors, oral acetazolamide, and alfa-2 agonists. Fixed combinations of eye drops were calculated as two separate drugs. The number of IOP-lowering medications was then calculated by adding the number of categories to one another [12]. Hypotony was defined as an IOP $\leq$ 5 mmHg at two or more consecutive postoperative visits (excluding one day postoperative).

2.4. Search Strategy, Study Eligibility and Quality Assessment

For the second part of the study, a systematic review and meta-analysis of the literature was conducted in which the Embase, Medline ALL Ovid (Pubmed), Web of science (SCI-EXPANDED & SSCI, 1975) and Cochrane CENTRAL register of Trials were searched up to 24 May 2022 (date last searched). Reporting of the systematic review was achieved by adhering to the Preferred Reporting Items for Systematic review and Meta-Analyses (PRISMA) and the Meta-analysis Of Observational Studies in Epidemiology (MOOSE) guidelines [13,14]. Firstly, studies with an available abstract, with human participants, and studies of which a full text was available in English were independently screened by two researchers (SSMP and NDP). Secondly, the full text was read to assess whether an article was eligible for inclusion and the reference list was scanned to find additional eligible studies. Finally, the results were compared, and discrepancies were discussed. If the two researchers could not reach consensus, a third researcher (WDR) was involved to clarify. Studies had to report on pre- and post-operative IOP and/or IOP-lowering medication. Exclusion criteria were case reports or a follow-up of less than 6 months. If the same study population was used in multiple studies, only one study was included. Next, relevant data was extracted from the articles which included author, sample size, publication year, diagnosis, study design, follow-up, number of secondary surgeries, occurrence of complications, pre- and post-operative IOP and IOP-lowering medications, and proportion of patients without any IOP-lowering medication at follow-up. To assess the methodological quality of the individual studies, the Newcastle–Ottawa Scale for assessing the quality of comparative non-randomized studies was used [15].

2.5. Statistical Analysis

Baseline characteristics were analyzed using the independent t-test for continuous data and the chi-square test (or Fisher's exact test if applicable) for categorical data. The paired samples t-test was used for within subgroup analysis (e.g., pre- and post-operative IOP).

Differences in IOP and IOP-lowering medication over time were assessed using linear mixed models. Two models were created both assuming an unstructured correlation matrix, in which one of the variables was fitted as the dependent variable with visit (fixed) as a factor. The models were adjusted for age and gender (both fixed) and accounted for using both eyes from the same individual. Kaplan–Meier analyses were performed in which failure was defined as requiring secondary surgery (i.e., bleb revision or placement of another glaucoma drainage device). Follow-up was counted as the date of first surgery until the date of requiring secondary surgery. If an eye did not require secondary surgery, follow-up was counted as the date of first surgery until the date of the last postoperative visit. A separate Kaplan–Meier analysis was performed in which failure was defined according to the criteria by the World Glaucoma Association (WGA) [16]. Surgery was considered a failure if a patient had <20% reduction in IOP from baseline or if the IOP was out of target range (5–18 mmHg, inclusive) for two consecutive visits. Both counted after the first month postoperative onwards. If an eye met the failure criteria as defined by the WGA, follow-up was counted as the day of surgery until the first day failure was noted. The log-rank test was used to assess statistically significant differences between PRESERFLO as a standalone procedure and PRESERFLO as a cataract-combined procedure.

Statistical analyses were performed using SPSS v.25 for Windows (SPSS Inc., Chicago, IL, USA). Statistical significance was considered if $p < 0.05$.

Meta-analyses were performed using Revman (RevMan 5.3 for Windows and Mac; The Cochrane Collaboration, Oxford, UK). The mean and standard deviations were extracted to calculate the weighted mean difference (WMD) with corresponding 95% CI and the pooled mean with standard deviation for the specified time intervals. For the meta-analyses, fixed-effect models were used to pool the results. I2 statistics were calculated to assess heterogeneity.

3. Results

A total of 72 eyes (of 60 patients) underwent PRESERFLO MicroShunt implantation of whom 59 underwent a standalone procedure. The median (interquartile range) follow-up was 0.72 (0.33–1.12) and 1.15 (0.65–1.66) years for the standalone procedure and the cataract-combined procedure, respectively. One patient in the standalone procedure group was lost to follow-up at 1 month. Patients who underwent a standalone procedure had a significantly higher central corneal thickness compared to patients who underwent a cataract-combined procedure ($p = 0.025$; Table 1).

Table 1. Baseline preoperative characteristics of the population presented as the mean ± standard deviation unless stated otherwise.

	PRESERFLO MicroShunt (n = 59 Eyes)	PRESERFLO MicroShunt Combined with Cataract Extraction (n = 13 Eyes)	p-Value
Age (years)	67.11 ± 10.4	70.32 ± 13.4	0.343
Gender, female (n,%)	24 (40.6)	3 (23)	0.346
Caucasian descent (n,%)	30 (50.8)	7 (53.8)	0.384
Untreated IOP at diagnosis (mmHg)	25.0 ± 10.7	24.9 ± 8.5	0.957
IOP (mmHg)	21.4 ± 8.8	23.4 ± 5.8	0.311
Number of IOP-lowering medication	3.5 ± 1.4	2.9 ± 1.4	0.106
Visual acuity	0.75 ± 0.41	0.75 ± 0.23	0.942
Central corneal thickness (μm)	542.3 ± 36.3	514.3 ± 45	0.025
Previous intraocular surgery (n,%) *	14 (23.7)	0 (0)	0.059
Follow-up (median [IQR])	0.72 (0.33–1.12)	1.15 (0.65–1.66)	0.111

* = cataract surgery (24 of 59 eyes) not counted; IOP = intraocular pressure; IQR = interquartile range.

The IOP-levels and number of IOP-lowering medications for the PRESERFLO MicroShunt as a standalone procedure and as a cataract-combined procedure are presented in Figure 1A. The differences in IOP for PRESERFLO MicroShunt as a standalone procedure and as a cataract-combined procedure are graphically presented in Figure S1. The mean reduction in preoperative IOP and IOP-lowering medication for the standalone and combined procedures were similar 5.07 mmHg (23.6%) and 8.92 mmHg (38.2%; $p = 0.234$), and 2.67 (75.5%) and 1.62 (56.8%; $p = 0.830$), respectively, at the last postoperative visit. Moreover, the linear mixed model showed no significant differences in IOP and IOP-lowering medication if the whole follow-up period was taken into account ($p = 0.176$ and $p = 0.548$, respectively). Figure 2A shows a Kaplan–Meier curve in which cumulative failure is defined as requiring secondary surgery. Secondary surgeries were required in 12 eyes (20.3%) with PRESERFLO MicroShunt as a standalone procedure and in 2 eyes (15.4%) with PRESERFLO as a cataract-combined procedure, respectively ($p = 1.000$). Of the 14 (19.4%) eyes that required secondary surgery, 10 (71.4%) underwent surgery within 6 months after primary surgery. Figure 2B shows the cumulative failure rate as defined by the WGA-criteria. Of all operated eyes, 66.7% did not require any IOP-lowering medication at the last follow-up. Hypotony was observed in 3 eyes (5.1%) with PRESERFLO MicroShunt as a standalone procedure and in 2 eyes (15.4%) with PRESERFLO as a cataract-combined procedure ($p = 0.219$). All hypotony cases resolved spontaneously. There were no significant differences in visual acuity pre- and post-operative within/between both groups. We observed no serious complications (i.e., endophthalmitis or blebitis).

As there were no significant differences between the standalone and the cataract-combined procedure, we merged both groups ($n = 72$) for further analysis. Figure 1B shows the IOP levels and IOP-lowering medication for the total study population and separately for the eyes that underwent secondary surgery ($n = 14$ of 72 eyes). Eyes that required secondary surgery had a similar preoperative IOP-level but a significantly lower number of IOP-lowering medications (mean ± standard deviation: 26.17 ± 11.73 mmHg and 21.72 ± 8.35 mmHg ($p = 0.67$) and 3.40 ± 1.37 vs. 1.61 ± 1.54 ($p < 0.001$), respectively) compared to eyes that did not require secondary surgery.

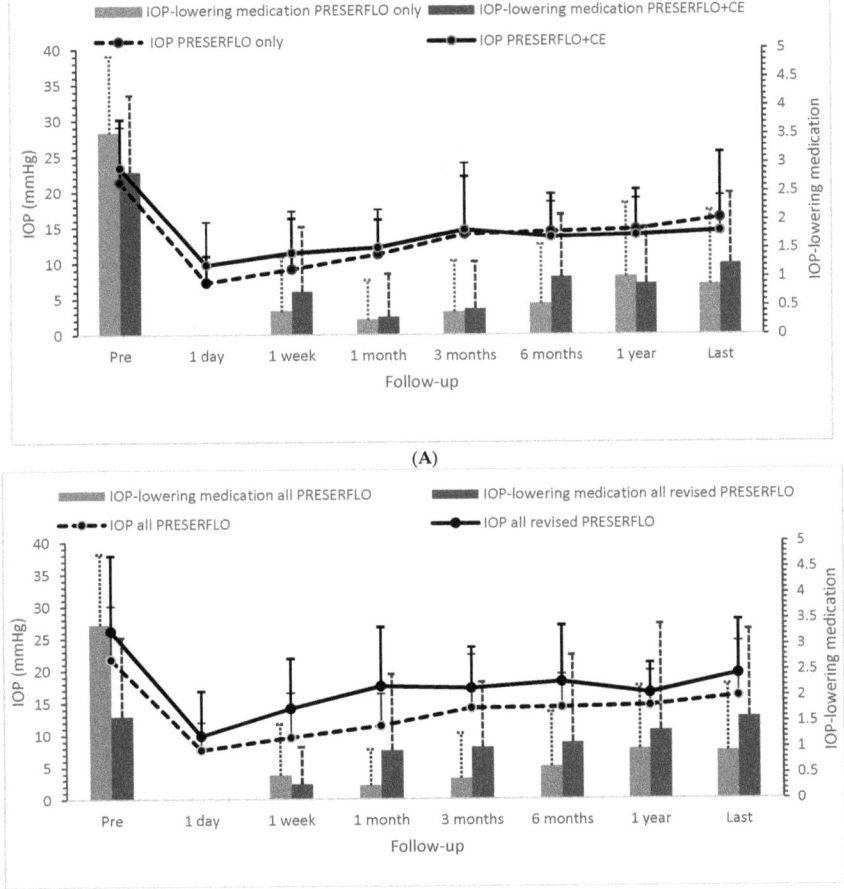

Figure 1. (**A**,**B**) Mean intraocular pressure (IOP, lines) and mean number of IOP-lowering medication (bars) for PRESERFLO as a standalone procedure vs. as a cataract-combined procedure (**A**) and all Preserflo surgeries (including combined procedures) vs. secondary surgeries (all revised Preserflo implants) (**B**). The "last" time interval had a median (interquartile range) follow-up of 1.02 (0.68–1.46) years. The vertical lines represent the standard deviation (SD). IOP = intraocular pressure; CE = cataract extraction.

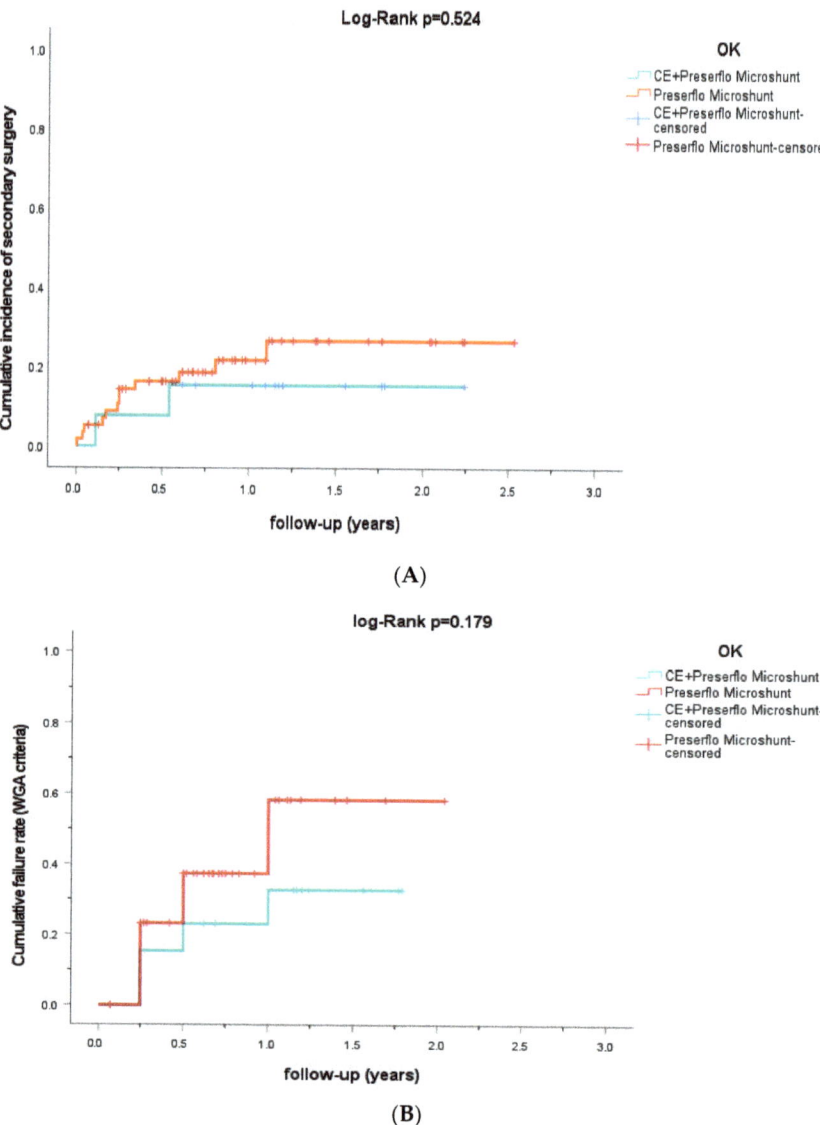

Figure 2. (**A**,**B**) Kaplan–Meier cumulative incidence curve for failure defined as requiring secondary surgery (**A**) and according to the WGA criteria (**B**) for PRESERFLO MicroShunt as a standalone procedure and as a cataract-combined procedure. Censored patients are represented by vertical tick marks. CE = cataractextraction, WGA = World Glaucoma Association.

The literature search yielded a total of 311 articles of which 14 studies (including 1213 PRESERFLO MicroShunt surgeries) were included in the current study and considered eligible for the meta-analysis (Table S1, Figure S2) [9,17–30]. Follow-up ranged from 12 months to 72 months. The median quality score (range) according to the Newcastle–Ottawa scale was 8 (7–8) on a scale from 0–9 (Table S2). Most studies included a mixture of different types of glaucoma with a majority having primary open-angle glaucoma (similar to our dataset). Table 2 shows the prevalence of complications across all included studies. The most common complications were hypotony (1.7–39%) and choroidal effusion/detachment (2.0–12.9%). Figure 3A,B show a summary of the meta-analysis for the performance of the PRESERFLO MicroShunt on the IOP and the IOP-lowering medication for all specified time intervals (for the full meta-analyses see Figures S3 and S4).

After 3 years of follow-up, the WMD (95%, CI; I2) IOP and IOP-lowering medication was 10.27 mmHg (8.23–12.32; 91%) and 1.77 (1.26–2.28; 0%), respectively. However, as only a few studies had such a long follow-up and to make the results more comparable to our data, we also report the 1 year WMD (95% CI; I2) for the IOP and IOP-lowering medication: 9.04 mmHg (8.46–9.63; 88%) and 2.67 (2.65–2.70; 89%) at 1 year, respectively.

Table 2. Prevalence of complications according to the systematic review.

Complications	Median (%)	Range(%)
Incorrect location/positioning	1.9	1.0–8.6
Choroidal effusion/detachment	8.9	2.0–12.9
Corneal dellen	1.2	1–1.2
Corneal edema	1.2	1–1.2
Hyphaema	6.8	2.5–22.7
Hypotony	11.1	1.7–39
Hypotonic maculopathy	1.1	0.8–6.9
Implant blocking/fracture/migration	2	1–4.3
Macula edema	1	0.6–3.6
Ptosis	2	1.2–2.4
Shallow/flat anterior chamber	5.7	2.5–13
Wound leak/seidel	4.9	0.6–8.9
Vitrious hemorrhage	1.2	0.6–4.3
Needling	12.2	1.6–62.5
Surgical revision	6.5	1.2–15.6

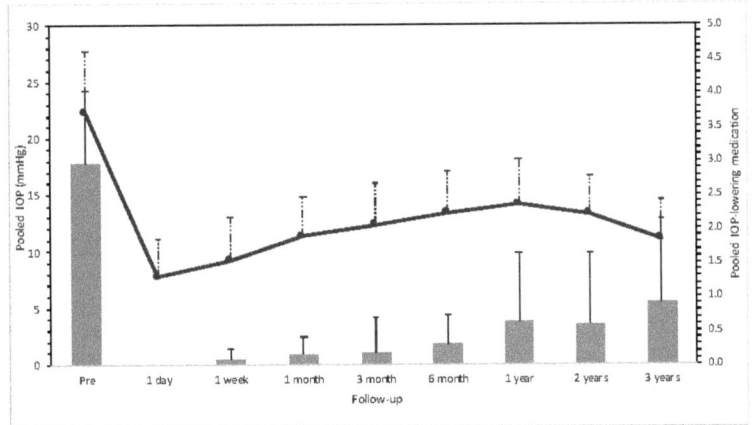

(A)

Figure 3. Cont.

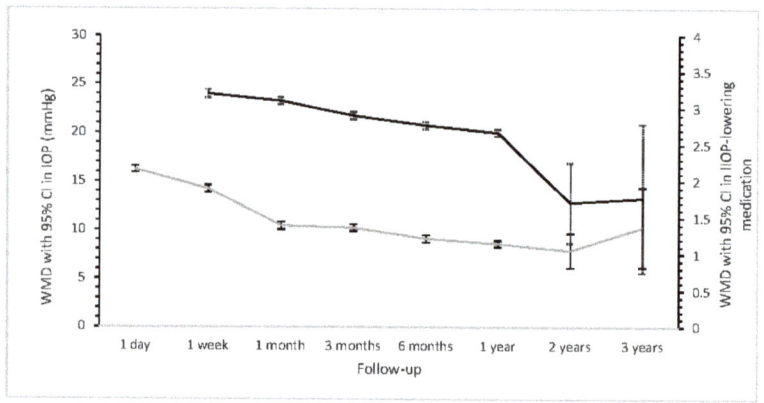

	1 day	1 week	1 month	3 months	6 months	1 year	2 years	3 years	
N (IOP)	366	419	419	410	390	846	104	30	grey
N (IOP-lowering medication)	272	267	267	258	241	801	105	30	black

(B)

Figure 3. (**A**,**B**) Meta-analyses for the change in intraocular pressure (IOP; grey) and number of IOP-lowering medications (black) after PRESERFLO MicroShunt surgery. Presented as the pooled mean with standard deviation (**A**) and weighted mean difference (WMD) with corresponding 95% confidence intervals (**B**). Table below gives the number of eyes.

The mean ± standard deviation preoperative IOP and IOP-lowering medication were 22.28 ± 5.38 mmHg and 2.97 ± 1.07, which declined to 14.09 ± 4.09 mmHg and 0.63 ± 1.00 at 1 year follow-up, respectively. Approximately 57% of eyes were free of any IOP-lowering medication after MicroShunt implantation. In our study population, eyes that underwent PRESERFLO MicroShunt surgery had a mean difference (95% CI) of 5.75 (3.19–8.30) mmHg and 2.47 (2.00–2.93) in IOP and IOP-lowering medication at the last postoperative visit, respectively.

4. Discussion

The PRESERFLO MicroShunt was found to significantly reduce IOP and number of IOP-lowering medications with 26.5% and 72.7%, respectively. At the end of follow-up, 66.7% of eyes did not require any IOP-lowering medication. As far as we know, the current study presents the first meta-analysis on the efficacy of the PRESERFLO MicroShunt. The total sample size included over one thousand PRESERFLO MicroShunt surgeries.

The preoperative IOP in the meta-analysis was higher than in the current study (22.28 vs. 21.70 mmHg). The preoperative number of medications were lower in the meta-analysis than in the current study (2.96 vs. 3.40). This may explain the finding that the absolute reduction in IOP was greater in the meta-analysis (11.21 mmHg vs. 5.75 mmHg) while the reduction in IOP-lowering medication was larger in our study population (2.47 vs. 2.06). The meta-analysis showed a WMD (95% CI; I2) for IOP of 9.04 mmHg (8.46–9.63; 88%) at 1 year, which is greater than the mean difference found in our study (5.56 mmHg [3.12–7.99]). The higher WMD in the meta-analysis is caused by a high WMD in four individual studies [18,20–22]. Additionally, the meta-analysis showed an interesting finding, namely that there was a decrease in IOP whilst also a slight increase of IOP-lowering medication use at 3 years postoperative. A possible explanation for this finding could be that only two studies reported on IOP and IOP-lowering medication at 3 years follow-up, of which one study reported a decrease in IOP whilst also reporting an increase in the number of IOP-lowering medications [18]. However, the authors of the study did not further discuss this finding.

The proportion of eyes requiring secondary surgery related to the PRESERFLO MicroShunt in our study population (19.4%) was higher than other studies reporting 1.2–15.6% (Table 2). It is important to note that studies used different surgical approaches when performing secondary surgery; some dissected the conjunctiva to remove overlying scar tissue with the Tenon's capsule and the PRESERFLO MicroShunt was replaced if needed, while others used needling with or without 5-fluorouracil (5FU) behind the slit lamp. An interesting finding was that if a patient required a secondary surgery, the surgery was usually performed within 6 months (71.4%; Figure 2A), which is comparable to the XEN-implants (63% within 6 months), another MIGS procedure [11]. Hypotony observed in our study (5 of 72 eyes (6.7%)) was in line with the literature; however, it is important to note that the reported range was wide (1.7–39%). There was an increase in number of IOP-lowering medications up to the "last" time interval (with a median [interquartile range] follow-up of 1.02 [0.68–1.46]); however, only the increases between 3 and 6 months and 6 months and 1 year were statistically significant. Similar to our study population, the meta-analysis also found a slight increase in the number of IOP-lowering medications at 2–3 years postoperative ($p = 0.41$).

A previously published study comparing trabeculectomy to the PRESERFLO MicroShunt found the MicroShunt to be inferior to trabeculectomy in regard to the proportion of eyes that met the criteria for surgical success (53.9% vs. 72.7%, respectively) [28]. Their study confirmed the favorable safety profile of the PRESERFLO MicroShunt, with patients in the MicroShunt group having a significantly lower incidence of hypotony compared to patients that underwent trabeculectomy (28.9% vs. 49.6%, respectively). Furthermore, fewer patients in the MicroShunt group required postoperative interventions compared to the trabeculectomy group (40.8% vs. 67.8%, respectively) [28]. Another study found that the XEN-implant did not show any significant differences between XEN-implant with or without a cataract-combined procedure for failure as requiring secondary surgery [11]. Similarly to its equivalent, we found that the PRESERFLO MicroShunt did not show significant differences between PRESERFLO MicroShunt as a standalone procedure and as a cataract-combined procedure for cumulative failure, defined as requiring secondary surgery (Figure 2A; log-rank $p = 0.524$) [11]. Nonetheless, it should be noted that it is difficult to compare the results of different (non-comparative) studies, because of different populations, surgery indications, and outcome criteria.

Our study has several limitations. Firstly, the surgeon may have a certain preference for a specific procedure in a particular situation (e.g., difference between standalone and combined procedure), which may result in selection bias. Secondly, the results of the cataract-combined procedures should be taken with caution, as the size of this subgroup was low and the indication to combine the surgery with cataract-extraction might be driven by the status of the anterior chamber angle. Thirdly, surgery was performed by two surgeons, which could contribute to variability in outcomes. However, no significant differences in outcomes were found for postoperative IOP and number of IOP-lowering medications between both surgeons. Moreover, the rates of secondary surgery between both surgeons were similar 16.1% and 22.0% ($p = 0.537$).

The arising question is: Will the PRESERFLO MicroShunt be able to replace trabeculectomy and glaucoma drainage devices (GDDs) in the near future? The answer is probably "no". The IOP decreasing efficacy seems less than, for example, the Ahmed or Baerveldt implant or a trabeculectomy. A recent study showed a 39.1% and 38% IOP reduction for the Baerveldt implant and trabeculectomy, respectively [31]. The safety profile of the PRESERFLO MicroShunt in terms of complications, however, seems better than traditional GDDs [32]. Therefore, MIGS might be a good first choice if a surgical intervention is required to lower IOP.

5. Conclusions

The PRESERFLO MicroShunt is effective in lowering IOP in patients with glaucoma. The IOP-lowering performance seems less than traditional surgical procedures; however, the MicroShunt seems to have a better risk profile than conventional glaucoma surgeries.

Future studies in the form of randomized controlled clinical trials with long follow-ups are needed to confirm the current results and to establish the place of the PRESERFLO MicroShunt within glaucoma treatment paradigm.

Supplementary Materials: The following supporting information can be downloaded at: https://www.mdpi.com/article/10.3390/jcm11237149/s1, Table S1: Summary of the retrieved studies from the systematic review; Table S2: Quality assessment of the included studies according to the Newcastle–Ottawa Scale; Figure S1: Scatterplot showing preoperative and postoperative IOP for PRESERFLO MicroShunt as a standalone procedure and as a cataract-combined procedure; Figure S2: Flowchart showing the selection process for inclusion of studies from our searches according to the PRISMA guidelines; Figure S3: Meta-analysis of the effect of the PRESERFLOMicroShunt on IOP for all specified time intervals; Figure S4: Meta-analysis of the effect of the PRESERFLO MicroShunt on IOP-lowering medication for all specified time intervals.

Author Contributions: S.S.M.P. and W.D.R. analyzed the data and wrote the main manuscript text. S.S.M.P., J.P., H.J.P. and V.A.d.V. collected the data. S.S.M.P., N.D.P. and W.M.B. performed the literature search. W.D.R. conceived and designed this study. R.C.W.W. critically reviewed the manuscript. All authors have read and agreed to the published version of the manuscript.

Funding: This research received no external funding.

Institutional Review Board Statement: Not applicable.

Informed Consent Statement: All procedures performed in studies involving human participants were in accordance with the ethical standards of the institutional and/or national research committee and with the 1964 Helsinki Declaration and its later amendments or comparable ethical standards. For this type of study, formal consent is not required.

Data Availability Statement: The data presented in this study are available on request from the corresponding author.

Conflicts of Interest: The authors declare no conflict of interest.

References

1. Weinreb, R.N.; Aung, T.; Medeiros, F.A. The pathophysiology and treatment of glaucoma: A review. *JAMA* **2014**, *311*, 1901–1911. [CrossRef] [PubMed]
2. Yadav, K.S.; Rajpurohit, R.; Sharma, S. Glaucoma: Current treatment and impact of advanced drug delivery systems. *Life Sci.* **2019**, *221*, 362–376. [CrossRef] [PubMed]
3. Gazzard, G.; Konstantakopoulou, E.; Garway-Heath, D.; Garg, A.; Vickerstaff, V.; Hunter, R.; Ambler, G.; Bunce, C.; Wormald, R.; Nathwani, N.; et al. Selective laser trabeculoplasty versus drops for newly diagnosed ocular hypertension and glaucoma: The LiGHT RCT. *Health Technol. Assess.* **2019**, *23*, 1–102. [CrossRef]
4. Gedde, S.J.; Feuer, W.J.; Shi, W.; Lim, K.S.; Barton, K.; Goyal, S.; Ahmed, I.I.K.; Brandt, J.; Primary Tube Versus Trabeculectomy Study, G. Treatment Outcomes in the Primary Tube Versus Trabeculectomy Study after 1 Year of Follow-up. *Ophthalmology* **2018**, *125*, 650–663. [CrossRef]
5. Saheb, H.; Gedde, S.J.; Schiffman, J.C.; Feuer, W.J.; Tube Versus Trabeculectomy Study Group. Outcomes of glaucoma reoperations in the Tube Versus Trabeculectomy (TVT) Study. *Am. J. Ophthalmol.* **2014**, *157*, 1179–1189.e1172. [CrossRef]
6. Francis, B.A.; Singh, K.; Lin, S.C.; Hodapp, E.; Jampel, H.D.; Samples, J.R.; Smith, S.D. Novel glaucoma procedures: A report by the American Academy of Ophthalmology. *Ophthalmology* **2011**, *118*, 1466–1480. [CrossRef] [PubMed]
7. Saheb, H.; Ahmed, I.I.K. Micro-invasive glaucoma surgery: Current perspectives and future directions. *Curr. Opin. Ophthalmol.* **2012**, *23*, 96–104. [CrossRef]
8. Pinchuk, L.; Riss, I.; Batlle, J.F.; Kato, Y.P.; Martin, J.B.; Arrieta, E.; Palmberg, P.; Parrish, R.K., 2nd; Weber, B.A.; Kwon, Y.; et al. The development of a micro-shunt made from poly(styrene-block-isobutylene-block-styrene) to treat glaucoma. *J. Biomed. Mater. Res. B Appl. Biomater.* **2017**, *105*, 211–221. [CrossRef]
9. Martinez-de-la-Casa, J.M.; Saenz-Frances, F.; Morales-Fernandez, L.; Perucho, L.; Mendez, C.; Fernandez-Vidal, A.; Garcia-Saenz, S.; Sanchez-Jean, R.; Garcia-Feijoo, J. Clinical outcomes of combined Preserflo Microshunt implantation and cataract surgery in open-angle glaucoma patients. *Sci. Rep.* **2021**, *11*, 15600. [CrossRef]
10. Al Habash, A.; Aljasim, L.A.; Owaidhah, O.; Edward, D.P. A review of the efficacy of mitomycin C in glaucoma filtration surgery. *Clin. Ophthalmol.* **2015**, *9*, 1945–1951.
11. Poelman, H.J.; Pals, J.; Rostamzad, P.; Bramer, W.M.; Wolfs, R.C.W.; Ramdas, W.D. Efficacy of the XEN-Implant in Glaucoma and a Meta-Analysis of the Literature. *J. Clin. Med.* **2021**, *10*, 1118. [CrossRef] [PubMed]

12. Ramdas, W.D.; Pals, J.; Rothova, A.; Wolfs, R.C.W. Efficacy of glaucoma drainage devices in uveitic glaucoma and a meta-analysis of the literature. *Graefes Arch. Clin. Exp. Ophthalmol.* **2019**, *257*, 143–151. [CrossRef] [PubMed]
13. Liberati, A.; Altman, D.G.; Tetzlaff, J.; Mulrow, C.; Gøtzsche, P.C.; Ioannidis, J.P.; Clarke, M.; Devereaux, P.J.; Kleijnen, J.; Moher, D. The PRISMA statement for reporting systematic reviews and meta-analyses of studies that evaluate health care interventions: Explanation and elaboration. *PLoS Med.* **2009**, *6*, e1000100. [CrossRef] [PubMed]
14. Stroup, D.F.; Berlin, J.A.; Morton, S.C.; Olkin, I.; Williamson, G.D.; Rennie, D.; Moher, D.; Becker, B.J.; Sipe, T.A.; Thacker, S.B. Meta-analysis of observational studies in epidemiology: A proposal for reporting. Meta-analysis Of Observational Studies in Epidemiology (MOOSE) group. *JAMA* **2000**, *283*, 2008–2012. [CrossRef]
15. Wells, G.A.; Shea, B.; O'Connel, D.; Peterson, J.; Welch, V.; Losos, M.; Tugwell, P. The Newcastle-Ottawa Scale (NOS) for Assessing the Quality of Nonrandomised Studies in Meta-Analyses. Available online: https://www.ohri.ca//programs/clinical_epidemiology/oxford.asp (accessed on 10 February 2022).
16. Shaarawy, T.; Grehn, F. *Guidelines on Design and Reporting of Glaucoma Surgical Trials*; Kugler Publications: Amsterdam, The Netherlands, 2009.
17. Ahmed, T.; Honjo, M.; Sakata, R.; Fujishiro, T.; Shirato, S.; Aihara, M. Long-term results of the safety and effectiveness of a novel microshunt in Japanese patients with primary open-angle glaucoma. *Jpn. J. Ophthalmol.* **2022**, *66*, 33–40. [CrossRef]
18. Batlle, J.F.; Fantes, F.; Riss, I.; Pinchuk, L.; Alburquerque, R.; Kato, Y.P.; Arrieta, E.; Peralta, A.C.; Palmberg, P.; Parrish, R.K., 2nd; et al. Three-Year Follow-up of a Novel Aqueous Humor MicroShunt. *J. Glaucoma* **2016**, *25*, e58–e65. [CrossRef]
19. Beckers, H.J.M.; Aptel, F.; Webers, C.A.B.; Bluwol, E.; Martinez-de-la-Casa, J.M.; Garcia-Feijoo, J.; Lachkar, Y.; Mendez-Hernandez, C.D.; Riss, I.; Shao, H.; et al. Safety and Effectiveness of the PRESERFLO R MicroShunt in Primary Open-Angle Glaucoma: Results from a 2-Year Multicenter Study. *Ophthalmol. Glaucoma* **2022**, *5*, 195–209. [CrossRef]
20. Durr, G.M.; Schlenker, M.B.; Samet, S.; Ahmed, I.I.K. One-year outcomes of stand-alone ab externo SIBS microshunt implantation in refractory glaucoma. *Br. J. Ophthalmol.* **2022**, *106*, 71–79. [CrossRef]
21. Fea, A.M.; Laffi, G.L.; Martini, E.; Economou, M.A.; Caselgrandi, P.; Sacchi, M.; Au, L. Effectiveness of MicroShunt in Patients with Primary Open-Angle and Pseudoexfoliative Glaucoma: A Retrospective European Multicenter Study. *Ophthalmol. Glaucoma* **2022**, *5*, 210–218. [CrossRef]
22. Quaranta, L.; Micheletti, E.; Carassa, R.; Bruttini, C.; Fausto, R.; Katsanos, A.; Riva, I. Efficacy and Safety of PreserFlo R MicroShunt After a Failed Trabeculectomy in Eyes with Primary Open-Angle Glaucoma: A Retrospective Study. *Adv. Ther.* **2021**, *38*, 4403–4412. [CrossRef]
23. Schlenker, M.B.; Durr, G.M.; Michaelov, E.; Ahmed, I.I.K. Intermediate Outcomes of a Novel Standalone Ab Externo SIBS Microshunt With Mitomycin C. *Am. J. Ophthalmol.* **2020**, *215*, 141–153. [CrossRef] [PubMed]
24. Scheres, L.M.J.; Kujovic-Aleksov, S.; Ramdas, W.D.; de Crom, R.; Roelofs, L.C.G.; Berendschot, T.; Webers, C.A.B.; Beckers, H.J.M. XEN R Gel Stent compared to PRESERFLO TM MicroShunt implantation for primary open-angle glaucoma: Two-year results. *Acta Ophthalmol.* **2021**, *99*, e433–e440. [CrossRef] [PubMed]
25. Scheres, L.M.J.; Kujovic-Aleksov, S.; De Crom, R.M.P.C.; Webers, C.A.B.; Beckers, H.J.M. Minimally invasive glaucoma surgery with the PRESERFLO™ MicroShunt: 3-year results. *Acta Ophthalmol.* **2021**, *99*, 21–22. [CrossRef]
26. Vastardis, I.; Fili, S.; Perdikakis, G.; Kontopoulou, K.; Balidis, M.; Gatzioufas, Z.; Kohlhaas, M. Preliminary results of Preserflo Microshunt versus Preserflo Microshunt and Ologen implantation. *Eye Vis.* **2021**, *8*, 33. [CrossRef]
27. Tanner, A.; Haddad, F.; Fajardo-Sanchez, J.; Nguyen, E.; Thong, K.X.; Ah-Moye, S.; Perl, N.; Abu-Bakra, M.; Kulkarni, A.; Trikha, S.; et al. One-year surgical outcomes of the PreserFlo MicroShunt in glaucoma: A multicentre analysis. *Br. J. Ophthalmol.* **2022**. [CrossRef]
28. Baker, N.D.; Barnebey, H.S.; Moster, M.R.; Stiles, M.C.; Vold, S.D.; Khatana, A.K.; Flowers, B.E.; Grover, D.S.; Strouthidis, N.G.; Panarelli, J.F.; et al. Ab-Externo MicroShunt versus Trabeculectomy in Primary Open-Angle Glaucoma: One-Year Results from a 2-Year Randomized, Multicenter Study. *Ophthalmology* **2021**, *128*, 1710–1721. [CrossRef]
29. Saletta, G.; Alexoudis, A.; Gkatzioufas, Z.; Grieshaber, M.; Papazoglou, A.; Tschopp, M.; Töteberg, M.; Gugleta, K. Retrospective Analysis of 12 Months Glaucoma Implant Efficacy: XEN45 and PreserFlo Microshunt. *Klin. Mon. Für Augenheilkd.* **2022**, *239*, 429–434. [CrossRef]
30. Ibarz Barberá, M.; Martínez-Galdón, F.; Caballero-Magro, E.; Rodríguez-Piñero, M.; Tañá-Rivero, P. Efficacy and Safety of the Preserflo Microshunt With Mitomycin C for the Treatment of Open Angle Glaucoma. *J. Glaucoma* **2022**, *31*, 557–566. [CrossRef]
31. Islamaj, E.; Wubbels, R.J.; de Waard, P.W.T. Primary Baerveldt versus trabeculectomy study after one-year follow-up. *Acta Ophthalmol.* **2018**, *96*, e740–e746. [CrossRef]
32. Poelman, H.J.; Wolfs, R.C.W.; Ramdas, W.D. The Baerveldt Glaucoma Drainage Device: Efficacy, Safety, and Place in Therapy. *Clin. Ophthalmol.* **2020**, *14*, 2789–2797. [CrossRef]

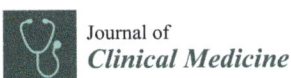

Article

Long-Term Changes in Corneal Endothelial Cell Density after Ex-PRESS Implantation: A Contralateral Eye Study

Xiaotong Ren [1], Jie Wang [2], Xuemin Li [1,*] and Lingling Wu [1,*]

[1] Department of Ophthalmology, Peking University Third Hospital, Beijing 100191, China
[2] Huangshan City People's Hospital, Huangshan 245000, China
* Correspondence: lxmlxm66@sina.com (X.L.); wullc@hotmail.com (L.W.); Tel.: +86-156-1190-8409 (X.L.); +86-135-2185-8359 (L.W.)

Abstract: Our purpose is to evaluate long-term changes in corneal endothelial cells after Ex-PRESS shunt implantation for the treatment of glaucoma in Chinese patients by comparison with the contralateral eye. In this retrospective observational study, glaucoma patients with a single eye undergoing Ex-PRESS shunt implantation surgery were consecutively enrolled. For each patient, the clinical assessment, including corneal endothelial cell density (CECD) before surgery and at 6, 12 months, and at last follow-up (2.43 ± 0.63 years) after surgery was reviewed. The operated eyes were in the study group and the unoperated contralateral eyes were used as the control group to compare the CECD change. A total of 48 subjects (age, 51.02 ± 17.96 years) were included. The follow-up period was 2.08~3.17 years, with an average of 2.43 ± 0.63 years. At the last follow-up after the surgery, the CECD decrease in the operated eyes (5.0%) was similar to that in the contralateral eyes (3.2%) (p = 0.130). There were no significant differences in CECD reduction between the two groups at baseline and each postoperative follow-up (6 months, 12 months and at the last follow-up) (all p > 0.05). The average IOP reduction after the surgery was 50.8%, and the number of IOP-lowering medications was significantly reduced (p < 0.05). In addition, visual acuity showed no significant differences during follow-up (p > 0.05). In this study, we found that the CECD reduction of Ex-PRESS shunt-implanted Chinese eyes was similar to that of contralateral eyes without surgery.

Keywords: corneal endothelial cell density (CECD); contralateral eyes; Ex-PRESS; glaucoma; intraocular pressure (IOP); long-term

Citation: Ren, X.; Wang, J.; Li, X.; Wu, L. Long-Term Changes in Corneal Endothelial Cell Density after Ex-PRESS Implantation: A Contralateral Eye Study. *J. Clin. Med.* **2022**, *11*, 5555. https://doi.org/10.3390/jcm11195555

Academic Editors: Michele Figus and Karl Mercieca

Received: 22 August 2022
Accepted: 18 September 2022
Published: 22 September 2022

Publisher's Note: MDPI stays neutral with regard to jurisdictional claims in published maps and institutional affiliations.

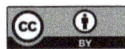

Copyright: © 2022 by the authors. Licensee MDPI, Basel, Switzerland. This article is an open access article distributed under the terms and conditions of the Creative Commons Attribution (CC BY) license (https://creativecommons.org/licenses/by/4.0/).

1. Introduction

Glaucoma is a group of heterogeneous diseases characterized by the gradual loss of retinal ganglion cells, cupping of the optic disc, and thinning of the retinal nerve fiber layer [1]. Epidemiological research data have shown that glaucoma is the main cause of irreversible vision loss worldwide [2]. Glaucoma has a worldwide prevalence of 3.5% of the population aged over 40 years, and 2.6% in China [2,3].

From a pathophysiological and therapeutic point of view, reducing IOP to reach the target IOP is the only evidence-based treatment, which can be achieved by the combination with drug, laser therapy, and surgical procedures [1]. Glaucoma filtration surgery is performed to reduce IOP and prevent further optic nerve damage or deterioration of the visual field when maximum tolerated drug and laser therapy does not adequately reduce IOP.

Filtration surgery is the most frequently used technique for surgical glaucoma treatment. At present, trabeculectomy is still the main operation [4]. In terms of safety, although significant progress has been made in trabeculectomy, complications such as hypotony, choroidal detachment, and anterior chamber collapse are still possible and problematic [5]. In addition, the loss of corneal endothelial cells has also gradually received attention. Corneal decompensation was reported as a late postoperative complication after trabeculectomy [6–8]. Furthermore, some shunt implantation surgery such as Baerveldt tube or

Ahmed glaucoma valve implantation also has been paid attention to for the corneal endothelium loss [6]. Corneal complication rates of 8–29% after aqueous shunt implantation were reported [6].

In recent years, some new microinvasive shunting devices as an alternative to trabeculectomy have been offered, such as Ex-PRESS implant, Xen Gel stent. The damage to corneal endothelium of these implants has always been concerned, even though Xen Gel stent caused little endothelial cell damage in some studies [9,10]. The Ex-PRESS shunt is a non-valved stainless steel tube that is inserted under a partial-thickness scleral flap to connect the anterior chamber (AC) to the subconjunctival space [11,12], which is prevalent worldwide and was approved in Japan in December 2011 [13], and used widely in China since 2012. Compared with trabeculectomy, it has the advantages of reduced trauma, simple operation, and improved safety. Most studies proved that the Ex-PRESS implantation had an equivalent curative effect to trabeculectomy [14–20], even with more complete success [21,22]; however, some literature argued that it was less effective than trabeculectomy [23–25]. Regarding corneal endothelial cells, some studies have proven their safety [12,13,26–28]. Previous studies reported no significantly faster loss in endothelial cell counts after Ex-PRESS implantation compared with trabeculectomy [14,17,29]. While other studies reported that corneal endothelial cell density (CECD) was significantly decreased after Ex-PRESS implantation [29–33]. However, these studies mainly done on the Japanese [28–30] and some on Korean [14], Italian [34] and American [18] populations. In addition, few studies reported longer assessments for CECD loss after Ex-PRESS implantation and no study compared with the contralateral eyes. Therefore, the aim of this study was to evaluate long-term changes in corneal endothelial cells after Ex-PRESS shunt implantation in Chinese patients by comparison with the contralateral eye.

2. Patients and Methods

2.1. Patients

In this retrospective observational study, patients with glaucoma and a single eye undergoing Ex-PRESS shunt implantation treatments at the Peking University Third Hospital Eye Center from October 2015 to June 2020 were included. The study was approved by the Ethics Committee of Peking University Third Hospital and adhered to the tenets of the Declaration of Helsinki. Unoperated contralateral eyes were used as controls to compare CECD changes.

All patients had unsatisfactory IOP control despite maximally tolerating topical medication before the surgery. We included patients who were over 18 years of age and completed regular postoperative follow-up for at least 2 years. Exclusion criteria include: (a) congenital glaucoma; (b) previous keratoplasty, preoperative corneal decompensation, corneal endothelial cell disease, and any other corneal epithelial or stromal disorders in either the operated eye or the contralateral eye; (c) patients who were performed glaucoma filtration surgery or other ocular surgery on the contralateral eye during follow-up; (d) patients with aphakic or pseudophakic eyes or other ocular disorders that would affect the corneal endothelium (including fellow eyes).

2.2. Surgical Procedure

All operations were performed by the same doctor (WLL, an experienced Chief Ophthalmologist). All eyes were administered retrobulbar anesthesia with lidocaine 2%. After a fornix-based conjunctival flap creation, a 0.2 mg/mL solution of mitomycin C (MMC) was applied for 3 min, followed by copious irrigation with a balanced salt solution. A rectangle scleral flap was developed, and the Ex-PRESS (model P50, Alcon Laboratories, Fort Worth, TX, USA) was introduced into the AC at the base of the scleral flap, midway between the iris periphery and the cornea. Finally, the flap was closed by 10-0 Nylon sutures combined with releasable sutures, and the conjunctiva was approximated sutured to the limbus also using 10-0 Nylon sutures. We used the balanced salt solution to reform the anterior chamber, and checked for wound leaks. A sterile eye shield was placed over the eye following the corticosteroid/antibiotic ointment. Postoperatively, topical antibiotics and steroid treatment were administered for approximately 4–6 weeks. The releasable sutures were removed within one week.

2.3. Preoperative and Postoperative Examinations

Age, sex, preoperative IOP, the number of IOP-lowering medications (a fixed combination agent was counted as two medications), and the diagnosis were reviewed for all patients. Apart from routine preoperative and postoperative examinations, specular microscopic examination of corneal endothelial cells was routinely performed by an experienced examiner using a noncontact specular microscope (Robo SP-8000; Konan Medical, Nishinomiya, Japan) immediately before surgery and at 6 months, 1 year and at the last follow-up ($\geq$2 years) after surgery. This instrument automatically captures images of the endothelium once the subject fixates on a target. Then, the CECD (cells/mm^2) and at least 50 contiguous endothelial cells centered on the screen were hand-marked, and a computer algorithm was used to calculate the values. The results on the central area of the cornea were analyzed.

The preoperative and postoperative IOPs were measured by Goldmann applanation tonometry (Haag-Streit AG, Bern, Switzerland). Types of IOP-lowering medications were recorded.

Complete success was defined as an IOP between 5 and 21 mm Hg without additional medications or/and procedures to reduce IOP, while the definition of qualified success was the same criteria mentioned above but with medications.

2.4. Statistical Analysis

SPSS software version 22 (SPSS Inc., Chicago, IL, USA) was used for statistical analysis. The Kolmogorov-Smirnov test was applied to determine data normality. The descriptive data are presented as the mean and standard deviation (SD). The mixed linear model was used to compare differences pre- and post-operate. To analyze repeated measurements, the eye was selected as the subject, and the time point was set as the repeated factor. For comparisons of the two groups, the paired *t*-test was used for normally continuous variables, and the Wilcoxon nonparametric test was applied for ordinal variables. *p* values less than 0.05 were considered statistically significant.

The sample size was estimated according to the standard formula for mean comparison. α and β were set as 0.05 and 0.1 respectively. Change rate of corneal endothelial cell density was selected as main outcome for sample size estimation. According to a previous study [31], it was estimated that 30 pairs of eyes were needed.

3. Results

A total of 48 subjects were eligible for the study. All patients were over 18 years of age, and the average age was 51.02 $\pm$ 17.96 years old. There were 36 males and 12 females. The general information of the patients is shown in Table 1. The follow-up period was 2.08~3.17 years, with an average of 2.43 $\pm$ 0.63 years.

3.1. Change in Clinical Parameters after Ex-PRESS Implantation

As shown in Table 2, compared with preoperative baseline, the average IOP and the number of IOP-lowering medications were significantly reduced at each follow-up time point (all *p* = 0.000). However, visual acuity (logMAR, BCVA) showed no significant differences (all *p* > 0.05).

Table 1. Patients' general information.

Characteristics	Number
Sex (M/F)	36/12
Age at surgery (years)	51.02 ± 17.96
Diagnosis, Number of eyes (rate)	
Primary open-angle glaucoma	42 (87.5%)
Secondary glaucoma	6 (12.5%)
pigmentary glaucoma	1 (2.1%)
angle-recession glaucoma	5 (10.4%)
Preoperative IOP (mm Hg)	27.42 ± 9.73
Number of preoperative IOP-lowering medications	2.79 ± 1.10
Preoperative corneal endothelial cell density (cells/mm^2)	2427.69 ± 473.82
The follow up period (years)	2.43 ± 0.63
Complete success eyes (rate) *	35 (73.1%)
Qualified success eyes (rate) *	44 (91.7%)

Data are presented as numbers or means ± standard deviations. M: male; F: female; IOP = intraocular pressure. *: at the final follow-up (>2 years). Complete success was defined as IOP between 5 and 21 mm Hg without additional medications or/and procedures to reduce IOP, while the definition of qualified success was the same criteria mentioned above with or without medications. During the follow-up, 4 patients were undergone bleb needling for IOP elevation.

Table 2. Changes in clinical parameters after Ex-PRESS implantation.

Clinical Parameters	Baseline	6 Months	12 Months	Final Follow up (>2 Years)
N (eyes)	48	42	32	48
LogMAR BCVA	0.45 ± 0.45	0.44 ± 0.39	0.42 ± 0.41	0.39 ± 0.36
p		0.564	0.577	0.169
IOP (mm Hg)	27.42 ± 9.73	14.31 ± 3.43	14.16 ± 2.98	13.49 ± 2.62
p		0.000	0.000	0.000
medications	2.79 ± 1.10	0.67 ± 1.00	0.71 ± 0.92	0.47 ± 0.69
p		0.000	0.000	0.000

Data are shown as the mean ± standard deviation. logMAR = logarithm of minimum angle of resolution; BCVA = best corrected visual acuity; IOP = intraocular pressure; medications: Number of preoperative IOP-lowering medications. p-valve: Compared to baseline (paired t test with Bonferroni correction). p values of less than 0.05 were considered statistically significant.

3.2. Comparison of CECD in Ex-PRESS-Implanted Eyes and Contralateral Eyes

At preoperative baseline, the CECD in the operated eyes were similar to that in the contralateral eyes. Compared with preoperative baseline, no significant difference existed in CECD at postoperative 6 and 12 months either in operated eyes or in contralateral eyes (Table 3). While at the last follow-up, CECD was significantly decreased both in operated eyes and in contralateral eyes compared with preoperative CECD ($p = 0.017$, $p = 0.012$). However, no statistically significant difference in the CECD decrease percentage was found between the two groups (5.0% vs. 3.2%, $p = 0.130$). Four patients underwent bleb needling for IOP elevation. Apart from that, neither patient had apparent tube-corneal contact nor required additional intraocular surgery, including the contralateral eyes.

Table 3. Comparison of CECD (cells/mm^2) in Ex-PRESS implanted eyes and contralateral eyes.

Follow-Up Period	N	Operated Eyes	p [a]	Contralateral Eyes	p [b]	p [c]
Baseline	48	2427.69 ± 473.82		2536.16 ± 435.36		0.879
6 months	31	2407.70 ± 593.91	0.384	2475.94 ± 292.94	0.978	0.523
reduction (%)		1.6 ± 12.6		1.0 ± 9.0		0.631
12 months	42	2364.28 ± 554.44	0.255	2417.18 ± 381.16	0.272	0.623
reduction (%)		2.2 ± 8.1		1.8 ± 5.0		0.572
Final	48	2316.70 ± 534.77	0.017	2401.47 ± 410.31	0.012	0.178
reduction (%)		5.0 ± 12.2		3.2 ± 7.8		0.130

Data are shown as the mean ± standard deviation. Operated eyes: Ex-Press implantation eyes; Final: final follow up (>2 years); reduction (%): Percentage decrease in CECD from baseline. p [a], p [b]: Compared to baseline (paired t test with Bonferroni correction). p [c]: Operation eyes vs. contralateral eyes (paired t test with Bonferroni correction). p values of less than 0.05 were considered statistically significant.

4. Discussion

This long-term follow-up study of more than 2 years showed that the CECD reduction of Ex-PRESS shunt-implanted eyes was similar to that of the contralateral eyes without surgery. To our knowledge, this was the first study to compare CECD reduction after Ex-PRESS shunt implantation between both eyes of patients. The mean CECD value is approximately 3000 cells/mm^2 in young adults and is reduced by 0.5 ± 0.6% due to aging every year [6]. POAG patients showed a reduction of 0.68–12.3% in CECD per year (the data include multiple treatment methods) [6,35]. Our study showed that the decrease was 2.2% in shunt-implanted eyes and 1.8% in contralateral eyes at the 12-month follow-up. At the last follow-up time point (>2 years), the decreases were 5.0% and 3.2%, respectively. We speculated that it was related to glaucoma itself but had little connection with Ex-PRESS shunt implantation, even though both groups had significant CECD loss at the last follow-up time point compared with the preoperative baseline.

This study showed that at 6 and 12 months postoperatively, the reduction in CECD in the operated eyes was not significant. This was a coincidence to a short-term prospective study in Italians [34], in which none of the endothelial cell parameters changed 1 and 3 months after Ex-PRESS implantation. Our results also showed that in shunt-implanted eyes, CECD loss (5.0%) was significant at the last follow-up (>2 years). This was consistent with some Japanese studies showing a 2.5~4% mean CECD decrease 2 years after surgery, [30,31] even though these studies did not compare it with the contralateral eyes. However, other Japanese studies showed that the mean CECD decrease reached 18.0% at 2 years [31] and 10.3~30.0% at 2~5 years after Ex-PRESS implantation [32]. One of the factors influencing the reduction in CECD after Ex-PRESS surgery might be the shunt inserted position. Tojo et al. found that the trabecular meshwork insertion group had a 5.2% decrease, while the corneal insertion group had a 15.1% reduction at 2 years after implantation [36]. A reported case of partial decompensation of the corneal endothelium adjacent to the filtering bleb pointed out that the Ex-PRESS was inserted from the cornea, not the trabecular meshwork [33]. Therefore, Ex-PRESS shunt insertion into the cornea was considered a risk factor for rapid CECD loss [36]. Other than the shunt inserted position, some factors may also contribute to CECD loss after implantation, such as iris–cornea contact, contact between the corneal endothelium and the Ex-PRESS, high IOP, cytotoxicity of IOP-lowering medications, inflammation, and glaucoma itself [6,14,26,33,36–38]. Ex-PRESS is a medical-grade stainless steel device that has the advantage of position stability, and it has been suggested to be suitable for patients with low corneal endothelium [14]. The Ahmed valve was reported to have more CECD reduction, which maybe because of its material [34,39]. The Xen Gel Stent is a hydrophilic tube and possessed no foreign body reaction [9], which may account for less CECD loss. In our study, no patient had apparent tube-corneal contact, required additional surgery for the IOP to be excessively increased or required other intraocular surgery, which helped us to better study the natural course.

The current study found that the average IOP had a dramatic decline after Ex-PRESS implantation, even though there was a reduction of 50.8% at the last follow-up after surgery. In addition, the use of IOP-lowering medications significantly decreased postoperatively. This was similar to previous studies by others [12,26,27], yet our IOP drop seemed even higher. Perhaps patient selection, the operation of different surgeons, and the control for target IOP caused the difference. In addition, visual acuity showed no significant differences during the follow-up, which was in accord with the research by Beatriz Puerto et al. [40].

There were several limitations of the study. First, it was a retrospective study, whose sample size was relatively small, and the time of follow-up was limited. However, our research was sufficiently innovative to compare shunt-implanted eyes with contralateral eyes, which made up for it to some extent. Second, the measurement records of corneal endothelial cells did not cover the coefficient of variation (CV) or the incidence of hexagonal cells (6A). Most previous studies focused on corneal endothelial cell density count, which has been considered the most important factor. However, further study is necessary to measure CV and 6A. Third, multiple directions or o'clock positions, especially the area of the shunt, were inserted where the CECD decreased significantly faster than other areas [31]. We did not measure CECD from multiple areas, and we determined that it was more comparable to select the same position compared with the contralateral eyes. Finally, data from several types of glaucoma were combined, which might have different pathogeneses (both primary and secondary glaucoma), so it may introduce potential bias to some extent.

In summary, the CECD reduction of Ex-PRESS shunt implanted eyes was similar to that of the contralateral eyes without surgery in this long-term follow-up study, which implied that there might be no obvious connection between CECD loss and Ex-PRESS shunt implantation. Further study would benefit from an enlarged sample size, a sufficiently long period, more rigorous inclusion standards, other additional examinations, and more parameter comparisons.

Author Contributions: X.R.: research design, data acquisition, data analysis, and manuscript preparation; J.W.: data acquisition; X.L.: research design; L.W.: research design, surgery perform, and manuscript amendment. All authors have read and agreed to the published version of the manuscript.

Funding: Publication of this article was supported by a grant from Natural Science Foundation of Beijing Municipality (7202229) and Cohort study of Peking University Third Hospital (BYSYDL20211015). The sponsor or funding organization had no role in the design or conduct of this research.

Institutional Review Board Statement: The study was approved by the Ethics Committee of Peking University Third Hospital (approval number M2022308) and adhered to the tenets of the Declaration of Helsinki.

Informed Consent Statement: Not applicable.

Data Availability Statement: The datasets generated and analyzed during the current study are not publicly available but are available from the corresponding author on reasonable request.

Conflicts of Interest: All authors declare that they have no conflict of interest.

References

1. Jonas, J.B.; Aung, T.; Bourne, R.R.; Bron, A.M.; Ritch, R.; Panda-Jonas, S. Glaucoma. *Lancet* **2017**, *11*, 390. [CrossRef]
2. Tham, Y.; Li, X.; Wong, T.Y.; Quigley, H.A.; Aung, T.; Cheng, C. Global Prevalence of Glaucoma and Projections of Glaucoma Burden through 2040. *Ophthalmology* **2014**, *121*, 2081–2090. [CrossRef] [PubMed]
3. Torabi, R.; Harris, A.; Siesky, B.; Zukerman, R.; Oddone, F.; Mathew, S.; Januleviciene, I.; Vercellin, A. Prevalence Rates and Risk Factors for Primary Open Angle Glaucoma in the Middle East. *J. Ophthalmic. Vis. Res.* **2021**, *16*, 644–656. [CrossRef]
4. Leske, M.C.; Heijl, A.; Hyman, L.; Bengtsson, B.; Dong, L.; Yang, Z. Predictors of Long-term Progression in the Early Manifest Glaucoma Trial. *Ophthalmology* **2007**, *114*, 1965–1972. [CrossRef] [PubMed]
5. Olayanju, J.A.; Hassan, M.B.; Hodge, D.O.; Khanna, C.L. Trabeculectomy-Related Complications in Olmsted County, Minnesota, 1985 Through 2010. *JAMA Ophthalmol.* **2015**, *133*, 574. [CrossRef] [PubMed]

6. Janson, B.J.; Alward, W.L.; Kwon, Y.H.; Bettis, D.I.; Fingert, J.H.; Provencher, L.M.; Goins, K.M.; Wagoner, M.D.; Greiner, M.A. Glaucoma-associated corneal endothelial cell damage: A review. *Surv. Ophthalmol.* **2018**, *63*, 500–506. [CrossRef] [PubMed]
7. Arnavielle, S.; Lafontaine, P.O.; Bidot, S.; Creuzot-Garcher, C.; D'Athis, P.; Bron, A.M. Corneal endothelial cell changes after trabeculectomy and deep sclerectomy. *J. Glaucoma* **2007**, *16*, 324–328. [CrossRef] [PubMed]
8. Hirooka, K.; Nitta, E.; Ukegawa, K.; Sato, S.; Kiuchi, Y. Effect of trabeculectomy on corneal endothelial cell loss. *Brit. J. Ophthalmol.* **2020**, *104*, 376–380. [CrossRef]
9. Olgun, A.; Duzgun, E.; Yildiz, A.M.; Atmaca, F.; Yildiz, A.A.; Sendul, S.Y. XEN Gel Stent versus trabeculectomy: Short-term effects on corneal endothelial cells. *Eur. J. Ophthalmol.* **2021**, *31*, 346–353. [CrossRef]
10. Oddone, F.; Roberti, G.; Posarelli, C.; Agnifili, L.; Mastropasqua, L.; Carnevale, C.; Micelli, F.T.; Pace, V.; Sacchi, M.; Cremonesi, E.; et al. Endothelial Cell Density after XEN Implant Surgery: Short-term Data from the Italian XEN Glaucoma Treatment Registry (XEN-GTR). *J. Glaucoma* **2021**, *30*, 559–565. [CrossRef]
11. Mermoud, A. Ex-PRESS implant. *Brit. J. Ophthalmol.* **2005**, *89*, 396–397. [CrossRef] [PubMed]
12. Fialová, V.; Váša, M. Use of ex-press®implant in glaucoma surgery–retrospective study. *Česká Slov. Oftalmol.* **2018**, *74*, 11–16. [CrossRef]
13. Gonzalez-Rodriguez, J.M.; Trope, G.E.; Drori-Wagschal, L.; Jinapriya, D.; Buys, Y.M. Comparison of trabeculectomy versus Ex-PRESS: 3-year follow-up. *Br. J. Ophthalmol.* **2015**, *100*, 1269–1273. [CrossRef]
14. Lee, G.Y.; Chong, E.L.; Kyoo, W.L.; Sam, S. Long-term efficacy and safety of ExPress implantation for treatment of open angle glaucoma. *Int. J. Ophthalmol.* **2017**, *10*, 1379–1384.
15. Wang, W.; Zhou, M.W.; Huang, W.B.; Gao, X.B.; Zhang, X.L. Ex-PRESS implantation versus trabeculectomy in Chinese patients with POAG: Fellow eye pilot study. *Int. J. Ophthalmol.* **2017**, *10*, 56–60.
16. Chen, G.; Li, W.; Jiang, F.; Mao, S.; Tong, Y. Ex-PRESS implantation versus trabeculectomy in open-angle glaucoma: A meta-analysis of randomized controlled clinical trials. *PLoS ONE.* **2014**, *9*, e86045. [CrossRef]
17. Bustros, Y.D.; Fechtner, R.; Khouri, A.S. Outcomes of Ex-PRESS and Trabeculectomy in a Glaucoma Population of African Origin: One Year Results. *J. Curr. Glaucoma Pract.* **2017**, *11*, 42–47. [CrossRef]
18. Wagschal, L.D.; Trope, G.E.; Jinapriya, D.; Jin, Y.; Buys, Y.M. Prospective Randomized Study Comparing Ex-PRESS to Trabeculectomy: 1-Year Results. *J. Glaucoma* **2015**, *24*, 624–629. [CrossRef]
19. Netland, P.A.; Sarkisian, S.R.; Moster, M.R.; Ahmed, I.I.K.; Condon, G.; Salim, S.; Sherwood, M.B.; Siegfried, C.J. Randomized, Prospective, Comparative Trial of EX-PRESS Glaucoma Filtration Device versus Trabeculectomy (XVT Study). *Am. J. Ophthalmol.* **2014**, *157*, 433–440. [CrossRef]
20. Moisseiev, E.; Zunz, E.; Tzur, R.; Kurtz, S.; Shemesh, G. Standard Trabeculectomy and Ex-PRESS Miniature Glaucoma Shunt. *J. Glaucoma* **2015**, *24*, 410–416. [CrossRef]
21. de Jong, L.; Lafuma, A.; Aguade, A.S.; Berdeaux, G. Five-year extension of a clinical trial comparing the EX-PRESS glaucoma filtration device and trabeculectomy in primary open-angle glaucoma. *Clin. Ophthalmol.* **2011**, *5*, 527–533. [PubMed]
22. Zhang, X.; Wang, B.; Liu, R.; Chen, Y.; Leng, X.; Wu, Y.; Lu, X. The effectiveness of AGV, Ex-PRESS, or trabeculectomy in the treatment of primary and secondary glaucoma: A systematic review and network meta-analysis. *Ann. Palliat. Med.* **2022**, *11*, 321–331. [CrossRef] [PubMed]
23. Kawabata, K.; Shobayashi, K.; Iwao, K.; Takahashi, E.; Tanihara, H.; Inoue, T. Efficacy and safety of Ex-PRESS®mini shunt surgery versus trabeculectomy for neovascular glaucoma: A retrospective comparative study. *BMC Ophthalmol.* **2019**, *19*, 75. [CrossRef] [PubMed]
24. Otsuka, M.; Hayashi, A.; Tojo, N. Ex-PRESS®surgery versus trabeculectomy for primary open-angle glaucoma with low preoperative intraocular pressure. *Int. Ophthalmol.* **2022**, *10*, Epub ahead of print. [CrossRef]
25. Hashimoto, Y.; Michihata, N.; Matsui, H.; Fushimi, K.; Yasunaga, H.; Aihara, M. Reoperation rates after Ex-PRESS versus trabeculectomy for primary open-angle or normal-tension glaucoma: A national database study in Japan. *Eye* **2020**, *34*, 1069–1076. [CrossRef]
26. Waisbourd, M.; Fischer, N.; Shalev, H.; Spierer, O.; Ben, A.E.; Rachmiel, R.; Shemesh, G.; Kurtz, S. Trabeculectomy with Ex-PRESS implant versus Ahmed glaucoma valve implantation-a comparative study. *Int. J. Ophthalmol.* **2016**, *9*, 1415–1420.
27. Wagdy, F.M.; Zaky, A.G. Comparison between the Express Implant and Transscleral Diode Laser in Neovascular Glaucoma. *J. Ophthalmol.* **2020**, *2020*, 3781249. [CrossRef]
28. Wang, L.; Sha, F.; Guo, D.D.; Bi, H.S.; Si, J.K.; Du, Y.X.; Tang, K. Efficacy and economic analysis of Ex-PRESS implantation versus trabeculectomy in uncontrolled glaucoma: A systematic review and Meta-analysis. *Int. J. Ophthalmol.* **2016**, *9*, 124–131.
29. Omatsu, S.; Hirooka, K.; Nitta, E.; Ukegawa, K. Changes in corneal endothelial cells after trabeculectomy and EX-PRESS shunt: 2-year follow-up. *BMC Ophthalmol.* **2018**, *18*, 243. [CrossRef]
30. Ishida, K.; Moroto, N.; Murata, K.; Yamamoto, T. Effect of glaucoma implant surgery on intraocular pressure reduction, flare count, anterior chamber depth, and corneal endothelium in primary open-angle glaucoma. *Jpn. J. Ophthalmol.* **2017**, *61*, 334–346. [CrossRef]
31. Arimura, S.; Miyake, S.; Iwasaki, K.; Gozawa, M.; Matsumura, T.; Takamura, Y.; Inatani, M. Randomised Clinical Trial for Postoperative Complications after Ex-PRESS Implantation versus Trabeculectomy with 2-Year Follow-Up. *Sci. Rep.* **2018**, *8*, 16168. [CrossRef] [PubMed]

32. Tojo, N.; Hayashi, A. Ex-Press®versus Baerveldt implant surgery for primary open-angle glaucoma and pseudo-exfoliation glaucoma. *Int. Ophthalmol.* **2021**, *41*, 1091–1101. [CrossRef] [PubMed]
33. Tojo, N.; Hayashi, A.; Miyakoshi, A. Corneal decompensation following filtering surgery with the Ex-PRESS®mini glaucoma shunt device. *Clin. Ophthalmol.* **2015**, *9*, 499–502. [PubMed]
34. Casini, G.; Loiudice, P.; Pellegrini, M.; Sframeli, A.T.; Martinelli, P.; Passani, A.; Nardi, M. Trabeculectomy Versus EX-PRESS Shunt Versus Ahmed Valve Implant: Short-term Effects on Corneal Endothelial Cells. *Am. J. Ophthalmol.* **2015**, *160*, 1185–1190. [CrossRef] [PubMed]
35. Cho, S.W.; Kim, J.M.; Choi, C.Y.; Park, K.H. Changes in corneal endothelial cell density in patients with normal-tension glaucoma. *Jpn. J. Ophthalmol.* **2009**, *53*, 569–573. [CrossRef]
36. Tojo, N.; Numata, A.; Hayashi, A. Factors influencing the reduction in corneal endothelial cells after Ex-Press surgery. *Int. Ophthalmol.* **2020**, *40*, 1201–1208. [CrossRef]
37. Storr-Paulsen, T.; Norregaard, J.C.; Ahmed, S.; Storr-Paulsen, A. Corneal endothelial cell loss after mitomycin C-augmented trabeculectomy. *J. Glaucoma* **2008**, *17*, 654–657. [CrossRef]
38. Abu, S.K.; Fernando, S.S.; Sarup, V. Decompression Retinopathy after ExPRESS Shunt Implantation for Steroid-Induced Ocular Hypertension: A Case Report. *Case Rep. Ophthalmol. Med.* **2011**, *2011*, 303287.
39. Kim, M.S.; Kim, K.N.; Kim, C.S. Changes in Corneal Endothelial Cell after Ahmed Glaucoma Valve Implantation and Trabeculectomy: 1-Year Follow-up. *Korean J. Ophthalmol.* **2016**, *30*, 416–425. [CrossRef]
40. Puerto, B.; López-Caballero, C.; Sánchez-Sánchez, C.; Oblanca, N.; Blázquez, V.; Contreras, I. Clinical outcomes after Ex-PRESS glaucoma shunt versus non-penetrating deep sclerectomy: Two-year follow-up. *Int. Ophthalmol.* **2017**, *38*, 2575–2584. [CrossRef]

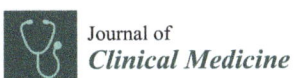

Article

Tube–Iris Distance and Corneal Endothelial Cell Damage Following Ahmed Glaucoma Valve Implantation

Yitak Kim [1], Won Jeong Cho [1], Jung Dong Kim [2], Hyuna Cho [2], Hyoung Won Bae [2], Chan Yun Kim [2] and Wungrak Choi [2,*]

1. Severance Hospital, Yonsei University College of Medicine, Seoul 03722, Korea
2. Department of Ophthalmology, Institute of Vision Research, Yonsei University College of Medicine, Seoul 03722, Korea
* Correspondence: wungrakchoi@hanmail.net or wungrakchoi@yuhs.ac; Tel.: +82-2-2019-3440; Fax: +82-2-3463-1049

Abstract: The most significant factor for endothelial cell loss should be readily identified, since prevention is the most crucial treatment. Here, we investigate risk factors for corneal endothelial cell density (ECD) decline following Ahmed glaucoma valve (AGV) implantation and determine the optimal cut-off values. This study included 103 eyes (95 patients) with glaucoma that underwent AGV implantation between January 2006 and January 2021 at a single medical center (Severance Hospital). We conducted consecutive *t*-tests between two groups separated by the ECD change rate to determine the survival state of the enrolled patients. Associations were evaluated using univariable and multivariable linear regressions. Optimal cut-off values for identified risk factors were analyzed using a Cox proportional hazards model and a receiver operating characteristic (ROC) curve based on logistic regression. Mean follow-up duration was 4.09 ± 2.20 years. After implementing consecutive *t*-tests, only patients with an ECD change rate greater than −6.1%/year were considered to have survived. Tube–iris distance (TID) was the only statistically significant factor identified in both the univariable and multivariable linear regressions. The cut-off value determined from the consecutive Cox regression method was 0.33 mm (smallest *p*-value of 0.0087), and the cut-off value determined from the ROC method was 0.371 mm (area under the receiver operating characteristic curve [AUC], 0.662). Patients with short TIDs showed a better ECD prognosis following AGV surgery; we suggest optimal TID cut-off values of 0.33 mm and 0.371 mm based on the implemented Cox regression and ROC methodology, respectively.

Keywords: glaucoma; endothelial cell density; Ahmed glaucoma valve

Citation: Kim, Y.; Cho, W.J.; Kim, J.D.; Cho, H.; Bae, H.W.; Kim, C.Y.; Choi, W. Tube–Iris Distance and Corneal Endothelial Cell Damage Following Ahmed Glaucoma Valve Implantation. *J. Clin. Med.* **2022**, *11*, 5057. https://doi.org/10.3390/jcm11175057

Academic Editors: Michele Figus and Karl Mercieca

Received: 8 July 2022
Accepted: 21 August 2022
Published: 28 August 2022

Publisher's Note: MDPI stays neutral with regard to jurisdictional claims in published maps and institutional affiliations.

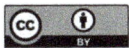

Copyright: © 2022 by the authors. Licensee MDPI, Basel, Switzerland. This article is an open access article distributed under the terms and conditions of the Creative Commons Attribution (CC BY) license (https://creativecommons.org/licenses/by/4.0/).

1. Introduction

Glaucoma drainage device (GDD) implantation is the preferred therapeutic choice for recalcitrant glaucoma patients who fail antiglaucoma medications or trabeculectomies [1–3]. The landmark Tube Versus Trabeculectomy Study demonstrated the superiority of GDD surgery over trabeculectomy with mitomycin C in terms of low failure and revision rates, while the ability to control intraocular pressure (IOP) as well as the number of necessary medications were comparable [2]. Consequently, the use of GDD surgeries has increased over the past two decades, and that of trabeculectomies with mitomycin C has decreased [3].

Endothelial cell density (ECD) damage is a long-term complication of GDD surgery observed at high rates in glaucoma patients [4–7]. The risks of consequent corneal edema and decompensation due to GDD implantation were twice as high as those associated with trabeculectomy, emphasizing the importance of identifying mediating mechanisms and preventing ECD damage [2,8,9].

Efforts with regard to ECD preservation include GDD insertion into the pars plana (PP) or ciliary sulcus (CS), in contrast to the conventional method of inserting it into the anterior chamber [10–13]. However, PP insertion requires vitrectomy and can cause additional complications in the posterior chamber [14]. Implantation in the CS also presents few limitations, including difficulty in localizing the tube during surgery (which requires the presence of pseudophakic or aphakic eyes) and the risk of incurring iris pigmentation due to friction [15].

Because of these constraints, most GDDs are inserted into the anterior chamber. Many studies have examined the optimal angle, depth, or location of tube insertion leading to the best surgical outcome [7,16–18]. Mendrinos et al. inspected the effects of intracameral tube length (TL), tube–corneal distance (TCD), and tube–iris distance (TID) on peripheral ECD reduction and did not find any significant correlations [7]. In contrast, later studies have consistently detected an association between a longer TCD and lower ECD change rates [16,17]. However, a recent study presented a strong association with the tube–corneal angle (TCA) but not with the TCD [18]. Another study did not target the change in ECD over time but instead determined that the existence of peripheral anterior synechiae (PAS) was associated with a lower ECD at a fixed time point [19].

Although many studies have attempted to discover the mechanisms mediating changes in ECD, to date, no research has comprehensively evaluated all tube and ocular parameters. Hence, we conducted the current study, which evaluated TL, TCA, TCD, TID, insertion–iris distance (IID), and other ocular parameters (such as PAS and angle parameters) and determined the optimal cut-off values for the identified risk factors when implanting an Ahmed glaucoma valve (AGV).

2. Materials and Methods

2.1. Study Population

This single-center retrospective case series study was approved by the Institutional Review Board of Severance Hospital (Seoul, Korea; IRB No. 4-2022-0043) and conducted in accordance with the requirements of the Declaration of Helsinki. The requirement for informed consent was waived due to its retrospective nature.

Patients with recalcitrant glaucoma unresponsive to maximal medical doses and who underwent AGV implantation (Model FP-7, New World Medical, Inc., Rancho Cucamonga, CA, USA) were reviewed from a prospectively maintained database at the Severance Hospital. A total of 692 patients underwent AGV implantation between January 2006 and January 2021 and at least one examination via specular microscopy before and after surgery. We excluded patients with a history of Descemet membrane endothelial keratoplasty, penetrating keratoplasty or any other baseline corneal disease affecting the corneal endothelium, cataract surgery, or any kind of vitrectomy. We also excluded patients in whom the AGV was not implanted into the anterior chamber (e.g., sulcus, pars plana). A total of 103 eyes were eligible.

These patients were followed up for more than 1 year. All patients had specular microscopy and anterior segment optical coherence tomography (AS-OCT) imaging findings of adequate quality. If additional intraocular surgery, including repositioning or removal of the valve, was required, follow-up was stopped to exclude possible effects on the corneal endothelium from the analysis.

2.2. Surgical Techniques

All surgeries were performed by glaucoma specialists. The tip of the AGV was placed in the anterior chamber, following its implantation which was performed as previously reported [20]. Briefly, a fornix-based conjunctival incision was made under sub-Tenon anesthesia, and the Tenon capsule was dissected using spring scissors. Two flaps, a 4 × 4 mm right-angled triangular-shaped partial-thickness scleral flap and a continuous 2 mm wide × 6 mm long bridge-shaped partial-thickness scleral flap, were constructed at the superotemporal or superonasal quadrant. Tube priming was performed using balanced salt solution irrigation, and the AGV body was placed 8–10 mm posterior to the limbus (between the rectus muscles). The tube tip was cut to an adequate length and placed in a bevel-up manner. Viscoelastic was injected to maintain the anterior chamber depth before tube insertion. Using a 23-gauge needle, a sclerotomy was created 1–2 mm posterior to the limbus under the scleral flap, entering the anterior chamber where the tube was inserted parallel to the iris plane. The scleral flap was adjusted over the tube and sutured using a 10–0 nylon suture, and the conjunctiva and Tenon's capsule were then secured at the limbus with interrupted 8–0 Vicryl sutures. Topical steroids and antibiotic eye drops were prescribed for eight weeks.

2.3. Examinations

Medical records were reviewed for preoperative clinical factors, including age at surgery, sex, laterality of the operated eye, past medical history (including hypertension [HTN], diabetes mellitus [DM], tuberculosis [TB], hepatitis, and cerebrovascular accidents [CVA]), glaucoma diagnosis, axial length (AXL), anterior chamber depth (ACD), IOP, postoperative data, and uveitis incidence. Other postoperative data, including ECD and ocular and tube parameters, were obtained as follows. Specular microscopic examination was performed by experienced examiners using a noncontact specular microscope (Topcon SP-3000P; Topcon Corp., Tokyo, Japan). The central area of the cornea was imaged while the patient gazed at the target. The manual center-dot method was used to evaluate central corneal ECD, marking at least 50 contiguous endothelial cells.

2.4. Anterior Segment Optical Coherence Tomography (AS-OCT)

The AS-OCT image (Casia SS-1000; Tomey, Nagoya, Japan) closest in time after the operation was used to measure ocular and tube parameters. Because the cross-sectional plane including the tube is not always parallel to the radial section of the eye, variables were evaluated in different cross-sections.

The TCD and TID were measured when the plane was positioned to involve the tube tip. TCD is defined as the distance between the anterior tip of the tube and the cornea (perpendicular to it). TID is defined as the distance between the posterior tip of the tube and the iris (perpendicular to it). The TCA and the IID were measured when the plane was placed to involve the insertion of the tube. The TCA is defined as the angle between the anterior surface of the tube and the posterior corneal surface. The IID is defined as the distance between the anterior insertion site of the tube and the iris (perpendicular to it). The intracameral length of the tube was not measured directly due to concerns regarding cross-sections and was instead computed by calculating the TCD/tan (TCA) ratio, assuming a right triangle (where TCD represents the length of the opposite side and TL represents the length of the hypotenuse). TCA was measured in degrees and then converted to a radian scale before applying tangent functions. The hypothesis is that the curvature of the posterior corneal surface in this triangle can be neglected (Figure 1). We also measured a range of other parameters, including the angle opening distance (AOD), angle recess area (ARA), trabecular iris space area (TISA), trabecular iris angle (TIA) from both the temporal and nasal sides, iris trabecular meshwork contact (ITC), and anterior chamber width (ACW). The central corneal thickness (CCT) was also determined by AS-OCT since the examination results of some patients were omitted from their medical records.

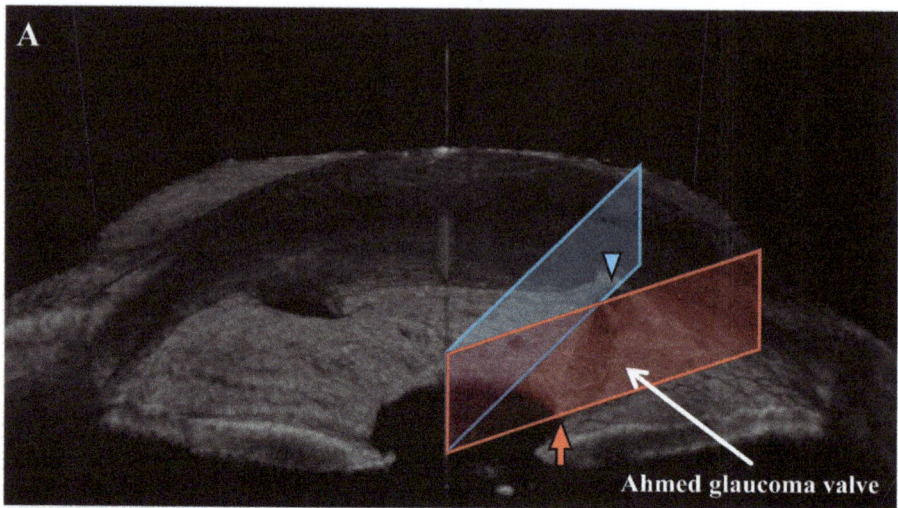
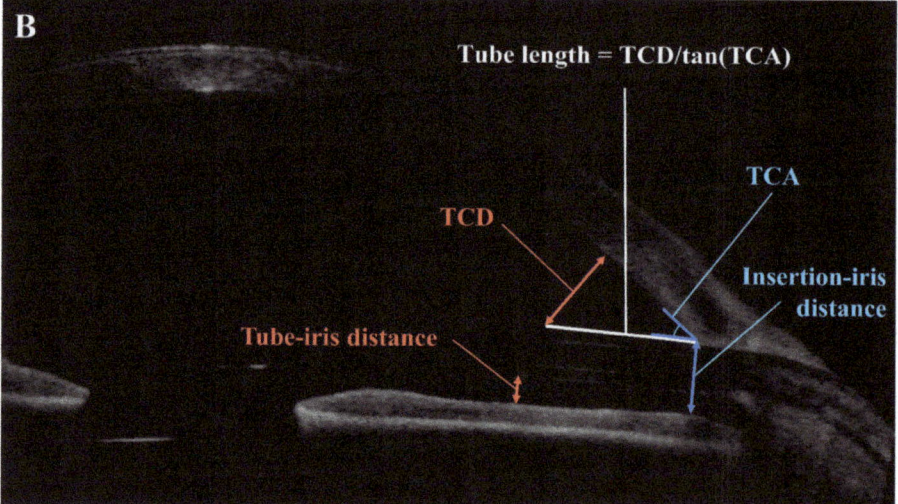

Figure 1. Measurement of tube parameters using anterior segment optical coherence tomography (AS-OCT). Two cross-sections either including depictions of the tube tip (red) or the tube insertion (blue), respectively, are shown in this 3D view. The red arrow indicates the tube tip, and the blue arrowhead shows the insertion site of the tube (**A**). Tube–corneal distance (TCD), tube–iris distance (TID), tube–corneal angle (TCA), and insertion–iris distance (IID) were measured directly, and tube length (TL) was computed as follows: TCD/tan (TCA). The cross-section in this figure was selected from a patient, wherein the tube tip and the insertion site could be seen in the same cross-section plane (**B**).

2.5. Statistical Analyses

Python (version 3.8.8 ; Fredericksburg, VA, USA) and statistical software package R (version 3.6.2; The R Project for Statistical Computing, Vienna, Austria) were employed for data manipulation, visualization, and conducting linear regressions.

Linear regression evaluating the association between ECD and time (years) was performed to derive the coefficient (i.e., the slope of ECD change, cells/mm^2 × year) for the examined patients. This slope was then divided by the preoperative ECD to derive the ECD change rate (%/year). If a patient had only two data points, the crude slope between them was used instead. ECD change rates were then separated into two groups using a single cut-off value, and *t*-tests were conducted to compare the means. The optimal cut-off value (i.e., the value associated with the smallest *p*-value) was determined from these *t*-tests. Groups A and B were defined as patients with small ECD change rates (less than 6.1% decrease) and with large ECD change rates (more than 6.1% decrease), respectively.

Continuous variables are presented as means ± standard deviations and categorical variables as numbers (percentages). We also compared baseline characteristics between Groups A and B using formal statistical tests. More specifically, continuous variables were subjected to Levene's test to examine the assumption of variance equality, and the associated *p*-values were derived using Student's *t*-test or Welch's *t*-test. Categorical variables were compared using either the chi-square test or Fisher's exact test. The tube parameters were compared in the same manner.

Univariable linear regressions evaluating associations between the ECD change rate (%/year) and each variable were performed. Selected factors were combined with data on TCD, TCA, and ITC, which were asserted to be significant with regard to ECD change based on previous results [16–19], in order to conduct a multivariable-adjusted linear regression analysis. A heatmap matrix evaluating Pearson's r correlations between independent variables was used to interpret collinearity. We prioritized achieving a lean model by excluding variables that showed a high correlation (r > 0.7) [21]. Accordingly, either TCD or TCA were always excluded from multivariable analysis models.

We used two different methods to determine the optimal cut-off value for the TID. First, to predict survival, hazard ratios (HRs, with a referent group defined as TID values less than the cut-off) and *p*-values were compared after running univariable Cox regression analyses over every potential cut-off value between 0.01 mm and 1.25 mm at 0.01 mm intervals (Figure 2A). Event state (y = 1) for this model was defined according to the patient's categorization into Group B (ECD change rate < −6.1%/year), survival state (y = 0) was defined according to the patient's categorization into Group A (ECD change rate > −6.1%/year), and follow-up years were used as the time variable.

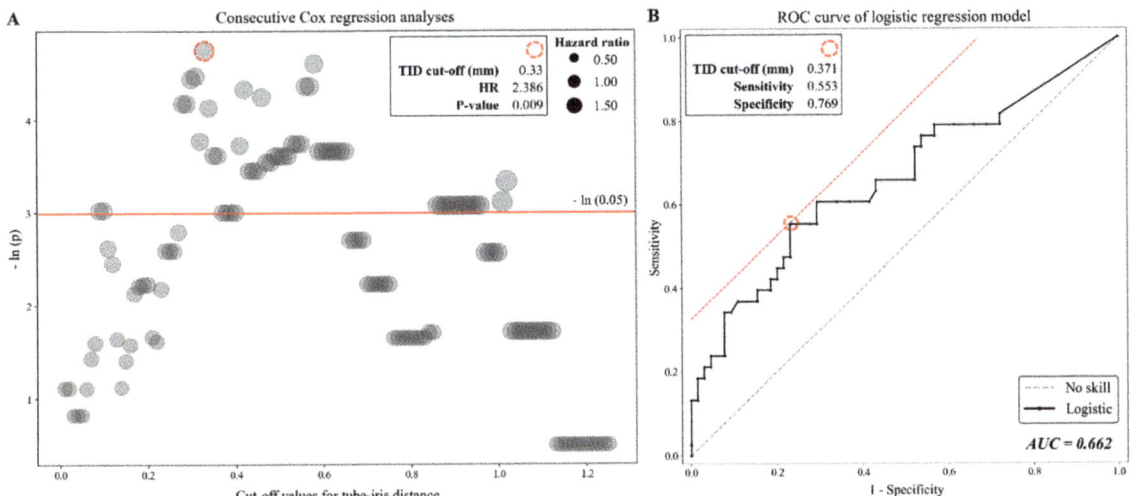

Figure 2. Determination of the optimal cut-off value regarding the tube–iris distance (TID). Consecutive Cox regression analyses were conducted for every potential cut-off value between 0.01 mm and 1.25 mm at 0.01 mm intervals. The x-axis indicates the evaluated TID cut-off values, the y-axis

indicates the −ln (*p*) of the *p*-value for each cut-off (and is demarcated by a red horizontal line showing the value of −ln (0.05)), and the circle size of the determined data points mark the values of the associated hazard ratios (HR) (**A**). A receiver operating characteristic (ROC) curve was plotted using an univariable logistic regression model employing TID as the independent variable, and the area under the ROC curve (AUC) was calculated (**B**).

Second, a receiver operating characteristic (ROC) curve was plotted and the area under the curve (AUC) was then calculated (Figure 2B). The model used to draw the curve was a univariable logistic regression model employing TID as the independent variable. Based on these cut-offs, patients were divided into two groups for constructing Kaplan–Meier (KM) curves, followed by a log-rank test (Figure 3A,B). Finally, we compared postoperative IOP and uveitis incidence between patients with short and long TID using Student's *t*-test and Fisher's exact test, respectively. Additionally, other combinations of variables were evaluated in univariable linear regression to support our interpretation of the results.

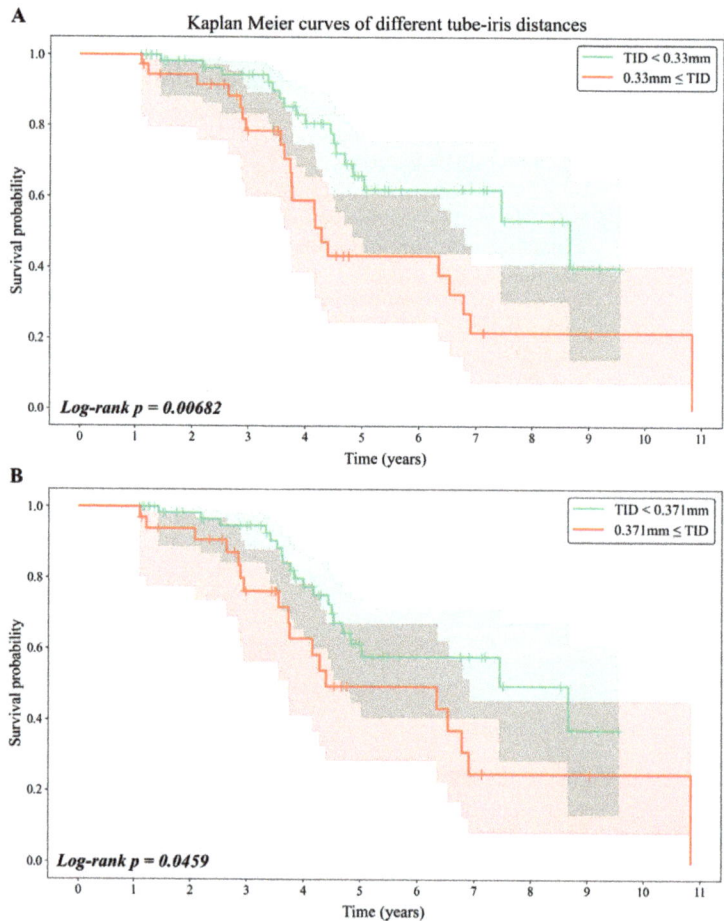

Figure 3. Kaplan–Meier curves of different tube–iris distances. Kaplan–Meier curves and log-rank tests were conducted for comparing patients with short or long tube–iris distances (TIDs), divided by the cut-off value determined from evaluations presented in Figure 2. Survival curves show significant difference with *p*-value of 0.00682 when 0.33 mm is used as the cut-off (**A**). When 0.371 mm is used as the cut-off, survival curves also show significant difference with *p*-value of 0.0459 (**B**).

3. Results

3.1. Patient Characteristics

Altogether, 103 eyes of 95 patients (mean age, 64.20 ± 13.85 years; 62% male) were included, 54% of the evaluated eyes were right eyes, none of the patients had complications such as tube–corneal touch or collapse of the anterior chamber, and patients were followed up for a mean of 4.09 ± 2.20 years. Primary open-angle glaucoma (POAG) was diagnosed in 55% of the glaucoma patients. The mean preoperative central ECD was 2183.42 ± 527.69 (cells/mm^2), the mean final ECD was 1765.49 ± 663.50 (cells/mm^2), and the mean ECD change rate was −4.26 ± 9.49 (%/year). Among 11 cases of neovascular glaucoma, diabetic retinopathy was the primary cause (four proliferative diabetic retinopathies and four non-proliferative diabetic retinopathies), while other three cases were caused by retinal vein occlusions. Additional treatments include panretinal photocoagulation and intravitreal anti-VEGF injections.

3.2. Comparison between Patients Separated by Low and High ECD Change Rates

We classified patients into two groups under the assumption that ECD does not decrease in all patients and conducted consecutive *t*-tests to determine the optimal cut-off value regarding the ECD change rate (Figure S1). The *p*-value continuously decreased as the cut-off increased, reaching a minimum point of 7.720×10^{-16}; the *p*-value continued to increase thereafter. Hence, we considered an ECD change rate of −6.1 (%/year) (i.e., where the *p*-value was the smallest) as the optimal cut-off value, and we thereby separated patients into Group A (with an ECD change rate of >−6.1%/year) and Group B (with an ECD change rate of <−6.1%/year). There were no significant differences in baseline characteristics between Groups A and B in terms of age, sex, laterality, follow-up years, or medical history of HTN, TB, DM, hepatitis, and CVA (Table 1). When tube parameters were compared, we found that TL was shorter, TID was shorter, and TCA was larger in Group A than in B (1.09 ± 0.37 mm vs. 1.27 ± 0.53 mm, *p* = 0.044; 0.23 ± 0.25 mm vs. 0.47 ± 0.46 mm, *p* = 0.004; 33.67 ± 11.24° vs. 28.73 ± 11.62°, *p* = 0.036, respectively; Table 2). In total, 51 out of 103 (50%) patients underwent hypertensive phase (HP), defined as IOP > 21 mmHg during the first 3 months after surgery, which was not associated with tube obstruction, retraction, or valve malfunction [22]. When IOP was above 21 mmHg during HP, glaucoma medications were added and we examined a significant decrease in final IOPs compared to preoperative IOPs (14.17 ± 4.51 vs. 26.02 ± 8.56 mmHg in overall patients, *p* < 0.001 from *t*-test).

Table 1. Patient medical and demographic characteristics (n = 103).

Baseline	Overall	Patients without an ECD Decline (Group A, n = 65)	Patients with an ECD Decline (Group B, n = 38)	*p*-Value
Age	64.20 ± 13.85	63.95 ± 13.79	64.63 ± 14.12	0.812
Sex (M/F)	64/39	40/25	24/14	0.963 *
Laterality (R/L)	56/47	38/27	18/20	0.376 *
AXL (mm)	24.80 ± 1.89	24.78 ± 1.86	24.82 ± 1.96	0.919
CCT (μm)	521.37 ± 51.27	518.60 ± 51.91	526.11 ± 50.49	0.476
Follow-up (years)	4.09 ± 2.20	4.02 ± 2.32	4.22 ± 2.01	0.663
Preoperative IOP (mmHg)	26.02 ± 8.56	25.56 ± 8.68	26.82 ± 8.41	0.475
Final IOP (mmHg)	14.17 ± 4.51	14.68 ± 4.56	13.30 ± 4.36	0.135
Preoperative ECD (cells/mm^2)	2183.42 ± 527.69	2215.87 ± 473.24	2127.90 ± 612.57	0.417
Final ECD (cells/mm^2)	1765.49 ± 663.50	2119.09 ± 494.94	1160.66 ± 441.07	<0.001
ECD change rate (%/year)	−4.26 ± 9.49	0.72 ± 5.42	−12.78 ± 8.9	<0.001

Table 1. Cont.

Baseline	Overall	Patients without an ECD Decline (Group A, n = 65)	Patients with an ECD Decline (Group B, n = 38)	p-Value
Systemic disease				
Hypertension	43 (41.75)	30 (46.15)	13 (34.21)	0.328 *
Tuberculosis	5 (4.85)	3 (4.62)	2 (5.26)	1.000 †
Diabetes mellitus	38 (36.89)	29 (44.62)	9 (23.68)	0.056 *
Hepatitis	2 (1.94)	2 (3.08)	0 (0.0)	0.530 †
Cerebrovascular accident	5 (4.85)	4 (6.15)	1 (2.63)	0.649 †
Glaucoma				
POAG	57 (55.34)	37 (56.92)	20 (52.63)	0.828 *
Chronic angle-closure glaucoma	3 (2.91)	2 (3.08)	1 (2.63)	1.000 †
Neovascular glaucoma	11 (10.68)	8 (12.31)	3 (7.89)	0.742 †
Pigmentary glaucoma	1 (0.97)	1 (1.54)	0 (0.0)	1.000 †
Pseudoexfoliation glaucoma	3 (2.91)	2 (3.08)	1 (2.63)	1.000 †
Secondary (d/t uveitis)	12 (11.65)	6 (9.23)	6 (15.79)	0.495 *
Secondary other	16 (15.53)	9 (13.85)	7 (18.42)	0.736 *

AXL, axial length; CCT, central corneal thickness; IOP, intraocular pressure; ECD, endothelial cell density; POAG, primary open angle glaucoma. * χ2 test; † Fisher's exact test; otherwise t-test.

Table 2. Comparison of tube parameters between the patients enrolled in Group A and Group B.

Tube Parameters	Overall	Patients without an ECD Decline (Group A, n = 65)	Patients with an ECD Decline (Group B, n = 38)	p-Value
Tube length (mm)	1.15 ± 0.44	1.09 ± 0.37	1.27 ± 0.53	0.044 *
Tube–corneal distance (mm)	0.77 ± 0.47	0.77 ± 0.40	0.76 ± 0.57	0.932
Tube–iris distance (mm)	0.32 ± 0.36	0.23 ± 0.25	0.47 ± 0.46	0.004 *
Tube–corneal angle (°)	31.85 ± 11.58	33.67 ± 11.24	28.73 ± 11.62	0.036 *
Insertion–iris distance (mm)	0.68 ± 0.27	0.66 ± 0.24	0.71 ± 0.32	0.372
Tube location (ST/SN) †	101/2	63/2	38/0	0.530

ECD, endothelial cell density; † Fisher's exact test; * $p < 0.05$ from t-test.

3.3. Tube–Iris Distance Was the Only Statistically Significant Factor Predicting the ECD Change Rate

Univariable linear regressions evaluating the association between the ECD change rate and independent factors revealed three statistically significant factors (Table 3): the final ECD ($\beta = 8.70 \times 10^{-5}$ $p < 0.001$), the TL ($\beta = -0.0422$, $p = 0.047$), and the TID ($\beta = -0.0722$, $p = 0.005$). We included the latter two parameters in the multivariable regression analysis but excluded the final ECD, since final values cannot be used to predict survival. We also included the parameters found to be statistically significant in previous reports (TCD, TCA, and ITC). The correlation matrix between independent variables showed a high correlation between TCD and TCA (r = 0.78 via the Pearson method), which was above our predetermined cut-off value of 0.7 (Figure S2). It was difficult to identify which variable to include when comparing TCD and TCA because both showed moderate correlations with TL (r = 0.55) and TID (r = −0.54), respectively. Hence, multivariable analyses were performed twice after excluding either of them. In both regressions, TID was the only factor that showed statistical significance regarding the ECD change rate ($\beta = -0.0684$, $p = 0.025$ when TCD was excluded; $\beta = -0.0743$, $p = 0.015$ when TCA was excluded; Table 4).

Table 3. Univariable linear regressions regarding associations with ECD change rates.

Variables	Univariable Analysis		
	β	95% Confidence Interval	p-Value
Age (years)	1.10×10^{-5}	$[-1.34 \times 10^{-3}, 1.36 \times 10^{-3}]$	0.987
Sex (M/F)	-4.30×10^{-3}	$[-4.27 \times 10^{-2}, 3.41 \times 10^{-2}]$	0.825
Laterality (R/L)	3.40×10^{-5}	$[-3.74 \times 10^{-2}, 3.74 \times 10^{-2}]$	0.999
AXL (mm)	1.70×10^{-4}	$[-9.74 \times 10^{-3}, 1.01 \times 10^{-2}]$	0.973
CCT (μm)	-7.70×10^{-5}	$[-4.42 \times 10^{-4}, 2.88 \times 10^{-4}]$	0.676
Follow-up (years)	-3.26×10^{-3}	$[-1.17 \times 10^{-2}, 5.21 \times 10^{-3}]$	0.447
Preoperative IOP (mmHg)	-2.52×10^{-4}	$[-2.44 \times 10^{-3}, 1.93 \times 10^{-3}]$	0.819
Final IOP (mmHg)	2.89×10^{-3}	$[-1.22 \times 10^{-3}, 7.00 \times 10^{-3}]$	0.166
Preoperative ECD(cells/mm^2)	-2.10×10^{-5}	$[-5.70 \times 10^{-5}, 1.40 \times 10^{-5}]$	0.232
Final ECD (cells/mm^2)	8.70×10^{-5}	$[6.40 \times 10^{-5}, 1.09 \times 10^{-4}]$	<0.001 *
Systemic disease			
Hypertension	2.01×10^{-2}	$[-1.75 \times 10^{-2}, 5.77 \times 10^{-2}]$	0.292
Tuberculosis	-6.50×10^{-3}	$[-9.32 \times 10^{-2}, 8.02 \times 10^{-2}]$	0.882
Diabetes mellitus	2.64×10^{-2}	$[-1.19 \times 10^{-2}, 6.47 \times 10^{-2}]$	0.174
Hepatitis	9.97×10^{-2}	$[-3.39 \times 10^{-2}, 2.33 \times 10^{-1}]$	0.142
Cerebrovascular accident	5.60×10^{-2}	$[-3.00 \times 10^{-2}, 1.42 \times 10^{-1}]$	0.199
Glaucoma			
POAG	7.25×10^{-3}	$[-3.02 \times 10^{-2}, 4.47 \times 10^{-2}]$	0.702
Chronic angle-closure glaucoma	9.86×10^{-3}	$[-1.01 \times 10^{-1}, 1.21 \times 10^{-1}]$	0.860
Neovascular glaucoma	2.99×10^{-2}	$[-3.02 \times 10^{-2}, 8.99 \times 10^{-2}]$	0.326
Pigmentary glaucoma	7.35×10^{-2}	$[-1.16 \times 10^{-1}, 2.63 \times 10^{-1}]$	0.443
Pseudoexfoliation glaucoma	-3.57×10^{-2}	$[-1.46 \times 10^{-1}, 7.49 \times 10^{-2}]$	0.524
Secondary (d/t uveitis)	-2.87×10^{-2}	$[-8.65 \times 10^{-2}, 2.91 \times 10^{-2}]$	0.326
Secondary other	-1.27×10^{-2}	$[-6.40 \times 10^{-2}, 3.87 \times 10^{-2}]$	0.626
Tube parameters			
Tube length (mm)	-4.22×10^{-2}	$[-8.38 \times 10^{-2}, -5.64 \times 10^{-4}]$	0.047 *
Tube–corneal distance (mm)	-4.04×10^{-3}	$[-4.41 \times 10^{-2}, 3.60 \times 10^{-2}]$	0.842
Tube–iris distance (mm)	-7.22×10^{-2}	$[-1.22 \times 10^{-1}, -2.23 \times 10^{-2}]$	0.005 *
Tube–corneal angle (°)	1.11×10^{-3}	$[-4.94 \times 10^{-4}, 2.71 \times 10^{-3}]$	0.173
Insertion–iris distance (mm)	-6.73×10^{-2}	$[-1.35 \times 10^{-1}, 5.87 \times 10^{-4}]$	0.052
Tube location (ST/SN)	-6.53×10^{-2}	$[-2.00 \times 10^{-1}, 6.91 \times 10^{-2}]$	0.337
Anterior chamber parameters			
ACD (mm)	-2.37×10^{-2}	$[-4.87 \times 10^{-2}, 1.33 \times 10^{-3}]$	0.063
ITC (%)	-9.30×10^{-5}	$[-7.19 \times 10^{-4}, 5.34 \times 10^{-4}]$	0.770
ACW (mm)	1.82×10^{-2}	$[-2.27 \times 10^{-2}, 5.91 \times 10^{-2}]$	0.379
nasal AOD500 (μm)	3.00×10^{-5}	$[-4.10 \times 10^{-5}, 1.01 \times 10^{-4}]$	0.405
nasal AOD750 (μm)	1.20×10^{-5}	$[-4.10 \times 10^{-5}, 6.60 \times 10^{-5}]$	0.650
nasal ARA500 (μm)	4.70×10^{-5}	$[-1.20 \times 10^{-4}, 2.15 \times 10^{-4}]$	0.576
nasal ARA750 (μm)	2.90×10^{-5}	$[-7.20 \times 10^{-5}, 1.30 \times 10^{-4}]$	0.575
nasal TISA500 (μm)	7.00×10^{-5}	$[-1.18 \times 10^{-4}, 2.59 \times 10^{-4}]$	0.461
nasal TISA750 (μm)	3.60×10^{-5}	$[-7.20 \times 10^{-5}, 1.44 \times 10^{-4}]$	0.510
nasal TIA500 (°)	3.25×10^{-4}	$[-7.94 \times 10^{-4}, 1.45 \times 10^{-3}]$	0.565
nasal TIA750 (°)	2.26×10^{-4}	$[-1.02 \times 10^{-3}, 1.47 \times 10^{-3}]$	0.719
temporal AOD500 (μm)	3.10×10^{-5}	$[-3.50 \times 10^{-5}, 9.80 \times 10^{-5}]$	0.350
temporal AOD750 (μm)	1.50×10^{-5}	$[-3.40 \times 10^{-5}, 6.50 \times 10^{-5}]$	0.540
temporal ARA500 (μm)	9.70×10^{-5}	$[-5.00 \times 10^{-5}, 2.43 \times 10^{-4}]$	0.194
temporal ARA750 (μm)	4.60×10^{-5}	$[-4.50 \times 10^{-5}, 1.37 \times 10^{-4}]$	0.317
temporal TISA500 (μm)	9.50×10^{-5}	$[-7.30 \times 10^{-5}, 2.62 \times 10^{-4}]$	0.264
temp_TISA_750 (μm)	4.70×10^{-5}	$[-5.00 \times 10^{-5}, 1.45 \times 10^{-4}]$	0.337
temp_TIA_500 (°)	3.73×10^{-4}	$[-6.68 \times 10^{-4}, 1.41 \times 10^{-3}]$	0.479
temp_TIA_750 (°)	4.02×10^{-4}	$[-7.94 \times 10^{-4}, 1.60 \times 10^{-3}]$	0.506

AXL axial length, CCT central corneal thickness, IOP intraocular pressure, ECD endothelial cell density, POAG primary open angle glaucoma, ACD anterior chamber depth, ITC iris trabecular meshwork contact, ACW anterior chamber width, AOD angle opening distance, ARA angle recess area, TISA trabecular iris space area, TIA trabecular iris angle, * $p < 0.05$

Table 4. Multivariable linear regressions regarding associations with endothelial cell density change rates. Due to the high collinearity between TCD and TCA, one or the other of these variables was excluded when conducting multivariable analyses.

Variables	Multivariable Analysis (TCD Excluded)			Multivariable Analysis (TCA Excluded)		
	β	95% CI	p-Value	β	95% CI	p-Value
Tube parameters						
Tube length (mm)	-3.71×10^{-2}	$[-7.80 \times 10^{-2}, 4.00 \times 10^{-3}]$	0.076	-3.00×10^{-2}	$[-8.40 \times 10^{-2}, 2.40 \times 10^{-2}]$	0.269
Tube–corneal distance (mm)				-1.13×10^{-2}	$[-6.60 \times 10^{-2}, 4.40 \times 10^{-2}]$	0.683
Tube–iris distance (mm)	-6.84×10^{-2}	$[-1.28 \times 10^{-1}, -9.00 \times 10^{-3}]$	0.025 *	-7.43×10^{-2}	$[-1.34 \times 10^{-1}, -1.50 \times 10^{-2}]$	0.015 *
Tube–corneal angle (°)	-3.52×10^{-5}	$[-2.00 \times 10^{-3}, 2.00 \times 10^{-3}]$	0.970			
Anterior chamber parameters						
ITC (%)	-6.25×10^{-5}	$[-1.00 \times 10^{-3}, 1.00 \times 10^{-3}]$	0.838	-7.03×10^{-5}	$[-1.00 \times 10^{-3}, 1.00 \times 10^{-3}]$	0.818

CI, confidence interval; ITC, iris trabecular meshwork contact; * $p < 0.05$.

3.4. Determination of the Optimal Cut-Off Value for TID

In our first approach, implemented to inspect the optimal cut-off values for TID, consecutive Cox proportional hazard analyses were conducted over every potential cut-off value between 0.01 mm and 1.25 mm at 0.01 mm intervals (Figure 2A). All cut-off values between 0.28 mm and 0.65 mm showed statistical significance regarding predicting survival ($p < 0.05$), while a TID of ≥ 0.33 mm showed the smallest p-value ($p = 0.0087$) and the largest impact (HR = 2.39). In our second approach, a univariable logistic regression model using TID as the independent variable showed an AUC of 0.662. An optimal cut-off value of 0.371 mm was determined by finding the point of contact of a line with a slope of 1 on the ROC curve. The sensitivity and specificity associated with this value were 0.553 and 0.769, respectively (Figure 2B).

3.5. Comparison between Patients with Short and Long TID

We also divided patients into two groups to draw KM curves based on TID values, with 0.33 mm and 0.371 mm as the respective cut-off values (Figure 3). The median survival times of patients with a TID of <0.33 mm, a TID of <0.371 mm, a TID of ≥ 0.33 mm, and a TID of ≥ 0.371 mm were 8.66 years (95% CI, 4.82–inf), 7.44 years (95% CI, 4.68–inf), 4.28 years (95% CI, 3.73–6.78), and 4.39 years (95% CI, 3.73–6.90), respectively. KM survival curves of short and long TID showed statistically significant differences regarding either cut-off value (cut-off, 0.33 mm, $p = 0.00682$ by the log-rank test; cut-off, 0.371 mm, $p = 0.0459$ by the log-rank test). Postoperative final IOP values were also compared via t-tests and did not show any differences between short and long TIDs (cut-off, 0.33 mm, 14.36 ± 4.01 mmHg vs. 13.83 ± 5.34 mmHg, $p = 0.569$; cut-off, 0.371 mm, 14.33 ± 4.03 mmHg vs. 13.84 ± 5.45 mmHg, $p = 0.612$; Table S1).

We also thoroughly reviewed medical records to examine uveitis onset after AGV implantation. Of those not initially diagnosed with secondary glaucoma due to uveitis, only one patient had postoperative uveitis, with a TID of 0.05 mm (Table S2). No significant differences in uveitis incidence between patients with short and long TID were identified ($p = 1.00$).

3.6. IID/TCA Was Significantly Associated with ECD Change Rate

We additionally conducted several univariable linear regressions to inspect associations between variables related to the tube–corneal angle or distance and the ECD change rate. Only IID/TCA was significantly associated with the ECD change rate, with a negative coefficient (β = −1.2467, $p = 0.021$, Table S2).

4. Discussion

In our study the mean ECD change rate after tube insertion was −4.26 ± 9.49 (%/year), showing similar or less ECD change rate with some minimally invasive glaucoma surgeries. For instance, Oddone et al. conducted a study regarding XEN implants and reported a mean ECD reduction of −5.6% per year and Ibarz-Barberá et al. reported −7.4% ECD loss after PRESERFLO implantation [23,24].

However, our study adopted the hypothesis that not all glaucoma patients show ECD decline after AGV implantation [18]. The proportion of patients classified into the ECD reduction group was 36.9%, comparable to that reported by Lee et al. (32.3%). The mean ECD change rate in those patients without ECD reduction was 0.72 ± 5.42 (%/year), which is similar to that of patients receiving glaucoma medication without undergoing surgery reported by previous studies from South Korea (−3.7 ± 5.2%/year and −0.1 ± 2.4%/year) [6,9]. This supported our a priori hypothesis. In agreement with a previous study [16], univariable linear regression showed no significant associations between the ECD change rate and glaucoma type, including uveitic glaucoma.

Several variables (TCD, TCA, ITC) that had a statistically significant effect on ECD loss in previous studies were found to be non-significant. A low TCD was correlated with increased ECD loss in a multivariable analysis performed by Koo et al. [17]. However, collinearity between independent variables was not checked in that study, although this is encouraged before applying linear regression analyses, especially when the purpose is to obtain a lean and operationalized model [25]. In our study, TCD and TCA showed a high correlation (r = 0.78), which surpassed our prespecified cut-off of 0.7 (adopted from Donath et al.) [21]. Thus, either variable was excluded from our multivariable-adjusted models, which might account for the differences between the study by Koo et al. and this one. Different TCD distributions could also underlie these contrasting findings. Secondly, unlike a recent study by Lee et al. in which TCA was found to be a strong factor for predicting ECD loss, our study did not find the significance of TCA in linear regressions. Only the statistical significance of TCA in a comparative t-test evaluating differences between Groups A and B demonstrated the same tendency. This discrepancy might arise from differences in the sample distribution. Our population showed a wider TCA distribution, with a standard deviation twice as large as that detected by Lee et al. Lastly, a higher PAS was previously reported to correlate with a smaller central ECD [19]. Therefore, we subjected the ITC variable to multivariable linear regression, but the results were non-significant. This implies that the ITC might show significance in cross-sectional but not in time-series data, but this should be confirmed in future research.

We used two different methods to determine the optimal cut-off value for TID for predicting endothelial cell damage. Both methods provided a similar value and the log-rank tests using either of them were significant. The median survival time of the short TID group showed an infinite upper limit for the 95% confidence interval (CI). However, we believe that this finding was due to only a few patients showing large ECD losses in the short TID group, and therefore spurious.

To the best of our knowledge, this study is the first to consider the AGV insertion site as a tube parameter. In a fixed ocular structure, the insertion–iris distance, tube–corneal angle, and tube length are the only variables necessary to calculate the distance from the tube tip to the iris. Therefore, we assert that the TID is an important endpoint variable that can be expressed as a function of eye structure, IID, TCA, and TL values. The fact that TCA does not show statistical significance regarding the ECD change rate can be understood in this context. With a fixed TCA, the TID increases or decreases with the IID. We investigated this issue by conducting univariable linear regressions using combinations of variables (Table S2). AXL and ACW were included as representations of the eye structure. Only the IID/TCA ratio showed a significant correlation with the ECD change rate. A negative coefficient regarding the IID/TCA ratio implies that, for the purpose of ECD preservation, when the IID is fixed, it is better to have a larger TCA, and when the TCA is fixed, it is better to have a smaller IID.

Our study has additional limitations. First, the sample enrolled comprised a relatively homogenous group of patients who were conservatively selected. However, the study was not pre-planned and selection bias could not be avoided due to its retrospective nature. Moreover, we did not include control groups but instead classified patients according to ECD change rates, which might have affected our result. This limitation was compensated by comparing the ratio of patient numbers and the mean ECD change rate in each group with findings from previous studies. Second, the frequencies and intervals of specular microscopic examinations differed among patients. Therefore, we calculated the slope of the ECD change over time using linear regression to compare the most appropriate ECD change rate between patients. Third, it has been reported that tube parameters in AS-OCT images can present differences over time [26]. Although we did not measure multiple AS-OCT images from each patient, further studies should consider this possibility. Lastly, we evaluated only the central region of the cornea for ECD calculation, but it has been shown that the peripheral area, especially the superotemporal area, is susceptible to greater ECD loss [6,17,18]. A plausible mechanism for this finding is that progenitor cells from the peripheral endothelium are more affected by jet flow or turbulence when the tube is inserted [27]. Additional prospective studies evaluating ECD in the entire cornea and considering the tube parameters evaluated here will provide more comprehensive insights.

Despite these limitations, the long follow-up duration, which is essential for observing ECD changes over time, is a substantial strength of our study. The mean follow-up time was 4.09 ± 2.20 years, which is higher than that from several previous studies (3 years, Tan et al.; 29.30 ± 14.67 months, Lee et al.; 2.5 ± 2.6 years, Koo et al.; 2 years, Lee et al.) [6,16–18].

5. Conclusions

In conclusion, our study suggests that TID is a feasible surrogate marker for surgeons to monitor during AGV implantations. We have shown that the TID can be determined as a function of the eye structure, the IID, the TCA, and the intracameral TL. The optimal cut-off value for the TID was found to be either 0.33 mm or 0.371 mm (depending on the methodology). Thus, our findings suggest that the tube should be inserted close enough to the iris to make the TID shorter than the cut-off value. Our findings guide future research directions and inform medical guidelines regarding surgical planning and follow-up protocols.

Supplementary Materials: The following supporting information can be downloaded at: https://www.mdpi.com/article/10.3390/jcm11175057/s1, Figure S1: Results of consecutive *t*-tests determining the optimal cut-off value for the endothelial cell density (ECD) change rate; Figure S2: Correlation heatmap matrix between a range of independent variables; Table S1: Comparison of postoperative IOP and uveitis incidence between patients with short TID and long TID; Table S2: Combinations of variables related to tube–corneal angle were used for additional univariable linear regression analyses.

Author Contributions: Y.K., W.J.C. and W.C. conceived of the study design. Y.K. and W.J.C. collected the study data. Y.K., W.J.C. and J.D.K. analyzed and interpreted the data. Y.K. and W.C. drafted this manuscript. Y.K., H.C., W.J.C., J.D.K., H.W.B., C.Y.K. and W.C. critically revised the manuscript. Y.K., W.J.C., J.D.K., H.C., H.W.B., C.Y.K. and W.C. approved the final version of the manuscript. All authors have read and agreed to the published version of the manuscript.

Funding: This work was supported by the Basic Science Research Program at the National Research Foundation of Korea (NRF-2022R1I1A1A01071919 & NRF-2019R1A2C1091089) and by a faculty research grant from the Yonsei University College of Medicine (6-2020-0139). The funding organizations had no role in the design or conduct of this study.

Institutional Review Board Statement: The study was conducted in accordance with the Declaration of Helsinki, and approved by the Institutional Review Board of Severance Hospital (Seoul, Korea; IRB No. 4-2022-0043).

Informed Consent Statement: Patient consent was waived due to due to its retrospective nature.

Data Availability Statement: The datasets used and/or analyzed during the current study are available from the corresponding author upon reasonable request.

Conflicts of Interest: The authors declare no conflict of interest.

References

1. Arora, K.S.; Robin, A.L.; Corcoran, K.J.; Corcoran, S.L.; Ramulu, P.Y. Use of Various Glaucoma Surgeries and Procedures in Medicare Beneficiaries from 1994 to 2012. *Ophthalmology* **2015**, *122*, 1615–1624. [CrossRef] [PubMed]
2. Gedde, S.J.; Schiffman, J.C.; Feuer, W.J.; Herndon, L.W.; Brandt, J.D.; Budenz, D.L. Treatment Outcomes in the Tube Versus Trabeculectomy (TVT) Study After Five Years of Follow-up. *Am. J. Ophthalmol.* **2012**, *153*, 789–803.e782. [CrossRef] [PubMed]
3. Vinod, K.; Gedde, S.J.; Feuer, W.J.; Panarelli, J.F.; Chang, T.C.; Chen, P.P.; Parrish, R.K., 2nd. Practice Preferences for Glaucoma Surgery: A Survey of the American Glaucoma Society. *J. Glaucoma* **2017**, *26*, 687–693. [CrossRef] [PubMed]
4. Topouzis, F.; Coleman, A.L.; Choplin, N.; Bethlem, M.M.; Hill, R.; Yu, F.; Panek, W.C.; Wilson, M.R. Follow-up of the original cohort with the Ahmed glaucoma valve implant. *Am. J. Ophthalmol.* **1999**, *128*, 198–204. [CrossRef]
5. Minckler, D.S.; Francis, B.A.; Hodapp, E.A.; Jampel, H.D.; Lin, S.C.; Samples, J.R.; Smith, S.D.; Singh, K. Aqueous shunts in glaucoma: A report by the American Academy of Ophthalmology. *Ophthalmology* **2008**, *115*, 1089–1098. [CrossRef]
6. Lee, E.-K.; Yun, Y.-J.; Lee, J.-E.; Yim, J.-H.; Kim, C.-S. Changes in Corneal Endothelial Cells after Ahmed Glaucoma Valve Implantation: 2-Year Follow-up. *Am. J. Ophthalmol.* **2009**, *148*, 361–367. [CrossRef]
7. Mendrinos, E.; Dosso, A.; Sommerhalder, J.; Shaarawy, T. Coupling of HRT II and AS-OCT to evaluate corneal endothelial cell loss and in vivo visualization of the Ahmed glaucoma valve implant. *Eye* **2009**, *23*, 1836–1844. [CrossRef]
8. Bailey, A.K.; Sarkisian, S.R., Jr. Complications of tube implants and their management. *Curr. Opin. Ophthalmol.* **2014**, *25*, 148–153. [CrossRef]
9. Kim, K.N.; Lee, S.B.; Lee, Y.H.; Lee, J.J.; Lim, H.B.; Kim, C.S. Changes in corneal endothelial cell density and the cumulative risk of corneal decompensation after Ahmed glaucoma valve implantation. *Br. J. Ophthalmol.* **2016**, *100*, 933–938. [CrossRef]
10. Qin, V.L.; Kaleem, M.; Conti, F.F.; Rockwood, E.J.; Singh, A.; Sood-Mendiratta, S.; Sears, J.E.; Silva, F.Q.; Eisengart, J.; Singh, R.P. Long-term clinical outcomes of pars Plana versus anterior chamber placement of Glaucoma implant tubes. *J. Glaucoma* **2018**, *27*, 440–444. [CrossRef]
11. Rososinski, A.; Wechsler, D.; Grigg, J. Retrospective review of pars plana versus anterior chamber placement of Baerveldt glaucoma drainage device. *J. Glaucoma* **2015**, *24*, 95–99. [CrossRef] [PubMed]
12. Weiner, A.; Cohn, A.D.; Balasubramaniam, M.; Weiner, A.J. Glaucoma tube shunt implantation through the ciliary sulcus in pseudophakic eyes with high risk of corneal decompensation. *J. Glaucoma* **2010**, *19*, 405–411. [CrossRef] [PubMed]
13. Maris, P.J., Jr.; Tsai, J.C.; Khatib, N.; Bansal, R.; Al-Aswad, L.A. Clinical outcomes of Ahmed Glaucoma valve in posterior segment versus anterior chamber. *J. Glaucoma* **2013**, *22*, 183–189. [CrossRef] [PubMed]
14. Kim, J.Y.; Lee, J.S.; Lee, T.; Seo, D.; Choi, W.; Bae, H.W.; Kim, C.Y. Corneal endothelial cell changes and surgical results after Ahmed glaucoma valve implantation: Ciliary sulcus versus anterior chamber tube placement. *Sci. Rep.* **2021**, *11*, 12986. [CrossRef]
15. Moon, K.; Kim, Y.C.; Kim, K.S. Ciliary Sulcus Ahmed Valve Implantation. *KJO* **2007**, *21*, 127–130. [CrossRef]
16. Tan, A.N.; Webers, C.A.; Berendschot, T.T.; de Brabander, J.; de Witte, P.M.; Nuijts, R.M.; Schouten, J.S.; Beckers, H.J. Corneal endothelial cell loss after Baerveldt glaucoma drainage device implantation in the anterior chamber. *Acta Ophthalmol.* **2017**, *95*, 91–96. [CrossRef]
17. Koo, E.B.; Hou, J.; Han, Y.; Keenan, J.D.; Stamper, R.L.; Jeng, B.H. Effect of glaucoma tube shunt parameters on cornea endothelial cells in patients with Ahmed valve implants. *Cornea* **2015**, *34*, 37–41. [CrossRef]
18. Lee, H.M.; Kim, K.N.; Park, K.S.; Lee, N.H.; Lee, S.B.; Kim, C.-S. Relationship between tube parameters and corneal endothelial cell damage after Ahmed glaucoma valve implantation: A comparative study. *J. Clin. Med.* **2020**, *9*, 2546. [CrossRef]
19. Hau, S.; Scott, A.; Bunce, C.; Barton, K. Corneal endothelial morphology in eyes implanted with anterior chamber aqueous shunts. *Cornea* **2011**, *30*, 50–55. [CrossRef]
20. Lee, C.K.; Ma, K.T.; Hong, Y.J.; Kim, C.Y. Long-term clinical outcomes of Ahmed valve implantation in patients with refractory glaucoma. *PLoS ONE* **2017**, *12*, e0187533. [CrossRef]
21. Donath, C.; Grässel, E.; Baier, D.; Pfeiffer, C.; Bleich, S.; Hillemacher, T. Predictors of binge drinking in adolescents: Ultimate and distal factors—A representative study. *BMC Public Health* **2012**, *12*, 263. [CrossRef] [PubMed]
22. Pakravan, M.; Rad, S.S.; Yazdani, S.; Ghahari, E.; Yaseri, M. Effect of early treatment with aqueous suppressants on Ahmed glaucoma valve implantation outcomes. *Ophthalmology* **2014**, *121*, 1693–1698. [CrossRef] [PubMed]
23. Oddone, F.; Roberti, G.; Posarelli, C.; Agnifili, L.; Mastropasqua, L.; Carnevale, C.; Micelli Ferrari, T.; Pace, V.; Sacchi, M.; Cremonesi, E.; et al. Endothelial Cell Density after XEN Implant Surgery: Short-term Data from the Italian XEN Glaucoma Treatment Registry (XEN-GTR). *J. Glaucoma* **2021**, *30*, 559–565. [CrossRef] [PubMed]
24. Ibarz-Barberá, M.; Morales-Fernández, L.; Corroto-Cuadrado, A.; Martinez-Galdón, F.; Tañá-Rivero, P.; Gómez de Liaño, R.; Teus, M.A. Corneal Endothelial Cell Loss After PRESERFLO™ MicroShunt Implantation in the Anterior Chamber: Anterior Segment OCT Tube Location as a Risk Factor. *Ophthalmol. Ther.* **2022**, *11*, 293–310. [CrossRef] [PubMed]
25. Vatcheva, K.P.; Lee, M.; McCormick, J.B.; Rahbar, M.H. Multicollinearity in Regression Analyses Conducted in Epidemiologic Studies. *Epidemiology (Sunnyvale)* **2016**, *6*, 227. [CrossRef] [PubMed]

26. Lopilly Park, H.; Jung, K.; Park, C. Serial intracameral visualization of the Ahmed glaucoma valve tube by anterior segment optical coherence tomography. *Eye* **2012**, *26*, 1256–1262. [CrossRef]
27. Joyce, N.C. Proliferative capacity of the corneal endothelium. *Prog. Retin. Eye Res.* **2003**, *22*, 359–389. [CrossRef]

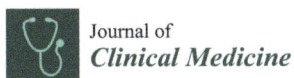

Article

Outcomes and Predictors of Failure of Ultrasound Cyclo Plasty for Primary Open-Angle Glaucoma

Faisal A. Almobarak [1,2,*], Ahmed Alrubean [1,3], Waleed Alsarhani [1,4,5], Abdullah Aljenaidel [1] and Essam A. Osman [1,2]

1. Department of Ophthalmology, College of Medicine, King Saud University, Riyadh 11451, Saudi Arabia
2. Glaucoma Research Chair, King Saud University, Riyadh 11451, Saudi Arabia
3. Department of Ophthalmology, College of Medicine, Al-Imam Muhammad Ibn Saud Islamic University, Riyadh 11564, Saudi Arabia
4. Department of Ophthalmology, King Faisal Specialist Hospital and Research Center, Riyadh 11564, Saudi Arabia
5. Department of Ophthalmology and Vision Sciences, University of Toronto, Toronto, ON M5T 3A9, Canada
* Correspondence: falmobarak@ksu.edu.sa

Abstract: Aims: To evaluate the outcomes of ultrasound cyclo plasty (UCP) for primary open-angle glaucoma (POAG) and identify the predictors of failure. **Methods:** This retrospective cohort study included patients with POAG who underwent UCP at King Abdul Aziz University Hospital, Riyadh, Saudi Arabia, between 2016 and 2021. The main outcome measures were the intraocular pressure (IOP), the number of antiglaucoma medications, and the presence of vision-threatening complications. The surgical outcome of each eye was based on the main outcome measures. Cox proportional hazard regression analysis was performed to identify the possible predictors of UCP failure. **Results:** Sixty-six eyes of fifty-five patients were included herein. The mean follow-up period was 28.95 (±16.9) months. The mean IOP decreased significantly from 23.02 (±6.1) to 18.22 (±7.0) and 16.44 (±5.3) mm Hg on the 12th and 24th months, respectively; the mean number of antiglaucoma medications decreased significantly from 3.23 (±0.9) to 2.15 (±1.5) and 2.09 (±1.6), respectively. The cumulative probabilities of overall success were 71.2 ± 5.6% and 40.9 ± 6.1% on the 12th and 24th months, respectively. High baseline IOP and the number of antiglaucoma medications were associated with a higher risk of failure (hazard ratio = 1.10 and 3.01, $p = 0.04$ and $p < 0.01$, respectively). The most common complications were cataract development or progression (30.8%) and prolonged or rebound anterior chamber reaction (10.6%). **Conclusions:** UCP reasonably controls the IOP and reduces the antiglaucoma medication burden in eyes with POAG. Nevertheless, the success rate is modest, with a high baseline IOP and number of medications.

Keywords: glaucoma; ciliary body; ultrasound cyclo plasty; primary open-angle glaucoma

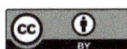

1. Introduction

Glaucoma is a group of ocular disorders characterised by progressive damage of retinal ganglion cells and the optic nerve. It is the leading cause of irreversible blindness, affecting nearly 80 million people worldwide, and this number is expected to reach 111.8 million by 2040 [1]. The significant morbidity of glaucoma presents remarkable health, societal, and economic burden [2]. Primary open-angle glaucoma (POAG) is the most common type of glaucoma, accounting for 60–90% of glaucoma cases across different ethnic groups but far less in the Saudi population (12.8%) [1,3,4]. Several studies have demonstrated that lowering the intraocular pressure (IOP) is the principal factor for reducing the glaucoma progression rate and for preserving sight. The traditional treatment algorithm aims to achieve a balance between aqueous humour inflow and outflow by decreasing production and/or increasing drainage and, therefore, IOP control. When topical medications or laser therapy do not achieve adequate IOP control, incisional surgery should be considered.

However, the postoperative complications should be taken into consideration before proceeding with such an option. Another option to reduce aqueous humour production is by destroying the ciliary body using different physical methods, such as laser therapy and cryotherapy [5,6]. However, the non-selective action of such cyclodestructive procedures over the target tissues and the arbitrary dose–effect relationship have resulted in significant risks of chronic hypotony, phthisis, uveal inflammation, macular oedema, and retinal detachment [7–9].

Ultrasound cyclo plasty (UCP) has been developed to achieve selective and controlled thermal effects on the ciliary body using high-intensity focused ultrasound. This procedure enables good tissue targeting and precise temperature control, resulting in the remodelling of the ciliary body by removing the epithelium and preserving the blood–aqueous barrier [10]. Both the miniaturised transducers and the circular-shaped probe matching the three-dimensional anatomy of the ciliary body allow correct focusing on the target tissue. Several studies reported encouraging results regarding the safety and efficacy of UCP [11–17]. Nevertheless, reports on the outcome of such a procedure in a major glaucoma type, such as POAG, which is a leading cause of blindness worldwide, are limited. We have previously described the outcomes of UCP in patients with different glaucoma types [16]. Since the literature lacks studies focusing on the outcomes of UCP in a major glaucoma type such as POAG, we were interested in evaluating the outcomes of UCP for uncontrolled POAG.

2. Materials and Methods

This retrospective study was approved by the institutional review board of King Saud University (E-22-6738), which is a part of a larger study on the outcomes of UCP, and all procedures adhered to the tenets of the Declaration of Helsinki. We reviewed the medical records of patients with POAG who underwent UCP between May 2016 and May 2021 at King Abdul Aziz University Hospital, Riyadh, Saudi Arabia. The inclusion criteria were as follows: medically uncontrolled IOP of ≥ 21 mm Hg despite maximum tolerated antiglaucoma medications; glaucomatous optic nerve head damage and open angle on gonioscopy; and a minimum follow-up period of 6 months. Meanwhile, the exclusion criteria were as follows: normal-tension glaucoma; secondary open-angle glaucoma; pregnancy; use of systemic medications that could affect the IOP; history of either refractive surgery, retinal detachment, or ocular tumour; and ocular infection 2 weeks prior to UCP. We followed the previous methods described by Almobarak et al. [16].

2.1. Surgical Methods

All procedures were performed using the EyeOP1 device (Eye Tech Care, Rillieux-la-Pape, France). The device consists of a single-use sterile pack, including a coupling cone and treatment probe of three sizes based on the biometric eye readings to best adapt to the eye, and a compact operator console. The surgeon's name and the patient's demographic data were registered, followed by the connection of the selected probe to the console. Thereafter, the machine automatically detected the probe, and the suction test began after clumping the suction probe. One of several staff glaucoma specialists credentialed for the procedure performed the surgery under peribulbar anaesthesia. The coupling cone was placed and adjusted on the centre of the patient's eye by visualising an equal white scleral ring surrounding the cornea. The coupling cone was kept in place via vacuum suction activated using a foot pedal and was then filled with a balanced salt solution to allow ultrasound transmission. A second-generation probe, consisting of six piezoelectric transducers, was used for all patients. The transducers were automatically activated at a frequency of 21 MHz and an acoustic power of 2.45 W, with an 8-s duration for each sector and a 20-s pause between each treatment to allow complete evacuation of heat. The UCP procedures were performed by authors FA, EO, and SA. Postoperatively, all patients were treated with topical prednisolone drops four times a day for 1 week, with the frequency tapered gradually on a weekly basis. Antiglaucoma drops were resumed postoperatively based on the surgeon's preference according to the case severity and IOP. The IOP was measured using the Goldmann applanation tonometer. The postoperative visits considered for this study were those conducted on the first postoperative day and at 2 to 4 weeks, 3 months, 6 months, 9 months, 12 months, 18 months, and 24 months.

2.2. Data Analysis

Pre- and postoperative data were collected for the following variables: age, sex, IOP, number of antiglaucoma medications, best-corrected visual acuity converted into logarithm of minimal angle of resolution (logMAR) format, time to failure, postoperative complications, and the need for subsequent pressure-lowering procedures to control the IOP. The variables were evaluated using Student's t-test and the Wilcoxon rank test. Kaplan–Meier life table analysis was performed to estimate the success rate over the postoperative period and is presented as percentages ± standard errors. Success was classified as follows: (i) overall success (IOP reduction of ≥20% from the baseline level and IOP between 6 and 21 mm Hg with or without antiglaucoma medications); (ii) complete success (IOP reduction of ≥20% from the baseline level and IOP between 6 and 21 mm Hg without antiglaucoma medications); (iii) qualified success (the same as absolute success but with antiglaucoma medications); and (iv) failure (when any of the following develops: IOP reduction of <20% from the baseline level and IOP of >21 mm Hg despite maximum tolerated antiglaucoma medications on two visits, persistent hypotony (IOP of ≤5 mm Hg) on two visits causing hypotony maculopathy, the need for a higher number of glaucoma medications compared with the preoperative baseline, loss of vision due to glaucoma progression, postoperative vision-threatening complications, or the need for further glaucoma procedures to control the IOP, including a repeat UCP). IOP spikes were considered when the IOP was more than 30 mm Hg or increased by >10 mm Hg compared with the preoperative baseline. Hazards ratios (HRs) and confidence intervals (CIs) were calculated using the Cox proportional hazard regression analysis to evaluate the impact of the baseline characteristics on survival. The variables were presented as means and standard deviations, and p-values of <0.05 were considered statistically significant. Statistical analyses were performed using SPSS version 23 (IBM Corp., Armonk, NY, USA).

3. Results

The study included 66 eyes of 55 patients. A flow chart is displayed in Figure 1. Twenty-nine eyes received previous glaucoma surgery, while 31 eyes received previous non-glaucoma surgery, mostly cataract surgery. The mean follow-up period was 28.95 (±16.9) months. Thirty-nine eyes were pseudophakic, while the remaining eyes were phakic and aphakic (Table 1). Among the 26 phakic eyes, 21 showed cataractous changes before surgery.

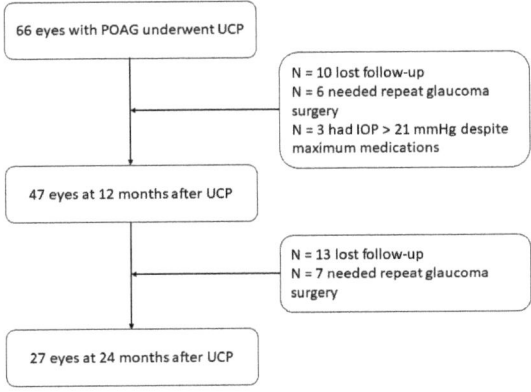

Figure 1. Flow chart of the study. UCP: Ultrasound cyclo plasty.

Table 1. Characteristics and ocular history *.

Variable	(N = 66)
Age at the time of surgery, year **	60.77 (±12.8)
Sex **	
Male	31 (53.0%)
Female	24 (47.0%)
Previous glaucoma surgery	
Yes	29 (43.9%)
No	37 (56.1%)
Frequency of glaucoma surgery	
1	27 (40.9%)
2	2 (3.0%)
Type of previous glaucoma surgery ǂ	
Trabeculectomy + MMC ± Phaco + PCIOL	11
Deep sclerectomy + MMC ± Phaco + PCIOL	11
Cyclophotocoagulation ± Phaco + PCIOL	5
Ahmed implant	2
Canaloplasty + MMC ± Phaco + PCIOL	1
Previous non-glaucoma surgery	
Yes	31 (47.0%)
No	35 (53.0%)
Type of previous non-glaucoma surgery ǂ	
Phaco + PCIOL	28
Pars plana vitrectomy	3
Lens status	
Phakic	26 (39.4%)
Pseudophakic	39 (59.1%)
Aphakic	1 (1.5%)
Axial length, mm	24.50 (±2.5)
White-to-white, mm	11.84 (±0.5)
Cone size used	
11	3 (4.5%)
12	32 (48.5%)
13	31 (47.0%)

* Data are presented as means (±SDs) and frequencies (%). Numbers are per eye. ** Numbers are per patient. ǂ Number represents the frequency of overall surgeries, including repeat surgeries. MMC: Mitomycin C. Phaco: Phacoemulsification. PCIOL: Posterior chamber intraocular lens implantation.

The mean IOP decreased significantly from 23.02 (±6.1) to 18.22 (±7.0), 16.39 (±4.4), and 16.44 (±5.3) mm Hg on the 12th, 18th, and 24th months, respectively; the mean number of antiglaucoma medications decreased significantly from 3.23 (±0.9) to 2.15 (±1.5), 2.00 (±1.6), and 2.09 (±1.6), respectively; both parameters decreased throughout the follow-up period ($p < 0.01$) (Figure 2). There was a significant change in the mean logMAR during the first day and the third month postoperatively (Table 2). The most common postoperative complications were cataract development or progression in 8 eyes out of 26 phakic eyes (30.8%), of which 6 eyes (23.1%) required cataract surgery; prolonged or rebound anterior chamber reaction in 7 eyes (10.6%); hypotony with choroidal detachment in 2 eyes (3.0%); and macular oedema in 2 eyes (3.0%) (Table 3).

Table 2. IOP, number of antiglaucoma medications, and logMAR.

Preoperative Baseline		p-Value
IOP, mm Hg	23.02 (±6.1)	-
No. of medications	3.23 (±0.9)	-
LogMAR	0.67 (±0.7)	-
No. of eyes	-	-
1 day postoperative		
IOP, mm Hg	15.10 (±6.1)	<0.01
IOP reduction (%)	34.82%	-
No. of medications	1.25 (±1.3)	<0.01
LogMAR	0.73 (±0.8)	0.02
No. of eyes	66	-
1 month postoperative		
IOP, mm Hg	16.54 (±5.5)	<0.01
IOP reduction (%)	28.84%	-
No. of medications	1.67 (±1.4)	<0.01
LogMAR	0.83 (±0.9)	0.12
No. of eyes	66	-
3 months postoperative		
IOP, mm Hg	17.20 (±6.7)	<0.01
IOP reduction (%)	32.36%	-
No. of medications	1.82 (±1.4)	<0.01
LogMAR	0.90 (±1.0)	0.03
No. of eyes	64	-
6 months postoperative		
IOP, mm Hg	17.04 (±5.5)	<0.01
IOP reduction (%)	41.07%	-
No. of medications	1.83 (±1.5)	<0.01
LogMAR	0.78 (±0.9)	0.16
No. of eyes	64	-
9 months postoperative		
IOP, mm Hg	15.60 (±4.8)	<0.01
IOP reduction (%)	42.03%	-
No. of medications	1.90 (±1.5)	<0.01
LogMAR	0.78 (±0.9)	0.18
No. of eyes	58	-
12 months postoperative		
IOP, mm Hg	18.22 (±7.0)	<0.01
IOP reduction (%)	35.51%	-
No. of medications	2.15 (±1.5)	<0.01
LogMAR	0.64 (±0.7)	0.55
No. of eyes	47	-
18 months postoperative		
IOP, mm Hg	16.39 (±4.4)	<0.01
IOP reduction (%)	39.57%	-
No. of medications	2.00 (±1.6)	<0.01
LogMAR	0.63 (±0.9)	0.37
No. of eyes	38	-
24 months postoperative		
IOP, mm Hg	16.44 (±5.3)	<0.01
IOP reduction (%)	38.04%	-
No. of medications	2.09 (±1.6)	<0.01
LogMAR	0.64 (±1.0)	0.7
No. of eyes	27	-

Data are presented as means (±SDs). P-values are calculated using the Wilcoxon test and Student's t-test. IOP: Intraoculr pressure, logMAR: logarithm of minimal angle of resolution.

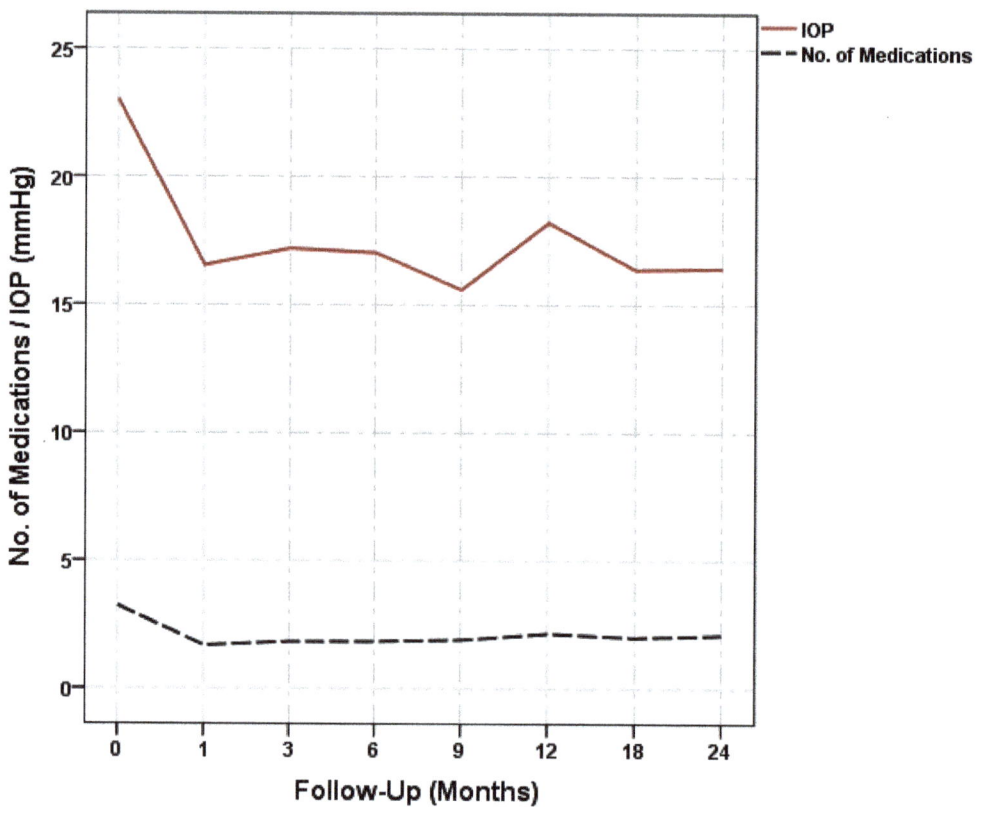

Figure 2. Changes in IOP and antiglaucoma medications.

Table 3. Postoperative complications following ultrasound cyclo plasty *.

Complication	Number (%)
Cataract development or progression ǂ	8 (30.8)
Prolonged or rebound anterior chamber reaction	7 (10.6)
Hypotony or choroidal detachment	2 (3.0)
Macular oedema	2 (3.0)
IOP spike of >30 mm Hg	1 (1.5)
Corneal abrasion	1 (1.5)

* Numbers are per eye. ǂ Percentage out of phakic eyes.

The cumulative probabilities of overall success were 71.2 ± 5.6%, 57.6 ± 6.1%, and 40.9 ± 6.1% on the 12th, 18th, and 24th months, respectively (Figure 3). The complete success rates were 78.6 ± 11.0%, 64.3 ± 12.8%, and 57.1 ± 13.2%, while the qualified success rates were 79.4 ± 6.9%, 67.6 ± 8.0%, and 50.0 ± 8.6% on the 12th, 18th, and 24th months, respectively. The Cox proportional hazard analyses of survival showed that the baseline IOP (HR = 1.10, 95% CI = 1.00–1.12, p = 0.04) and number of antiglaucoma medications (HR = 3.01, 95% CI = 1.61–5.60, p < 0.01) were both significant risk factors for failure. Age, sex, axial length, white-to-white diameter, history of old glaucoma surgery, and history of old non-glaucoma surgery were not significant risk factors for failure (Table 4).

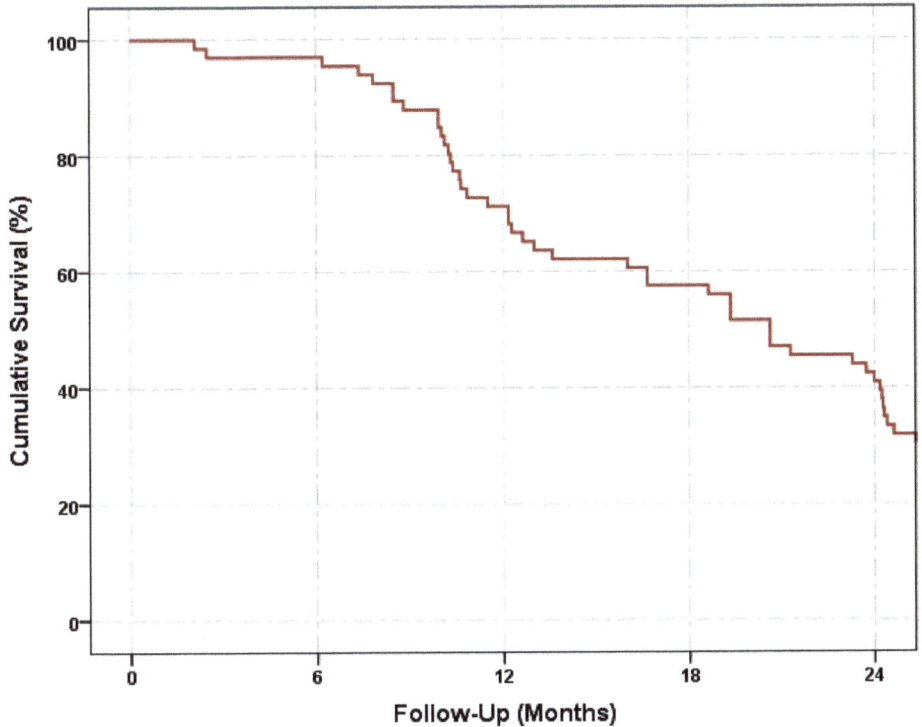

Figure 3. Kaplan–Meier survival curve showing the cumulative probability of success.

Table 4. Cox proportional hazard regression analysis.

Predictor	HR	95% CI	p-Value
Age	0.99	0.97–1.01	0.62
Sex	1.16	0.69–1.97	0.58
Baseline IOP	1.10	1.00–1.12	0.04
Baseline no. of medications	3.01	1.61–5.60	<0.01
Old glaucoma surgery	1.18	0.70–1.98	0.54
Old non-glaucoma surgery	0.64	0.37–1.10	0.11
Axial length	0.99	0.85–1.15	0.92
White-to-white-diameter	0.78	0.40–1.50	0.78

HR: Hazard ratio; CI: Confidence interval; IOP: Intraocular pressure.

In total, 16 eyes (24.2%) failed because of the following: 13 eyes (19.7%) had an uncontrolled IOP requiring further glaucoma surgery (3 eyes required a second glaucoma surgery to control the IOP), and 3 eyes (4.5%) had glaucoma progression with an uncontrolled IOP (1 eye had complete loss of vision) (Table 5). The mean time to failure was 11.73 (±6.2; range = 2.10–23.98) months. Most failures occurred 6 months after UCP.

Table 5. Eyes needing repeat glaucoma surgery.

First Repeat Surgery	Time Since the First Procedure (Month)	Second Repeat Surgery	Time Since the First Repeat Procedure (Month)
Ahmed implant	19.3		
Phaco + PCIOL * + ECP **	8.8	Micropulse cyclophotocoagulation	12
Ahmed implant	19.3		
Deep sclerectomy + MMC ǂ	11.5		
Trabeculectomy + MMC	7.8		
Ahmed implant	19.3		
Deep sclerectomy + MMC	12.7		
Deep sclerectomy + MMC	12.2	Ahmed implant	24
Phaco + PCIOL + trabeculectomy + MMC	6.2	Trabeculectomy + MMC	6
Micropulse cyclophotocoagulation	8.8		
Express shunt + MMC	12.3		
Express shunt + MMC	10.1		
Cyclophotocoagulation	23.9		

* Phacoemulsification with posterior chamber intraocular lens implantation; ** Endoscopic cyclophotocoagulation; ǂ Mitomycin C.

4. Discussion

The current study showed that UCP was safe and effective for significantly reducing the IOP in patients with POAG. There were significant differences in the IOP and antiglaucoma medication burden on the 6th, 12th, 18th, and 24th months after a single UCP. The rate of IOP reduction ranged between 28.8% and 42.0% throughout the follow-up period, and the IOP was <18 mm Hg. Although the number of antiglaucoma medications decreased significantly after UCP, a gradual increment was needed to maintain a controlled IOP. We have previously described the outcomes of UCP in patients with different glaucoma types [16]. However, we were interested in evaluating the outcomes in POAG, a major and leading type of blindness worldwide. Certain variations in the IOP reduction and success rates might exist among different glaucoma entities. Giannaccare et al. reported a 37.8% IOP reduction in eyes with angle-closure glaucoma compared with 20.0% in eyes with POAG and 26.2% in eyes with neovascular glaucoma (NVG) after 6 months [15]. Meanwhile, Hu et al. reported higher IOP reduction and success rates in eyes with primary angle-closure glaucoma (PACG) (36.1% reduction and 80.0% success) than in eyes with POAG (17.7% reduction and 55.6% success), NVG (18.6% reduction and 29.2% success), and traumatic glaucoma (21.6% reduction and 50.0% success) after 3 months [18]. Our 3rd- and 6th-month IOP reduction and success rates are higher than those in both of these studies. Nevertheless, both studies included eyes with refractory glaucoma, and such differences in the IOP reduction and success rates might be attributed to the differences in the ultrasound exposure, number of treated sectors, and baseline IOP. On the contrary, Torky et al. reported a 100% success rate of UCP as a primary intervention for both PACG (10 eyes) and POAG (13 eyes) after 12 months in a group subjected to the same treatment conditions; this rate was lower than that for NVG and uveitic glaucoma, suggesting that secondary glaucoma would have less IOP control [13]. The reduction in aqueous production in secondary glaucoma seems insufficient to compensate for the impaired trabecular drainage pathway. However, the outcomes of UCP seem to be comparable with those of interventions for heterogeneous groups of glaucoma entities. Moreover, the differences in success rates between eyes with POAG and our study is attributed to the big difference in sample size. In their study that included 52 eyes, Denis et al. reported comparable 12-month IOP reduction and success rates of the entire group (36.0% reduction and 48.0% success) compared with those for eyes with POAG (33.9% reduction and 45.0% success) at a 6-s exposure time [12]. Rouland et al. compared the IOP reduction rate between their overall study population and POAG groups, including patients with eyes with refractory glaucoma; they showed 31.0% and 29.0% 12-month IOP reduction rates and a 33.0% 24-month IOP reduction rate in both groups [19]. The IOP reduction rate in our study is comparable with that in previous studies; nevertheless, both studies maintained the same protocol of antiglaucoma medications, and there was no significant change in the burden of medications. The IOP reduction rate in our study is also comparable with that in other studies that included patients with POAG as the majority of their study population. In their study that included 26 patients with POAG, Aptel et al. reported a 30% IOP reduction at 12 months, where the IOP decreased from 28.8 to 19.6 mm Hg, while the number of antiglaucoma medications decreased from 3.6 to 3.1 [11]. Sarmento et al. reported a 12-month IOP reduction rate of 45.6% and an overall success rate of 100% in 14 eyes, where UCP was repeated for better IOP control [20]. Indeed, the IOP control and success rates vary among different studies, which is understandable owing to the differences in the study protocols, success criteria, glaucoma types included, baseline IOP and maintenance of antiglaucoma medications, and acceptance of repeat UCP as an enhancement rather than a failure of the initial UCP procedure. However, UCP seems to yield favourable outcomes for POAG. Notably, eyes with higher baseline IOP and antiglaucoma medication burdens are more prone to failure than their counterparts. Indeed, most previous studies have shown a high IOP reduction rate, reaching 30–40%, while almost maintaining the same antiglaucoma medications. However, such reductions might not be sufficient to reduce the IOP to a level deemed safe to prevent further glaucomatous progression and disc damage in the case of a high baseline IOP, even while maintaining antiglaucoma medications. It is not clearly known if subjecting more ciliary epithelium to ultrasound exposure would result in better IOP control. Hu et al. reported an initial better IOP reduction when exposing the ciliary epithelium to eight sectors of ultrasound than to six sectors; however, such an effect disappeared immediately thereafter and became insignificant [18]. Exposing more ciliary epithelium to coagulative necrosis would further decrease aqueous production, but such an effect is temporary, and the remaining epithelium would compensate for such production. Interestingly, most failures occurred after 6 months because of the high IOP. An explanation is that UCP might yield better initial coagulation of the ciliary body, while inflammatory mediator release would stimulate the uveoscleral pathway; therefore, UCP better reduced the IOP and burden of medications. Nevertheless, re-epithelisation and gradual narrowing of the stimulated uveoscleral pathway will contribute to failure in the future [10,11,21,22].

The most common postoperative complications in our study were cataract development or progression, prolonged or rebound anterior chamber reaction, hypotony with choroidal detachment, and macular oedema. All these complications were non-vision-threatening complications and shared a common predisposing factor, which is the release of inflammatory mediators after the disruption of the blood–aqueous barrier induced by ciliary epithelium coagulative necrosis. Such inflammatory mediators will spread to the anterior chamber and result in inflammation and cataract development or progression, stimulate the uveoscleral pathway and result in choroidal detachment with hypotony, or spread to the vitreous humour and result in the development or aggravation of macular oedema [16,17].

5. Conclusions

Although the current study had the limitations inherent in any retrospective study, it is the first to evaluate the outcomes of UCP for a major glaucoma entity, such as POAG. A significant IOP control and reduction of the antiglaucoma medication burden can be achieved with UCP. However, such effects could be less in cases of higher baseline IOP and antiglaucoma medication burden. Therefore, counselling patients with such conditions regarding the need for enhancement or other surgical modalities is recommended.

Author Contributions: All authors contributed to the study conception, design, and data collection. F.A.A. wrote the initial draft and undertook the analysis. All authors have read and agreed to the published version of the manuscript.

Funding: This research received no external funding.

Institutional Review Board Statement: The study was approved by the institutional review board (E-22-6738) of King Saud University, and all procedures adhered to the tenets of the Declaration of Helsinki.

Informed Consent Statement: All patients given informed consent.

Data Availability Statement: All data are available from the corresponding author upon request.

Conflicts of Interest: All authors declare no competing interest.

References

1. Tham, Y.C.; Li, X.; Wong, T.Y.; Quigley, H.A.; Aung, T.; Cheng, C.Y. Global prevalence of glaucoma and projections of glaucoma burden through 2040: A systematic review and meta-analysis. *Ophthalmology* **2014**, *121*, 2081–2090. [CrossRef] [PubMed]
2. Wang, W.; He, M.; Li, Z.; Huang, W. Epidemiological variations and trends in health burden of glaucoma worldwide. *Acta Ophthalmol.* **2019**, *97*, e349–e355. [CrossRef] [PubMed]
3. Friedman, D.S.; Wolfs, R.C.; O'Colmain, B.J.; Klein, B.E.; Taylor, H.R.; West, S.; Leske, M.C.; Mitchell, P.; Congdon, N.; Kempen, J.; et al. Prevalence of open-angle glaucoma among adults in the United States. *Arch. Ophthalmol.* **2004**, *122*, 532–538. [CrossRef] [PubMed]
4. Al Obeidan, S.A.; Dewedar, A.; Osman, E.A.; Mousa, A. The profile of glaucoma in a Tertiary Ophthalmic University Center in Riyadh, Saudi Arabia. *Saudi J. Ophthalmol.* **2011**, *25*, 373–379. [CrossRef] [PubMed]
5. Ansari, E.; Gandhewar, J. Long-term efficacy and visual acuity following transscleral diode laser photocoagulation in cases of refractory and non-refractory glaucoma. *Eye* **2007**, *21*, 936–940. [CrossRef]
6. Iliev, M.E.; Gerber, S. Long-term outcome of trans-scleral diode laser cyclophotocoagulation in refractory glaucoma. *Br. J. Ophthalmol.* **2007**, *91*, 1631–1635. [CrossRef]
7. Frezzotti, P.; Mittica, V.; Martone, G.; Motolese, I.; Lomurno, L.; Peruzzi, S.; Motolese, E. Longterm follow-up of diode laser transscleral cyclophotocoagulation in the treatment of refractory glaucoma. *Acta Ophthalmol.* **2010**, *88*, 150–155. [CrossRef]
8. Kirwan, J.F.; Shah, P.; Khaw, P.T. Diode laser cyclophotocoagulation: Role in the management of refractory pediatric glaucomas. *Ophthalmology* **2002**, *109*, 316–323. [CrossRef]
9. Vernon, S.A.; Koppens, J.M.; Menon, G.J.; Negi, A.K. Diode laser cycloablation in adult glaucoma: Long-term results of a standard protocol and review of current literature. *Clin. Exp. Ophthalmol.* **2006**, *34*, 411–420. [CrossRef]
10. Mastropasqua, R.; Fasanella, V.; Mastropasqua, A.; Ciancaglini, M.; Agnifili, L. High-Intensity Focused Ultrasound Circular Cyclocoagulation in Glaucoma: A Step Forward for Cyclodestruction? *J. Ophthalmol.* **2017**, *2017*, 7136275. [CrossRef]
11. Aptel, F.; Denis, P.; Rouland, J.F.; Renard, J.P.; Bron, A. Multicenter clinical trial of high-intensity focused ultrasound treatment in glaucoma patients without previous filtering surgery. *Acta Ophthalmol.* **2016**, *94*, e268–e272. [CrossRef] [PubMed]
12. Denis, P.; Aptel, F.; Rouland, J.F.; Nordmann, J.P.; Lachkar, Y.; Renard, J.P.; Sellem, E.; Baudouin, C.; Bron, A. Cyclocoagulation of the ciliary bodies by high-intensity focused ultrasound: A 12-month multicenter study. *Invest. Ophthalmol. Vis. Sci.* **2015**, *56*, 1089–1096. [CrossRef]
13. Torky, M.A.; Al Zafiri, Y.A.; Hagras, S.M.; Khattab, A.M.; Bassiouny, R.M.; Mokbel, T.H. Safety and efficacy of ultrasound ciliary plasty as a primary intervention in glaucoma patients. *Int. J. Ophthalmol.* **2019**, *12*, 597–602. [CrossRef] [PubMed]
14. Melamed, S.; Goldenfeld, M.; Cotlear, D.; Skaat, A.; Moroz, I. High-intensity focused ultrasound treatment in refractory glaucoma patients: Results at 1 year of prospective clinical study. *Eur. J. Ophthalmol.* **2015**, *25*, 483–489. [CrossRef] [PubMed]
15. Giannaccare, G.; Vagge, A.; Gizzi, C.; Bagnis, A.; Sebastiani, S.; Del Noce, C.; Fresina, M.; Traverso, C.E.; Campos, E.C. High-intensity focused ultrasound treatment in patients with refractory glaucoma. *Graefes Arch. Clin. Exp. Ophthalmol.* **2017**, *255*, 599–605. [CrossRef] [PubMed]
16. Almobarak, F.A.; Alrubean, A.; Alsarhani, W.K.; Aljenaidel, A.; Osman, E. Ultrasound Cyclo Plasty in Glaucoma: Two-Year Outcomes. *J. Glaucoma* **2022**, *31*, 834–838. [CrossRef]
17. Almobarak, F.A.; Alrubean, A.; Alsarhani, W.K.; Aljenaidel, A.; Osman, E. Ultrasound Cyclo Plasty after Failed Glaucoma Surgery: Outcomes and Complications. *Ophthalmol. Ther.* **2022**, *11*, 1601–1610. [CrossRef]
18. Hu, D.; Tu, S.; Zuo, C.; Ge, J. Short-Term Observation of Ultrasonic Cyclocoagulation in Chinese Patients with End-Stage Refractory Glaucoma: A Retrospective Study. *J. Ophthalmol.* **2018**, *2018*, 4950318. [CrossRef]
19. Rouland, J.F.; Aptel, F. Efficacy and Safety of Ultrasound Cycloplasty for Refractory Glaucoma: A 3-Year Study. *J. Glaucoma* **2021**, *30*, 428–435. [CrossRef]

20. Morais Sarmento, T.; Figueiredo, R.; Garrido, J.; Passos, I.; Rebelo, A.L.; Candeias, A. Ultrasonic circular cyclocoagulation prospective safety and effectiveness study. *Int. Ophthalmol.* **2021**, *41*, 3047–3055. [CrossRef]
21. Aptel, F.; Charrel, T.; Palazzi, X.; Chapelon, J.Y.; Denis, P.; Lafon, C. Histologic effects of a new device for high-intensity focused ultrasound cyclocoagulation. *Invest. Ophthalmol. Vis. Sci.* **2010**, *51*, 5092–5098. [CrossRef] [PubMed]
22. McKelvie, P.A.; Walland, M.J. Pathology of cyclodiode laser: A series of nine enucleated eyes. *Br. J. Ophthalmol.* **2002**, *86*, 381–386. [CrossRef] [PubMed]

MDPI
St. Alban-Anlage 66
4052 Basel
Switzerland
www.mdpi.com

Journal of Clinical Medicine Editorial Office
E-mail: jcm@mdpi.com
www.mdpi.com/journal/jcm

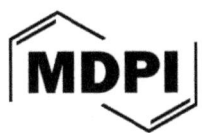

Disclaimer/Publisher's Note: The statements, opinions and data contained in all publications are solely those of the individual author(s) and contributor(s) and not of MDPI and/or the editor(s). MDPI and/or the editor(s) disclaim responsibility for any injury to people or property resulting from any ideas, methods, instructions or products referred to in the content.

www.ingramcontent.com/pod-product-compliance
Lightning Source LLC
LaVergne TN
LVHW070139100526
838202LV00015B/1852